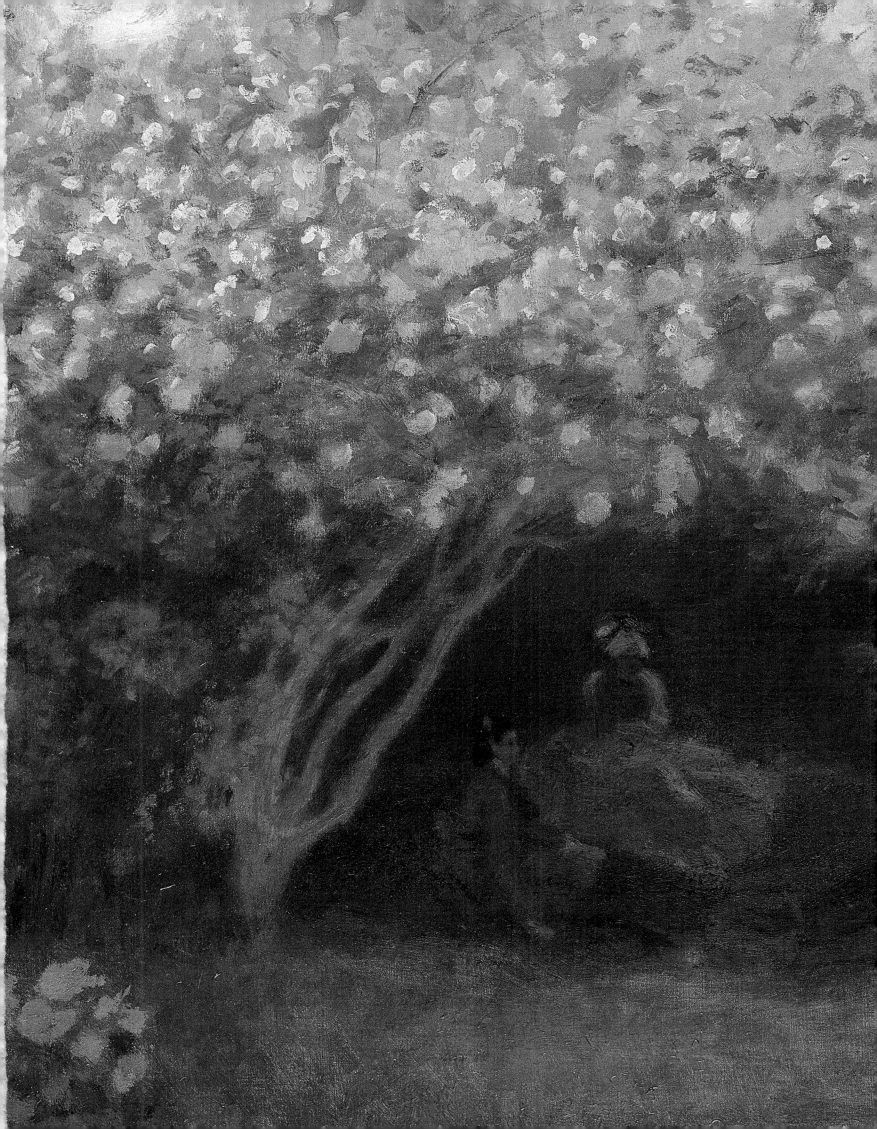

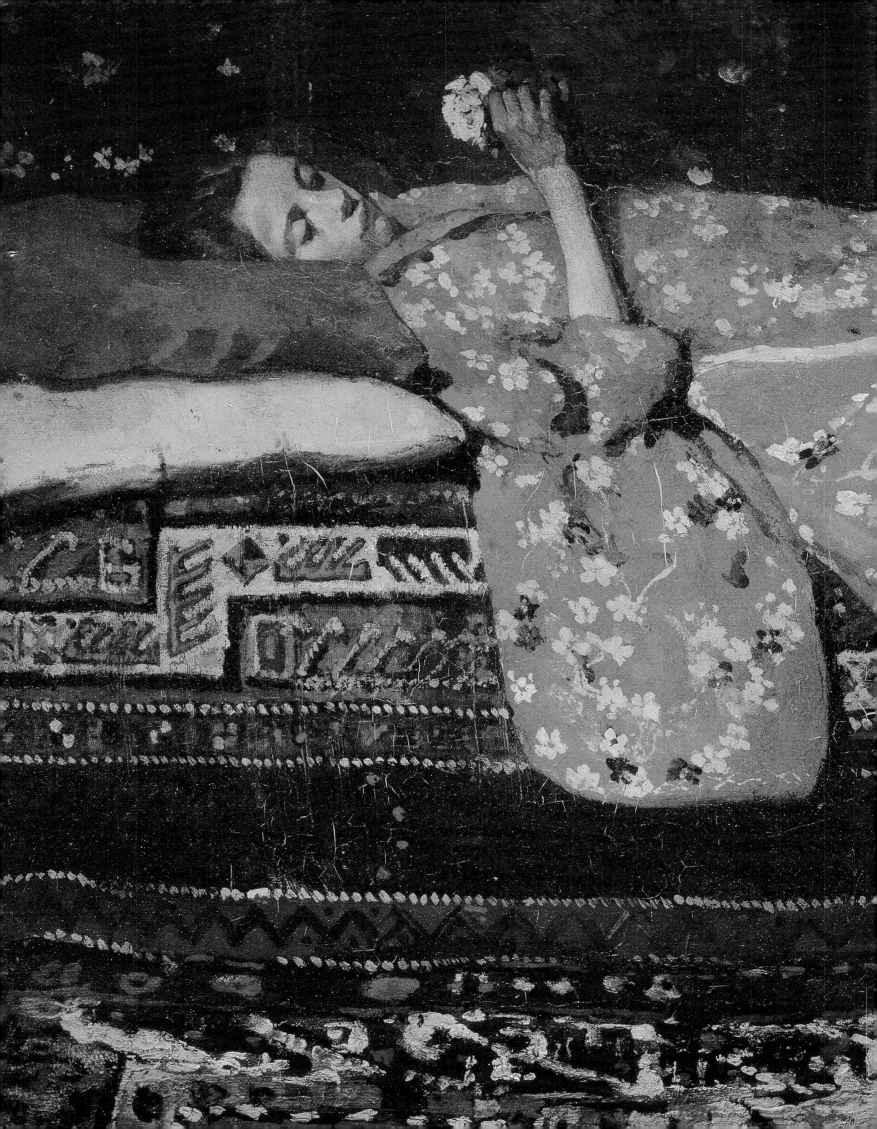

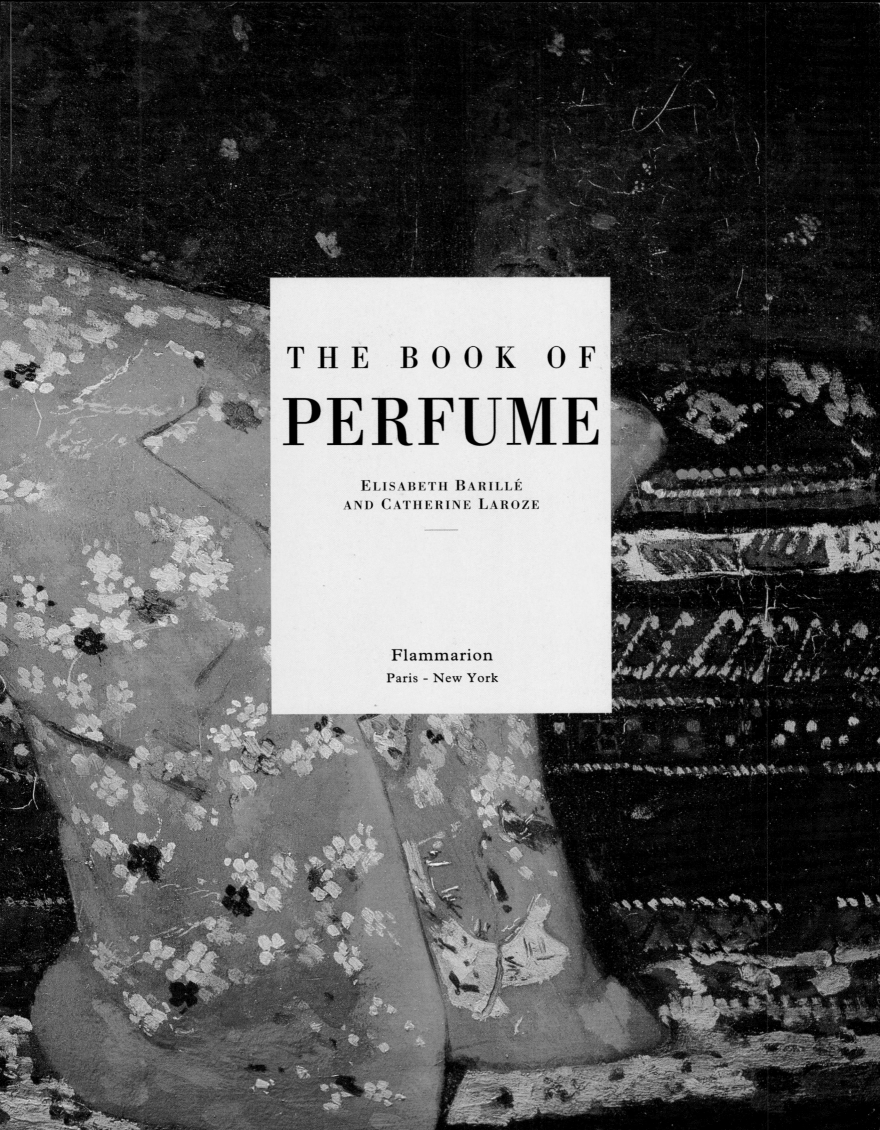

THE BOOK OF
PERFUME

ELISABETH BARILLÉ
AND CATHERINE LAROZE

Flammarion

Paris - New York

For Joël and Hilbrand—
for their kind support
and for being there.

Editorial Direction
GHISLAINE BAVOILLOT

Artistic Direction
MARC WALTER

Picture Research
RUTH EATON

Translation from the French
TAMARA BLONDEL

Editing
SOPHY THOMPSON

Typesetting : Octavo Editions, Paris

Origination : Colourscan, France

Printing : Canale, Turin

Flammarion
26, rue Racine, 75006 Paris

ISBN: 2-08013-590-2
Numéro d'édition: 3171
Dépôt légal: October 1995
Printed in Italy

CONTENTS

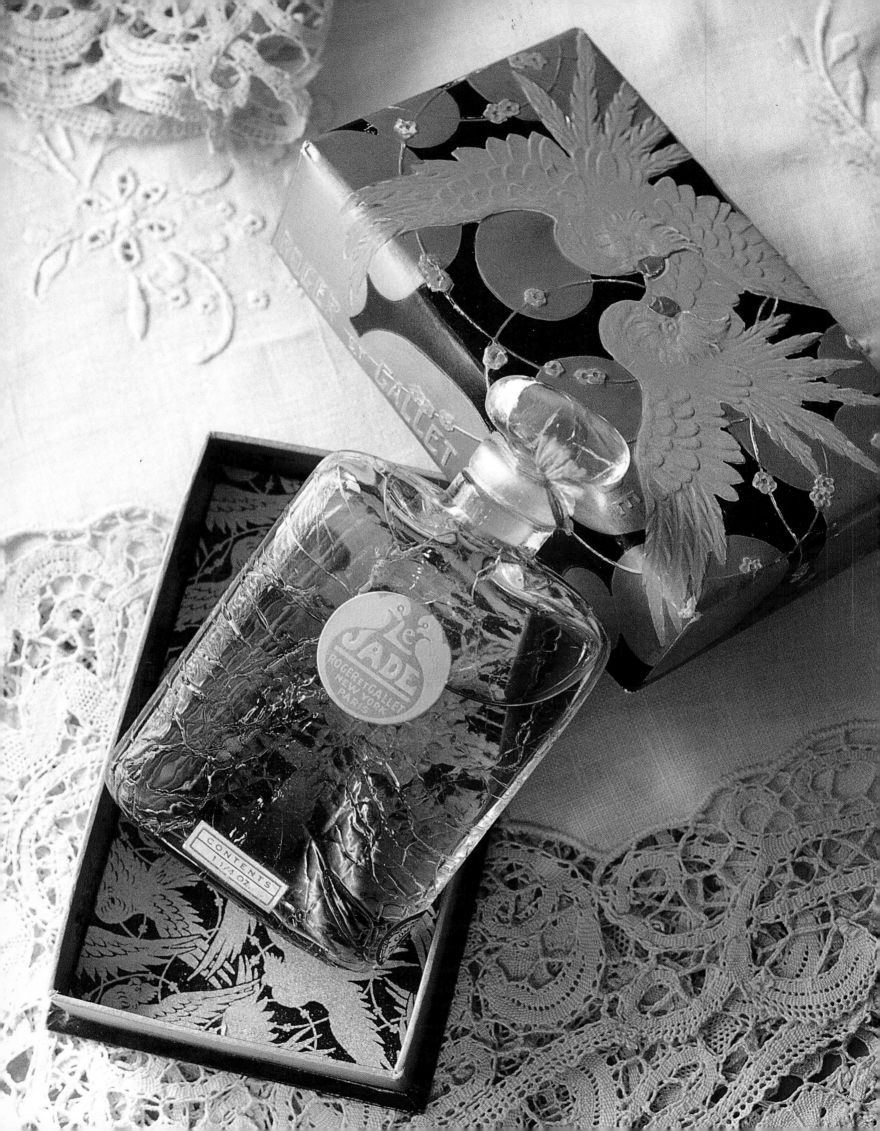

IN PRAISE
OF PERFUME

What would the world be like without scent or smell? Unbearable! When we set out to write this book, we discovered that we were both food-lovers by nature and so our thoughts first turned to the peaches we surreptitiously pick from the trees in August, to the sharp yet sweet-tasting wild strawberries and vanilla-scented pears which would be nothing without their enticing aroma. What about the desserts which remind us of our childhood? And the spring, the summer and the fall? The budding leaf would no longer smell of hazelnuts, the sand on the beach would no longer leave that briny, holiday smell of seaweed on our skin, the November bonfires would no longer leave their slightly acrid but reassuringly soft smell hanging in the air. And where would desire be without the whispered fragrance of the one you love?

According to Baudelaire, "Odors . . . possess the power of infinite things." But isn't it really our own infinity that they reveal, instilling new energy in that which delights us, that which we hope for and remember?

At one time or another in our lives, we have all experienced those sudden, unexpected moments when you catch a whiff of a fragrance which reminds you of an episode from your childhood, a forgotten landscape or the presence of an intimate friend. The memory becomes stronger than reality. Suddenly we are no longer thirty, but ten years old and back in that holiday house where we used to play, in that bedroom with its wall hangings impregnated with the heat of summer and the slightly musty smell of children's books.

For the author Marcel Proust, each hour of our life, as soon as it passes, is stored away in a smell, a taste, a sensation which, found again, can trigger a memory. His entire work was built on this belief. *Remembrance of Things Past* is a vast cathedral of words built to the glory of these sensations which, no matter how insignificant, cause "the tottering partitions of memory" to collapse.

Odors possess that rare power of capturing the precise essence of happiness, so difficult to define or formulate. The same is true of love. Like a melody written for a poem, odors often accompany our first romances or our most secret turmoils. Isn't love in fact a question of letting oneself be captivated by another's perfume? That is certainly what Pierre Bezukhov, the hero of Tolstoy's *War and Peace*, experiences: "He was conscious of the warmth of her body, the scent of perfume . . . And at that moment, Pierre felt that Hélène not only could, but must, be his wife, and that it could not be otherwise."

Marcel Proust, who so admirably evoked the richness of memories, wrote, "Let a noise or a scent, once heard or once smelt, be heard or smelt again . . . and immediately the permanent and habitually concealed essence of things is liberated and our true self which seemed to be dead but was not altogether dead, is awakened and reanimated." Le Jade by Roger & Gallet, created in 1923, with its decoration portraying a bird of paradise in full flight (opposite). Sumptuous abandon in *The Red Kimono*, painted by the Dutch Impressionist G.H. Breitner in around 1893 (previous double page). Claude Monet's *Under the Lilacs*, a richly perfumed setting (page 1).

The distinctive and irresistible odor of another becomes part of our existence. Even if we have never smelled it before, it is as though it has always been with us, as familiar and mysterious as the person we have chosen. The perfumes associated with wonderful meetings are never forgotten and when they are associated with falling in love they remain engraved in our memory. Who among us has never kept the perfume of a first love?

What is it we are looking for when we wear perfume? What impulse takes hold of us when we open the perfume bottle and spray on a well-loved fragrance? One thing is certain and that is we wish to attract. The art of seduction becomes like playing a game of hide-and-seek with our appearance and letting the other person get lost among all the facets of our character. If someone is shy, perfume helps them to appear daring and in control. Some perfumes are deliciously seductive, some frivolous, others like a meaningful glance, or a subtle gesture. Some sharpen and excite curiosity and, when worn with a certain degree of audacity, can be remarkably striking. For the fashion designer Karl Lagerfeld, "Perfume is a provocation."

We are well aware, of course, that far more than this is involved. Sometimes we put perfume on when we are alone to experience a hedonistic moment of joy or nostalgia. The perfume we never tire of is like a mirror reflecting our moods. It comforts and soothes us with its familiar, fragrant accords. It knows everything about us, it has been a part of our joys and sorrows and our most hidden secrets. It will not betray us, something that Bérénice, whom the hero of Louis Aragon's novel *Aurélien* secretly loves, understands: "Do not ask me the name of my perfume!" she cries. "It would mean our friendship would have to start with a refusal on my part and that would be a bad sign! A woman's perfume is her secret. To reveal it would be like taking one's clothes off in front of a stranger . . ."

A much-loved perfume, chosen in preference to all the others, holds, like children, an infinite capacity to amaze us. We tirelessly search for the right perfume, often finding it where we least expected to. "The search for perfume, which is a pleasure, but also an affliction of the noblest of our senses, follows no other path but that of obsession," explains the expert in this domain, Colette.

Those of us who have long been following the enchanted trail of fragrances know that the love of perfume is an all-consuming passion. One can of course make a career out of it. The perfumer seeking to enrich his palette ventures far afield to the most unexpected destinations, in the hope of discovering a fragrance unlike any other. A poet of the intangible, he often follows a lonely road, robbed of a normal routine by his olfactory dreaming. He might seem austere, but speak to him about fragrances and he will suddenly revive, like a lover talking about his fiancée. Perfumes are his obsession.

Then there are those who spend their time and fortune collecting perfume bottles. Although some may be experienced aesthetes, others start their collection with the first bottle of perfume they were given when young, or by the bust of Femme by Rochas, found in an antique shop. Some pursue their hobby on a small scale, just for pleasure, picking bottles up as they go along without ruining themselves. Others get caught up in a dangerous

Photographers (opposite), like authors, like to portray the subtleties of the senses: "Each body has its odor, just as each town has its silence, and like silence, it exists even when we are not aware of it. Perfume floats, motionless. It personifies the impossible and the sacred . . . For some, like Paul Valéry, it becomes synonymous with the divine," wrote Diane de Margerie.

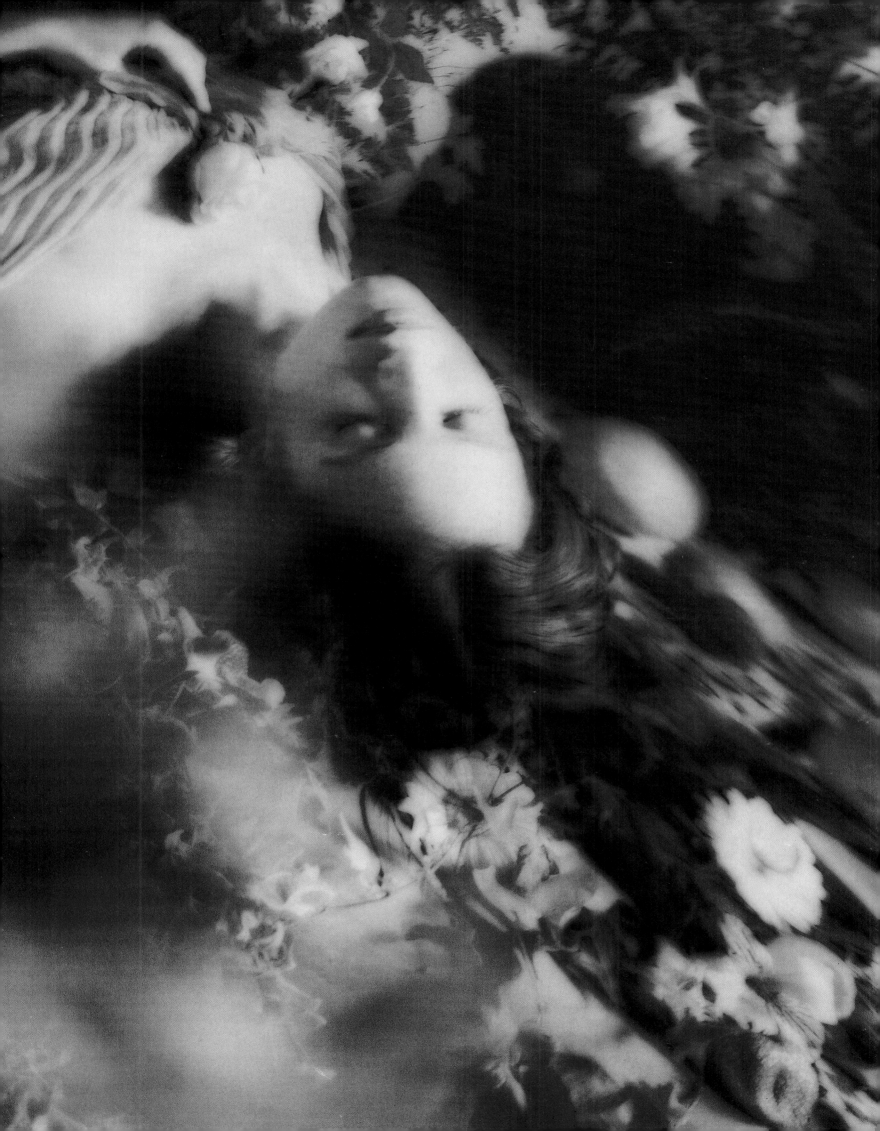

game, that of hunting down the rare object at any price. The perfume bottle which was so desirable yesterday fades into the background when a new one is discovered, even more precious than the last. Some collectors do not hesitate to jump on a plane in order to bid for a rarity to be auctioned at Christie's in London, or the Hôtel Drouot in Paris. Once bought, it will find its place among thousands of other perfume bottles, hoarded up like booty. How many do they actually own? They do not know. In fact, the question seems irrelevant. The only thing that interests them is the perfume bottle they have yet to acquire.

Many other people also have a passion for fragrances. There are, of course, the fashion designers, like Guy Laroche, who discovered a domain as fascinating as fashion itself when he launched his first perfume: "When I created my perfumes for men . . . I wanted to capture the fundamental, violent, sensual and eternal fragrances of nature in a bottle. To me nothing conjures up journeys better than perfumes. I am always ready to travel, and I can remember every olfactory detail of every country, landscape and town I have visited. Marrakech, that great jewel of the desert, overwhelmed me with its ardent fragrances. Everything merged into one: the lazy, immobile, blue tones of the lofty skies, the diamond-like Atlas Mountains, the gardens hiding behind the high red walls, the roads leading to the Sahara desert,

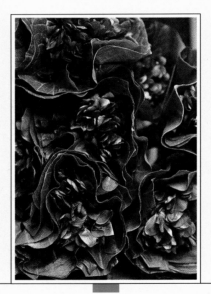

the burnt, musky and wild perfumes of this gateway to Africa."

There are many others who are as passionate about perfume as the fashion designers. Gardeners, for example, who compose gardens like bouquets, cooks, those virtuosos of subtle combinations such as consommé of crab and *langoustine* flavored with neroli essence, or wine experts, with their sensitive taste buds and acute sense of smell, who can recognize the infinite nuances of the famous vintage wines. Writers should also be included, like Didier Decoin for example, for whom the description of odors represents the summit of the art of writing. He admits, "Sometimes I spend long hours assembling the words which will enable me to reproduce the tantalizing fragrances you inhale when laying your cheek against that of a young girl in a garden in summer. In actual fact, it is probably easier to describe the great Cornelian agitation of the soul than the simple scent of a violet."

Therein, perhaps, lies the secret of the magic of perfumes. We think we possess them, but they constantly bring us new delights. We think we know them well, but they remain elusive. They are part of us and yet they escape us. They speak to us but we are unable to transcribe their imperceptible harmonies. Perfumes tell of childhood, distant lands, of ecstasy and of the secret rhythms of the world. Perfumes enable us to hear the deafening silence of love.

"The smell of violet, hidden in the green / Pour'd back into my empty soul and frame / The times when I remember to have been / Joyful and free from blame," *A Dream of Fair Women*, Alfred Lord Tennyson (1809–1892). Like the delicate violet (above), perfumes bring back lost paradises and the nonchalance of bygone days, as in this scene by the American photographer Seeley (opposite).

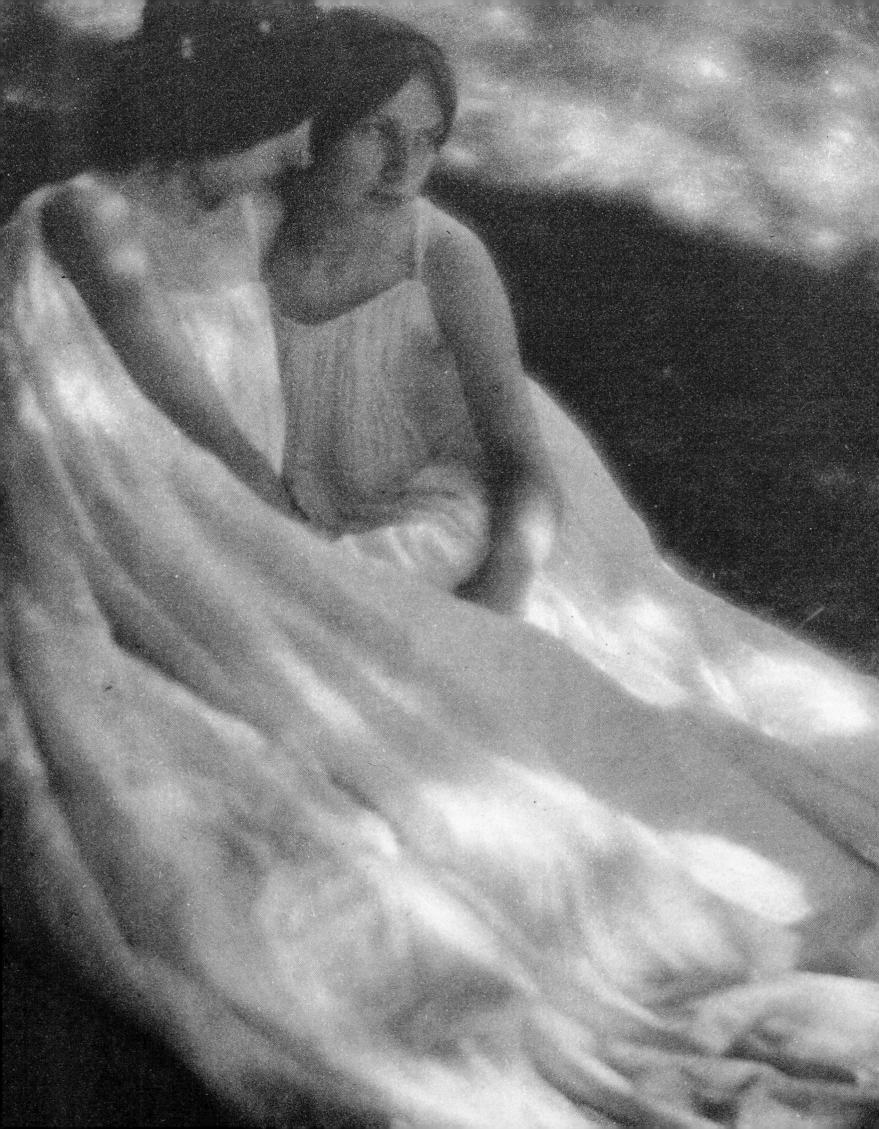

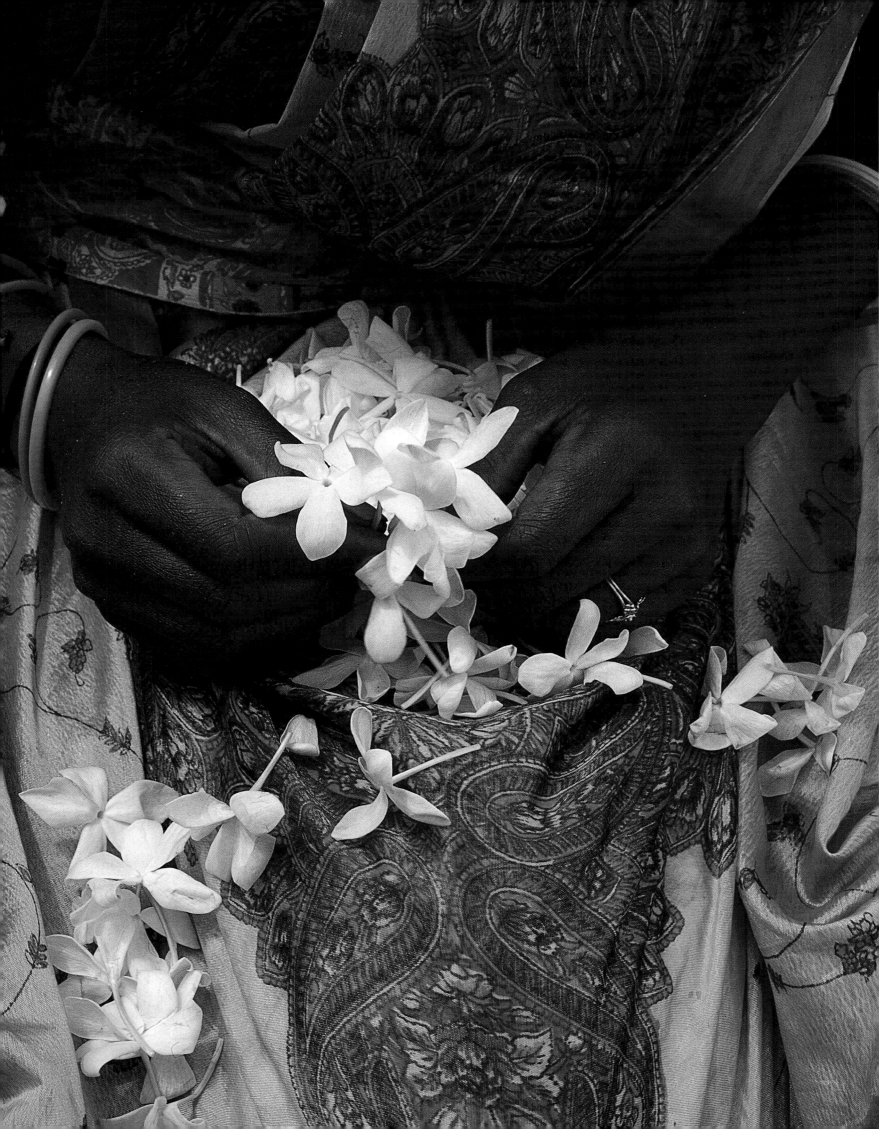

F R O M
FLOWER
· TO ·
ESSENCE

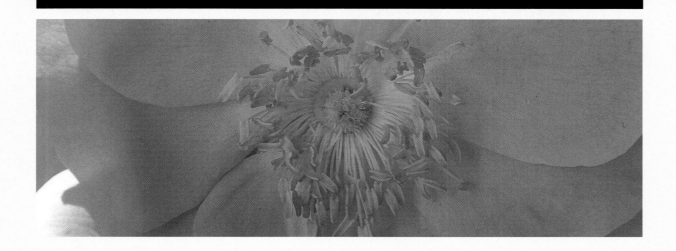

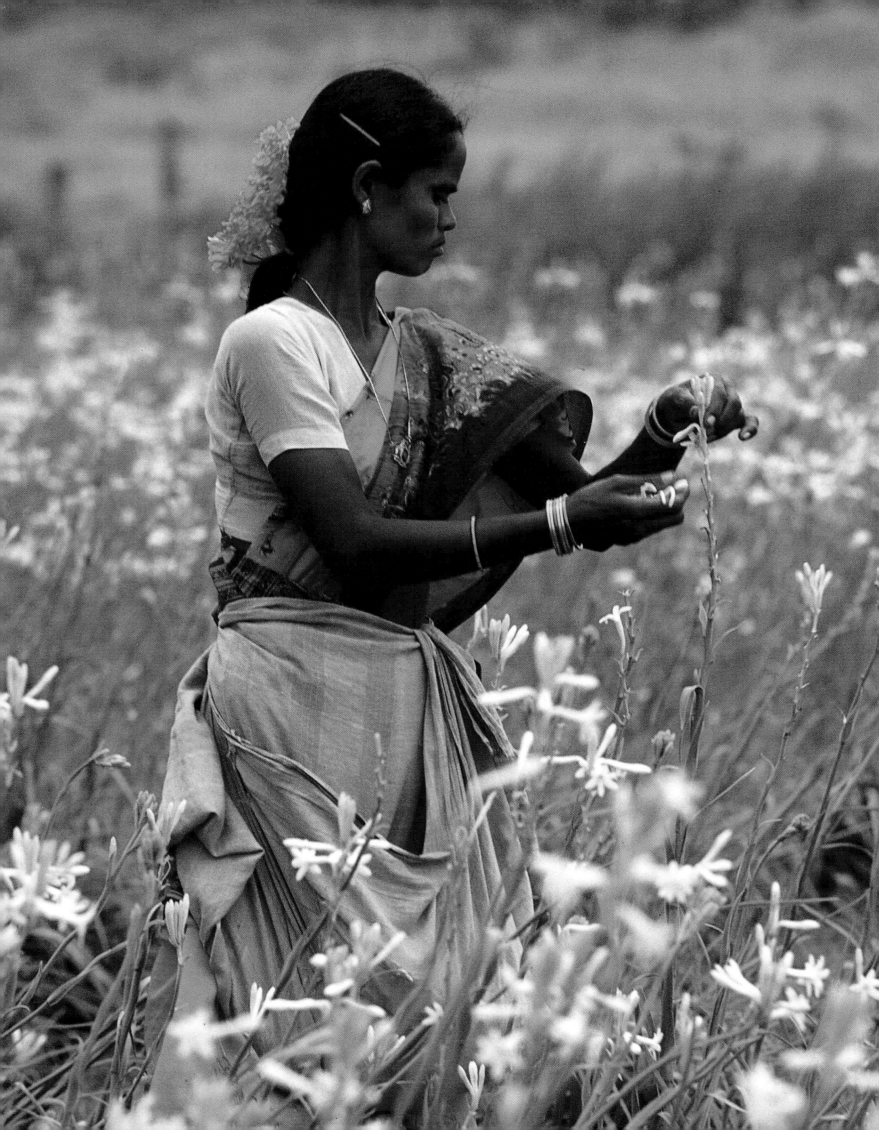

Capturing nature's fragrant secrets, transforming them into precious essences and blending them perfectly to compose a new melody, unknown to man, such is the mysterious art of the perfumer. To create a perfume, which involves emotion and intuition, is to perpetuate our sense of wonder before the beauty of nature.

It is still dark. Dawn is just breaking. Stooping between the jasmine bushes, the pickers are already busy gathering, one by one, the minute flowers which sparkle between their fingers and gradually fill their cotton aprons in a weightless load. The perfumer, half intoxicated by the vibrant fragrances, nevertheless keeps a close watch on the gathering of these flowers which will provide the precious essence for his perfume. "Does someone who has never experienced the magic of a field of jasmine or roses at the break of dawn really know what perfume is?" asks Jean-Paul Guerlain, the fourth creator in the Guerlain dynasty. Strolling in the scented atmosphere of a field of flowers, caressing the tender, velvety petals of a rose, treading the soft, warm earth and abandoning oneself to the heat and the pungent fragrances of the distilleries, these are some of the unforgettable moments which give the perfumer the impression of returning to the heart and soul of his profession.

The magic of fragrances lies in the ancestral links between man and nature and in his age-old interest in these sweet-smelling gifts, which express all the beauty of the world. As Jacques Polge, Chanel's perfume creator, puts it, "The day when, in the chain of events from the flower to the perfume, the flower is no longer picked, perfume will have lost its power. Capturing the flower, taking possession of its soul in order to transform it, is a way of uniting ourselves with the earth and of giving perfume its place in a mysterious and unique process . . . when perfume is worn by men and women, they take on an essential role in this process."

Perfumers are modern-day magicians. They alone know the mystery of the metamorphosis of flowers. They alone are able to detect the infinite nuances of an essence and to imagine the role they might play in the olfactory picture they paint.

The more privileged among them are the perfumers employed by the prestigious perfume houses, who travel the world in search of the finest essences. Jacques Polge for Chanel, Jean Kerléo, the perfume creator for Jean Patou, and Jean-Paul Guerlain visit the plantations several times a year to do their "shopping" and are constantly crisscrossing the world. Every country and every region produces very different flowers and essences, just as the character of grapes destined for famous wines varies according to where they are grown.

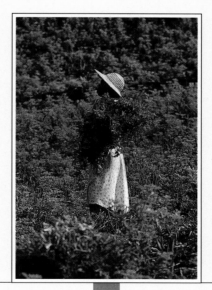

Ritual movements and ancestral elegance of the pickers in harmony with the precious flowers. Armfuls of geraniums are gathered in Réunion (above). Tuberose blooms are delicately removed from their stems in India (opposite). Jasmine flowers, as light as feathers, are gathered one by one (page 12). The scent of the Damask rose (*Rosa damascena*) will remain intact thanks to the practiced skill of the pickers (page 13).

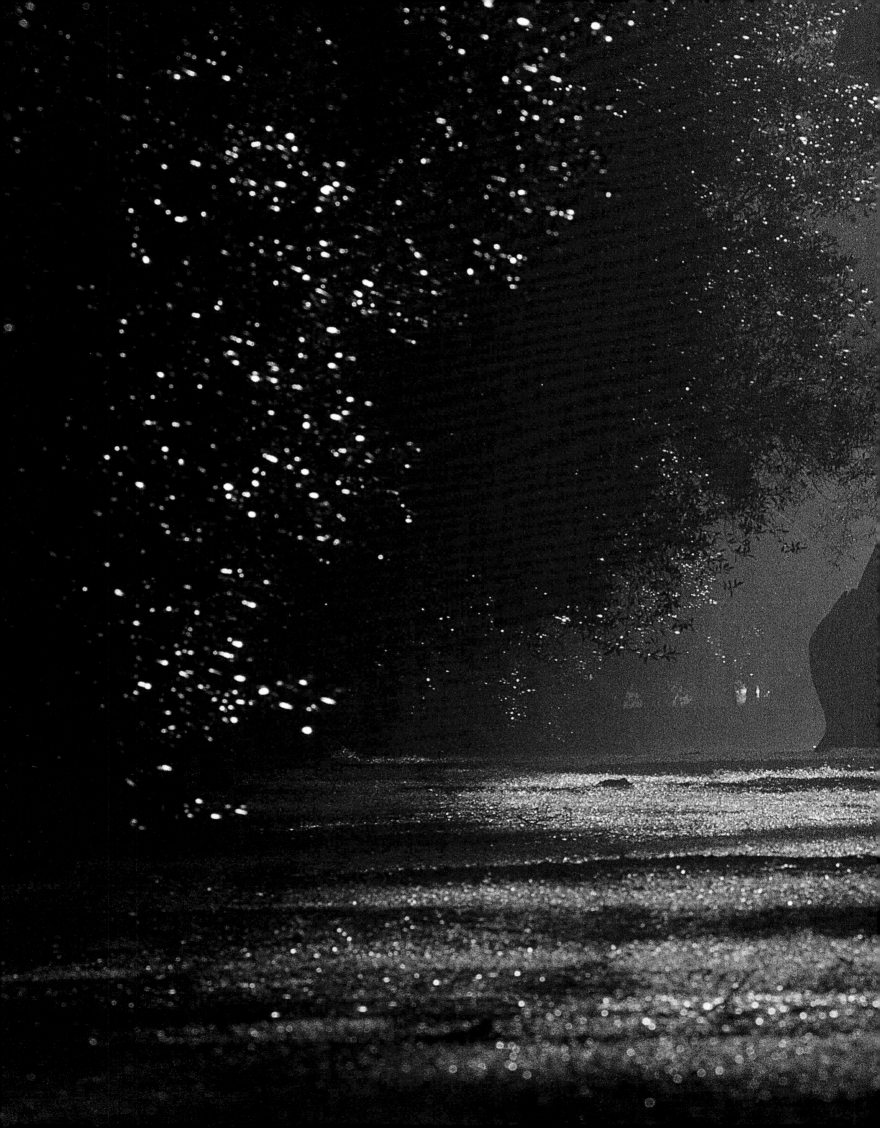

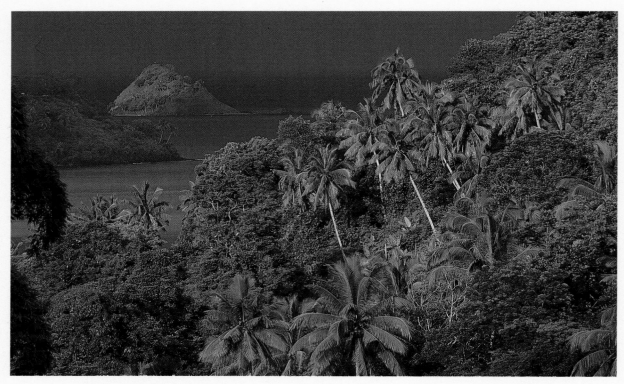

Jean-Paul Guerlain practices this art with a pleasure he readily communicates. According to him, "A perfumer has to go out in search of new fragrances." From India to Turkey, from the Indian Ocean to Italy, he jealously guards his protégés: "My sandalwood, roses and bergamot are the most precious assets I have. I never hesitate to jump on a plane to go and see for myself whether the jasmine I intend to use for Samsara is as perfect as I need it to be."

A badly organized harvest is sufficient to spoil the scent of a flower. Careful control of how and when the crop is picked and maintaining high standards in the distillation and extraction factories are the best guarantees for the perfumer for obtaining the highest quality essences and absolutes, worthy of being used for the perfumes which have made Guerlain its reputation.

Although Jean Kerléo often goes to Singapore to choose his patchouli and nutmeg essences and likes to immerse himself in the atmosphere of the rose plantations in Egypt, and despite the fact that his best memories are of a 150-acre jasmine orchard in Morocco, the fragrance of which enchanted him, leaving an indelible mark on his memory, his favorite moment of all is when he selects the rose essences destined for the Jean Patou perfumes. Once a year, in September, in the

Ylang-ylang flowers nonchalantly diffuse their vanilla scent in the Comoro Islands, in the Indian Ocean (above). In the Vittoria gardens in Calabria, Italy, one-hundred-year-old olive trees are interspersed with mandarin trees laden with golden, aromatic fruit (previous double page).

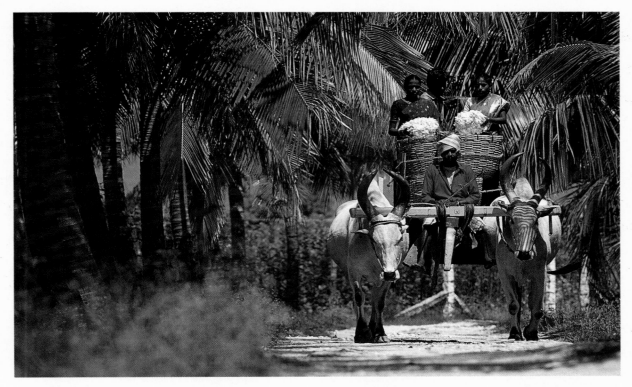

serenity of his office in Levallois, in the suburbs of Paris, he compares, assisted only by his nose, the thirty-odd samples from Grasse, Turkey, Bulgaria or Russia and picks out the smoothest and richest essences, those which are worthy of being used in Jean Patou's most prestigious perfumes, such as Joy, 1000 or Sublime.

However, not all perfumers are lucky enough to be able to go in search of their flowers. In fact, most of them work for large international companies dealing in raw materials and compositions, such as Quest, IFF (International Flavours and Fragrances), Givaudan-Roure, Haarmann & Reimer,

Takasago, Firmenich, Dragoco and Robertet, and are employed exclusively for the creation of perfumes. The windows of their laboratories no longer look out onto fields of roses or jasmine and nowadays computers have replaced the weighing scales. Nevertheless, as the perfumer Maurice Maurin, creator of Amazone for Hermès and the uncontested specialist of odorous plants, observes, "Although a certain amount of knowledge has disappeared and nowadays we are scarcely capable of recognizing the origin and altitude of a lavender plantation, in the way a wine expert can identify a vine, each perfumer instinctively recognizes the aura and

Odorous treasures, the raw materials used to make perfume come from all over the world. In India, before the heat becomes too torrid, baskets laden with fresh jasmine flowers are taken along fragrant paths to the distillation sites (above).

the vital energy of an essence obtained from the best fragrant flowers."

Françoise Caron, a perfume creator for Quest, is constantly lured by the charm of natural raw materials: "Each time you choose ginger, narcissus or mimosa, you are perpetuating the tradition and beauty of an ancient craft. At the same time, it is like going on a wonderful journey. Natural materials invoke a change of scenery, they conjure up their country of origin, the pickers, the atmosphere of the extraction factories and, above all, a wealth of colors and fragrances of breathtaking beauty."

FRAGRANT TREASURES FROM THE WORLD OVER

Every perfumer is, in fact, an armchair traveler. Alone in his laboratory, he sits surrounded by hundreds of perfume bottles, containing fragrant treasures from the world over. The suave, smooth perfume of the rose takes him to the precious fields around Grasse in the Provence region in the south of France, where the Provence rose, *Rosa* × *centifolia*, blooms in the month of May (hence its common French name, rose de mai). As one of the girl pickers remarks, "You have to love

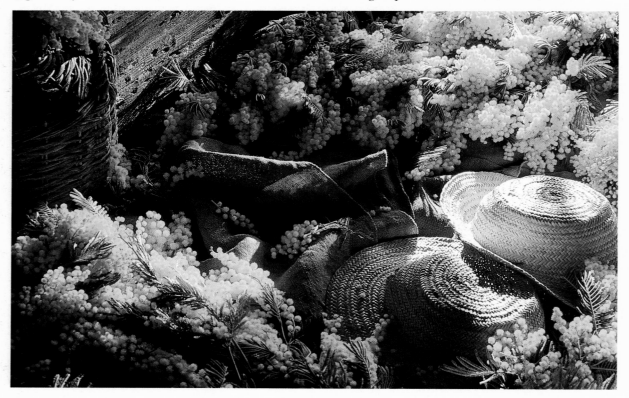

The intoxicating fragrances of plants haunt the region around Grasse like a melody. Mimosa, which originates from Australia, produces a suave, powder-scented essence (above). At the end of July, fresh, stimulating lavender, the fragrance of which has become identified with the Provence region, perfumes the hills, painting them a marvelous purple (opposite).

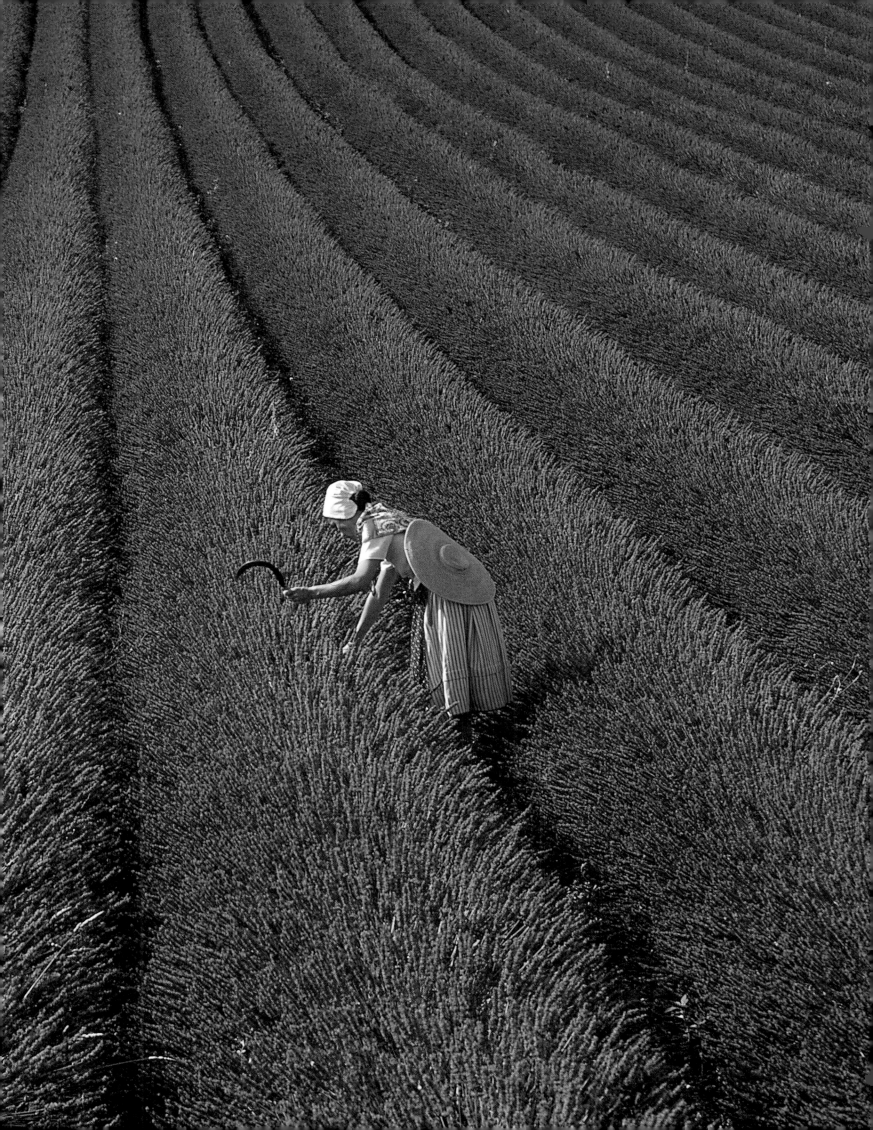

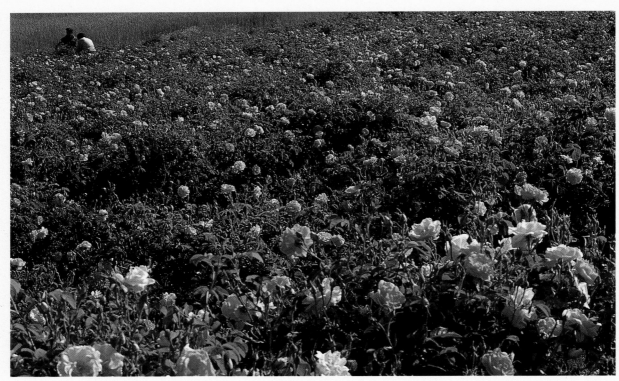

these roses to want to go and pick them every morning, in all weathers." It is true: these flowers are magnificent. The absolute extracted from them is so subtle and rich that it is a perfume all to itself. The Provence rose is also grown in Morocco, in the biblical landscape of the Dades valley, where it spreads its fragrant, colorful carpets as far as the eye can see. Their perfume changes, however, depending on the quality of the soil. Originally from Damascus, the Damask rose, *Rosa damascena*, is cultivated in Turkey and Bulgaria. After distillation, it produces a very delicate essence which is greatly prized by perfumers.

The delicate jasmine, which the inhabitants of Grasse refer to with a mixture of affection and respect as *la fleur* (the flower), has a magnificent, heady and sensual perfume. When the small, white, star-shaped flowers with their red hearts are picked they make a little squeaking noise, and are said to be "complaining." They are gathered at dawn, in July, in the fields around Grasse. They are so light that one metric ton of petals (eight million flowers) is needed to make just five and a half pounds of concrete and obtain just over two pounds of the fabulous *jasmin pays*, otherwise known as the *jasmin de Grasse* (Grasse jasmine). In olden times,

The Damask rose is cultivated on the plateaux of Bulgaria and Turkey. Its bushes grow to the height of a man and the roses produce a delicate rose-water and a fine, ethereal and slightly musky essence, the harmonious accompaniment to perfume head notes (above).

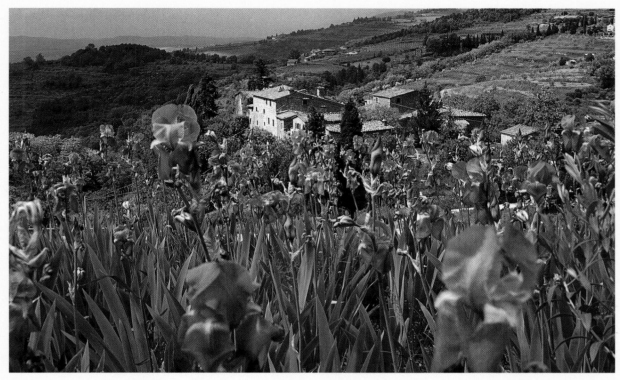

young girls were warned never to inhale the perfume of the tuberose in the evening, for fear of sinking into a state of voluptuous intoxication. This slender, elegant flower, reminiscent of the lily, diffuses a tantalizing scent. It has been cultivated in Grasse for many years and is now also found in Italy, Morocco and India.

In the July heat the beautiful bluish waves of lavender undulate across the mountainous landscapes of Provence. Its warm aromatic perfume is an inextricable part of the lives of the region's inhabitants. The delicate violet, which prefers the shade of the olive trees, deigns to flower in Bar-sur-Loup and Tour-

rettes-sur-Loup, near Grasse. Its precious scent is extracted from its leaves rather than from its flowers.

The fresh perfumes of bitter orange blossom, lemon and bergamot draw the perfumer to plantations in Calabria in southern Italy and in Sicily. The glossy leaves and the virginal flowers with their intoxicating perfumes are reminiscent of the mythical garden of the Hesperides.

In the eighteenth century, fashionable women were extremely fond of the iris, which is still cultivated on terraces near Florence, in Italy. The chalk-colored rhizomes have to be left to dry for several years before its powder-

Perfumers use the majestic, pale-colored iris (*Iris fiorentino*), which is cultivated at an altitude of 90 to 200 feet in the rocky soil of Tuscany in Italy. Their rhizomes are gathered every three years in the spring (above).

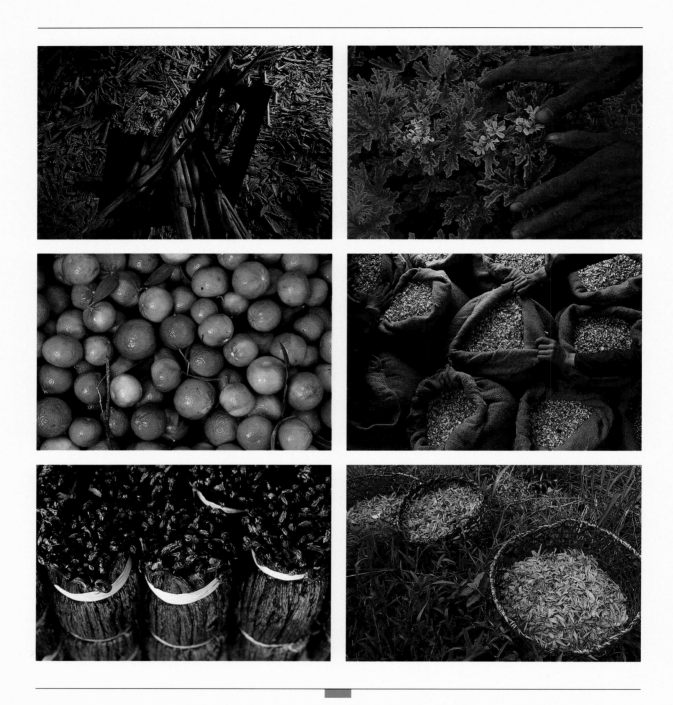

Barks, petals and aromatic fruits, gathered from the four corners of the earth, impart an attractive and exotic aura to perfumed compositions. Top (left to right): cinnamon from the island of Mayotte, geraniums from Réunion. Middle: green mandarins from Sicily, orange blossom from Tunisia. Bottom: vanilla from Madagascar and ylang-ylang from the Comoro Islands.

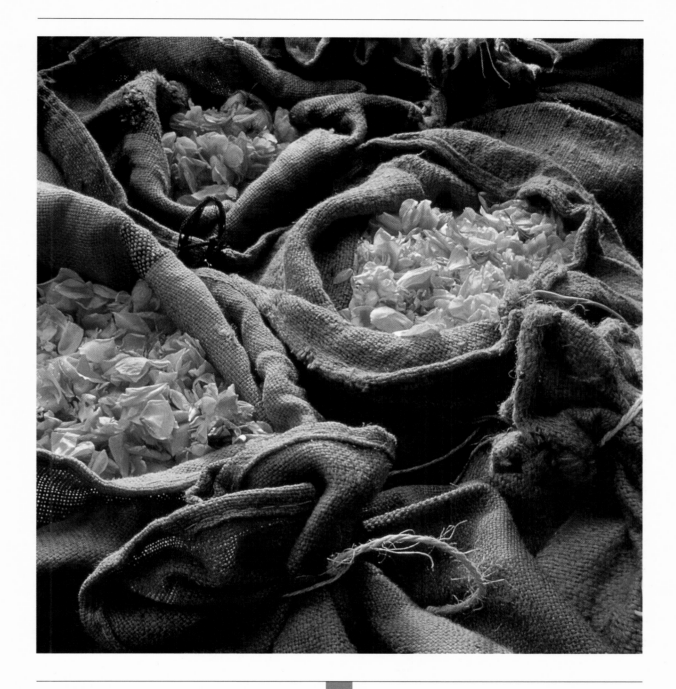

The rose, the undisputed queen of flowers, harbors the richest and most complex of fragrances in the softness of its delicate petals. More than four hundred volatile components contribute to its unique, rich, suave perfume. These cloth bundles contain fresh rose petals from the region around Grasse (above).

scented essence can be extracted. Myrrh, also known as the balm of Mecca, which is said to have been the perfume of Poseidon and the Nereids, is a suavely fragrant gum, produced by trees growing in the vicinity of the Red Sea. It is still used—mixed with two oriental-fragranced resins, opopanax and incense, which grow in the arid soil of Somalia and Ethiopia—to implore the favor of the gods. Vetiver, a perennial and particularly hardy plant, comes from the island of Réunion in the Indian Ocean, where its tufts of fine, long grass dance in the wind. A bitter, herbaceous essence is extracted from *khus-khus*, its roots. The scent of the nonchalant, white corollas of the ylang-ylang flowers pervades the atmosphere of the island of Mayotte, also in the Indian Ocean. The delicate green pods of vanilla, a member of the orchid family, only release their fragrance after they have "sweated" for months under covers. The best vanilla essence is also from Réunion and is known as Bourbon vanilla, after the island's former name.

Sandalwood has a warm, milky fragrance and is obtained from the majestic, odorous santal, a sacred tree in India from the southern state of Mysore, which is also grown in Australia. Sri Lanka is the land of spices, where barks, kernels, roots and plants offer their fragrant tributes. The dried leaves of patchouli, a small tree native to Indonesia but also grown in India and South America, are widely used in the perfume industry. They have a surprising scent with rough earthy notes, which was used to perfume cashmere garments to protect them from insects during long journeys. Patchouli oil is usually used in conjunction with vetiver. A smoky-smelling essence is extracted from the bark of the silver birches which rustle on the plains of Russia. Oakmoss, which is impregnated with the fragrance of the trees under and on which it grows, is found in the forests of former Yugoslavia, in Morocco and in the Massif Central region in France. Among the most noble of perfumery's absolutes, it has a rich, woody smell with an oceanic note, a distant reminder of the sea which once covered the forests.

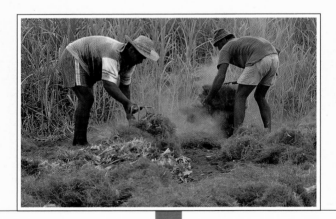

Vetiver is gathered in Réunion in the dry season from July to December (above). The rhizomes of Tuscan irises are preserved in sacks and are only distilled four or five years after picking (opposite, top). Bergamot, which comes from Bergamo in northern Italy, is grown in Sicily. It imparts a soft, suave essence to perfumes for example Cristalle by Chanel (opposite, bottom).

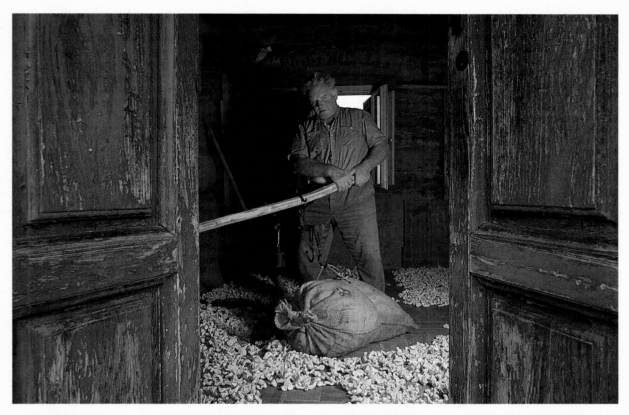

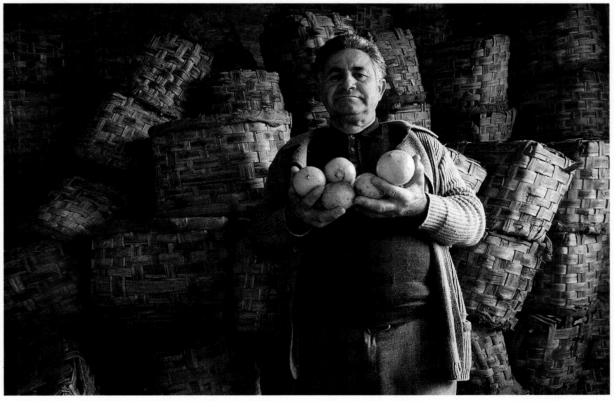

Oakmoss is often used in perfumes with heavy bouquets. The cedar trees growing in the Moroccan Atlas Mountains produce a warm, intense fragrance which provides one of the world's finest essences. The best varieties of ginger are found in Jamaica, but it also grows in the vast territories of China.

Although these particular raw materials are considered the most noble by perfumers, they should not overshadow the many odorous plants, the essences of which complete the creator's palette. These include aromatic plants such as basil, mint, coriander, tarragon and sage, and flowers such as mimosa, jonquil, broom, narcissus and, in the past, carnation.

Whereas flowers bring a soft and gentle femininity to perfumes, it is the animal notes which are responsible for their power and occasionally rough sensuality which give them their depth. Although they are not numerous, they are vital for the richness and body they give to a perfume. And although their intensity may shock more delicate nostrils, when combined with other ingredients they become incomparably soft and tenacious.

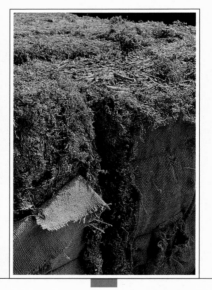

Musk comes from the musk deer which lives in the Himalayas and in Siberia, and produces a suave, very sensual animal essence which is known to have been a special favorite of Napoleon's first wife, Joséphine de Beauharnais. Ambergris, a form of calculus expelled naturally by the sperm whale into the sea, is mainly found on the shores of Portugal. Its light, oceanic scent is one of the warmest and subtlest of all. The civet cat, a small animal about the size of a fox which originates from Ethiopia, produces a strong, warm perfume which lends a composition a honeyed, animal note. Castoreum, a substance with a strong leathery smell, is obtained from the beavers native to Russia and Canada.

For some years now, however, the manufacture of these products has been curbed and their use has significantly diminished due to new legislation protecting these animals. The attitude of certain countries, such as Great Britain, who categorically refuse to use them in their compositions, has forced perfumers to turn increasingly to synthetic animal notes, such as the "modern musks" which now substitute natural musk.

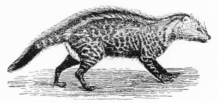

The strong animal odor of the civet cat marries well with the tender fragrances of flowers (opposite). Oakmoss, compressed into bales, provides a strong, green fragrance, reminiscent of the forest floor (above). Ylang-ylang trees in the Comoro Islands are regularly pruned so that the flowers are easily accessible to the pickers (opposite).

VIVERRA CIVETTA.

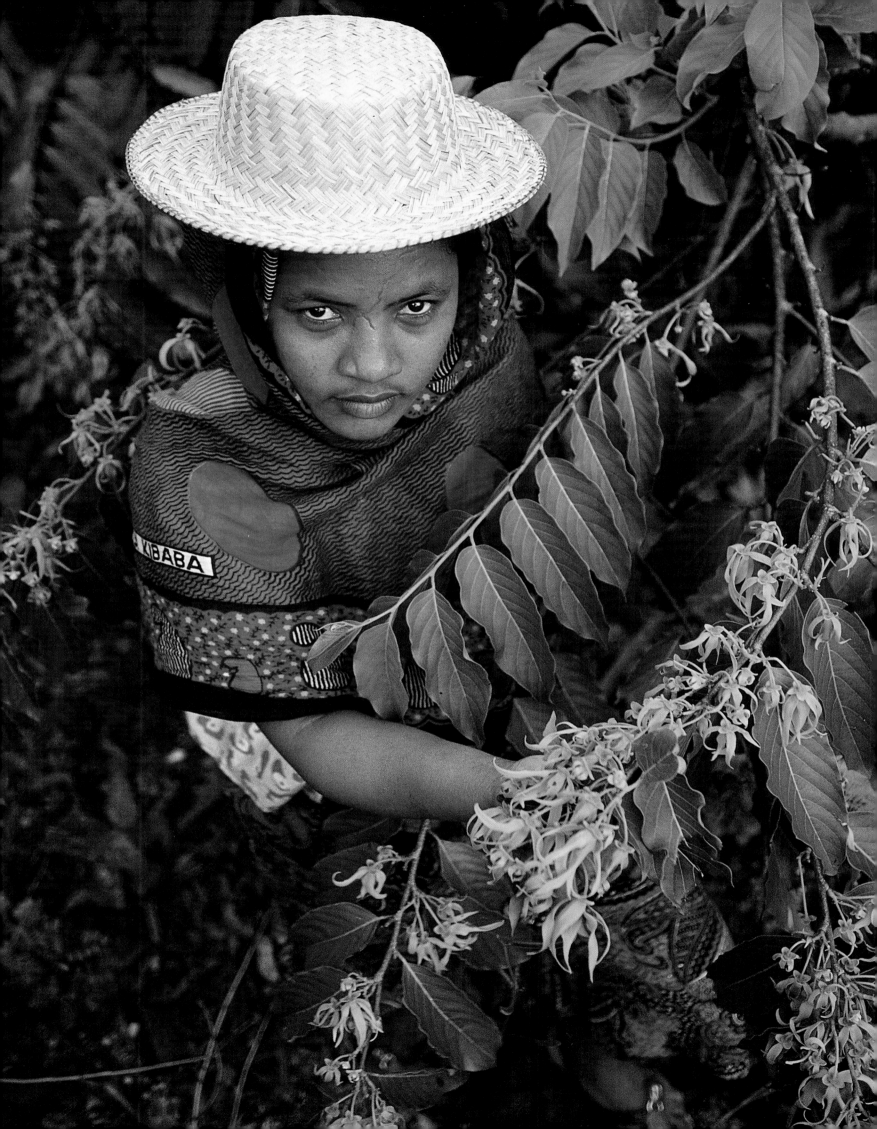

EXTRACTING AN ESSENCE

The privileged visitor who crosses the threshold of the perfumer's laboratory might well be somewhat disappointed. One has visions of an alchemist's cavern, full of iridescent, colored phials and a confusion of fragrances, where in actual fact one is confronted with hundreds of identical bottles lined up on shelves, differentiated only by the names on their labels. The fleshy, fragrant petals, the rough barks and the crystallized resins have all been transformed into essential oils, absolutes and infusions, the forms required for them to be used in the preparation of a perfume.

The writer Maurice Maeterlinck, a lover of flowers and nature, evokes with a certain degree of emotion in *L'Intelligence des fleurs* the "Processes by which the fragrant secret of a flower is torn from its heart and imprisoned in crystal."

Over the centuries, the various extraction techniques have undergone constant evolu-tion, which has enabled the finest and purest ingredients to be obtained.

Distillation, a process whereby odorous molecules are evaporated with steam by means of an alembic (a steam still), is one of the oldest methods and even now one of the most widely used. Until the Middle Ages, this activity merely served to recover the water distilled from flowers and plants, such as roses or orange blossom. During the Renaissance, however, the Catalan, Arnold de Villanova, and later the Swiss, Paracelse, proved that the residue oil, until then considered undesirable, in fact contained the quintessence of the plant's odorous principles. Henceforth it was these precious oils that perfumers strived to obtain, and gradually the process was developed industrially. Although the apparatus has become more sophisticated, the basic principles have remained the same. Swathes of lavender, rose petals or oakmoss lie in heaps on the ground before being transferred into one of the numerous boilers in the distillation factory. The odorous material to be

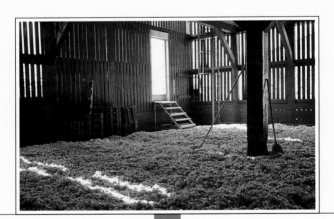

In the Givaudan-Roure factory in Grasse, rose petals are thoroughly aired in hangars before being poured into the distillation vats. Five metric tons of flowers yield little more than two pounds of essential oil (above and opposite).

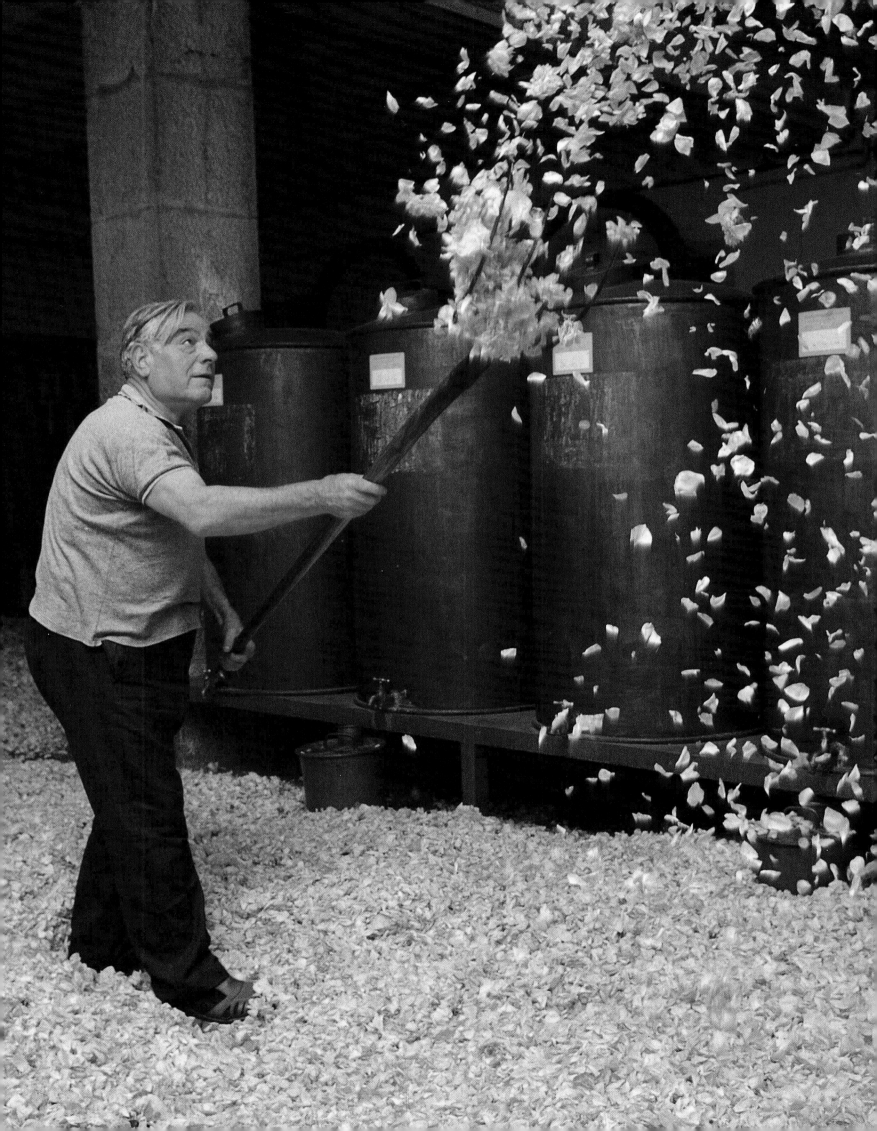

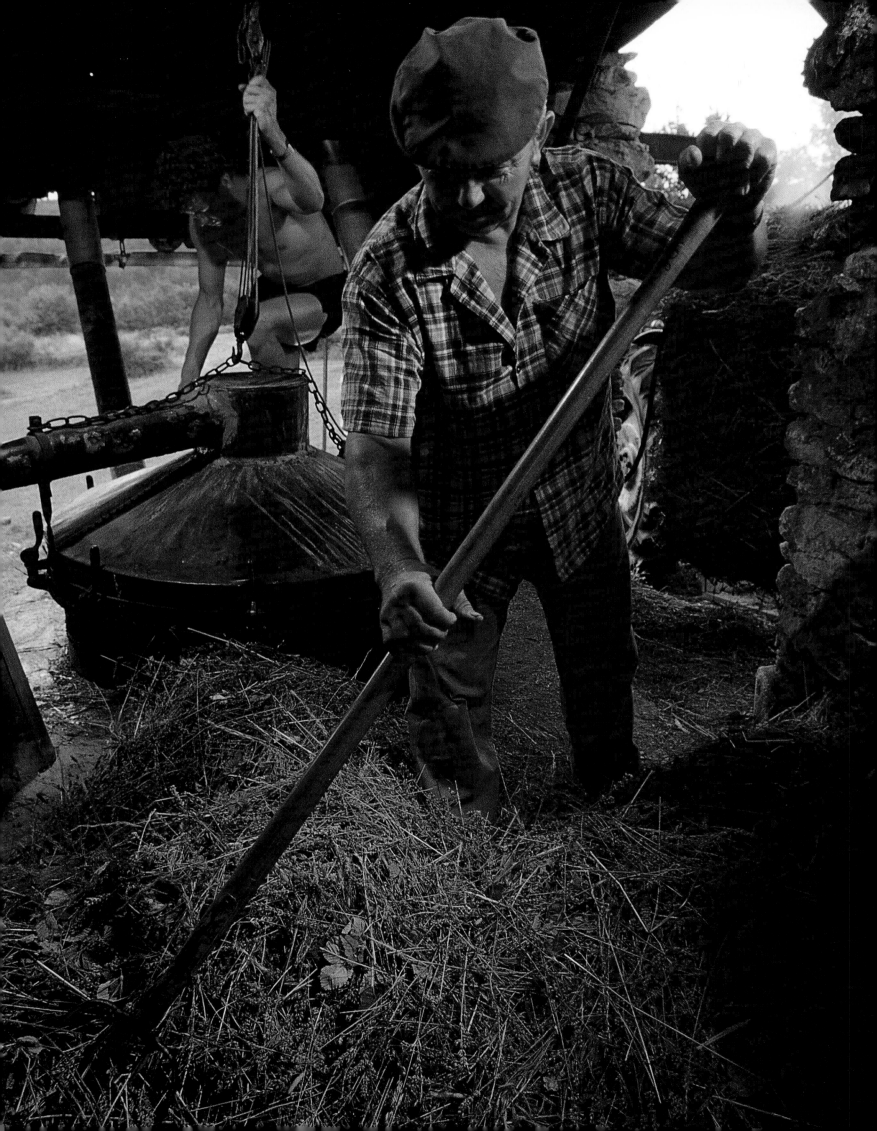

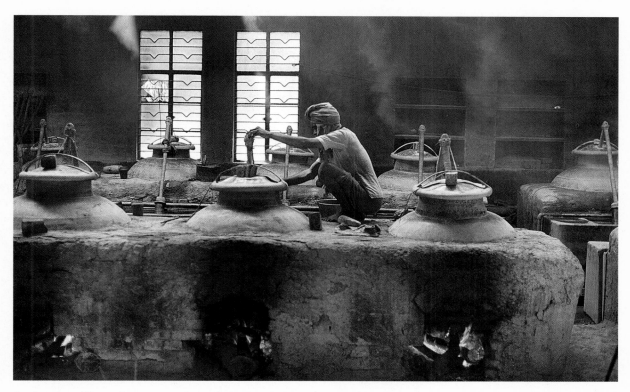

"exhausted" is then mixed in the apparatus with five times its weight of boiling water. The resulting steam containing the aromas passes through a gooseneck and is cooled. The mixture of condensed steam and oil is finally collected in a Florence flask, which is designed to allow the essential oils to be separated off from the water.

Whereas, as Maurice Maeterlinck remarks, once in the gigantic boilers the "complacent" rose gives up its aroma in all simplicity, other flowers are not at all suited to this method. This is the case, for example, of the tuberose, which, after distillation, provides a somewhat crude essence which is of no use in perfumery,

or of jasmine, from which nothing can be extracted by this method. It became clear that new techniques were needed. At the beginning of the nineteenth century, the inhabitants of Grasse developed a method known as *enfleurage*, an ancient process used first by the Egyptians, which consists of exploiting the capacity of absorption of odors by fat. *Enfleurage* was to revolutionize the art of perfumery as it made it possible to extract the odorous principles from flowers such as tuberose or jasmine, which cannot be treated by any of the other methods. Freshly picked flowers are carefully laid out on glass frames which have been coated with a layer of odor-

Often odorous raw materials are distilled at the place where they have been gathered. Here, in Réunion, the geraniums go straight into the vats, following a tradition which has remained unchanged since the nineteenth century (above). In the Cassan-Simiane la Rotonde distillery in Provence, a similar fate awaits the fragrant lavender, which produces a powerfully aromatic essence (opposite).

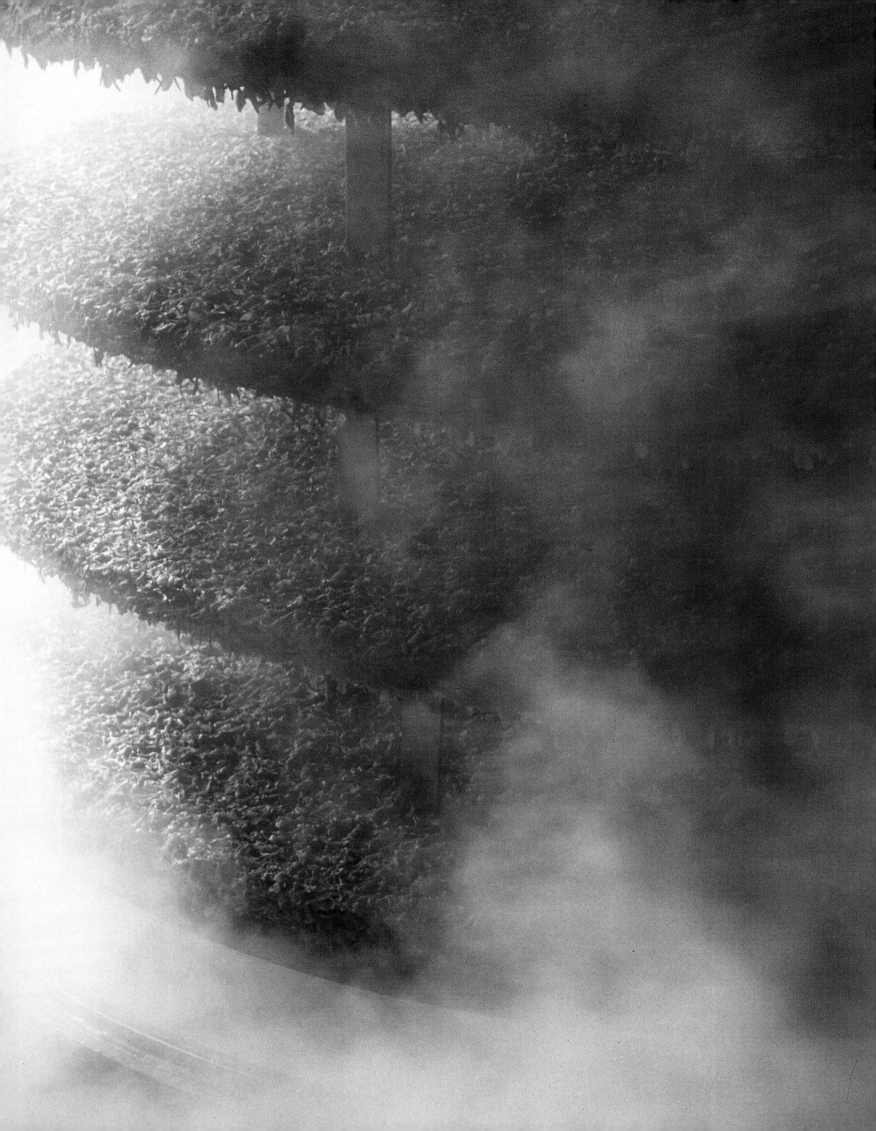

less fat and are replaced at regular intervals (every twenty-four hours for jasmine) until the fat is saturated with the flower's fragrance. Grenouille, the hero of Patrick Süskind's novel *Perfume*, becomes a master of this process, and uses it to extract the odorous "essence" of the loveliest young girls in the town of Grasse, thus obtaining a perfume, the essence of seduction, which gives him, the man born without human odor, a supernatural, diabolical power of attraction.

In 1880, a new type of extraction was developed. The steam used in distillation was replaced by volatile solvents, hence the term—volatile solvent extraction. This more powerful method made it possible to obtain essences from plants which have only a faint aroma, such as dry materials, bark, roots and animal products. Perforated trays covered with a thick layer of raw materials are placed inside extractors, then a solvent is run through them which draws off the odorous molecules. Once this perfumed fat, known as pomade, has been treated with alcohol, the perfumed mixture undergoes various processes until a waxy material, known as a concrete, is obtained. When further purified by alcohol, this produces the absolute, which has an extremely fine perfume, rather like that of a freshly picked flower. Gums and resins when treated by this method produce a substance known as resinoid.

Essential oils are extracted from citrus fruit by a very simple process known as citrus extraction. The peel is removed and pressed so as to rupture the minute pockets containing the essential oils. Nowadays cylinders equipped with special blades are used, but formerly the extraction was carried out by hand using a sponge and an *écuelle* (a hollow vessel with spikes inside), or a leather glove with inlaid stone chips.

The contrast between the imposing machines, the complex techniques and the delicacy of the flowers and evanescence of their perfumes is certainly striking. Maurice Roucel, a perfumer employed by Quest, explains, "The thermal and physical shocks undergone by the plants during the various stages of the production of the essence, considerably modify the quality of the odorous molecules."

The object of a study carried out by the company IFF was to prove that a flower's perfume is modified immediately after being picked. As soon as the "umbilical cord" linking the flower or fruit to the plant is cut, the fragrance deteriorates rapidly. Some twenty years ago, researchers developed a very simple yet revolutionary process known as headspace. A fresh flower, still attached to its roots, is placed in the center of a bell jar through which a neutral gas is passed, which captures its scent. A molecular identity card is established according to the analysis of the gas containing the odorous molecules and given to the perfumer, who then reconstitutes the perfume with the help of natural raw materials and synthetic products. The substance thus obtained reproduces the freshness and lightness of the perfumes of living plants in a very natural manner. This technique can be applied to numerous plants and enables one not only to capture the fragrance of those which flower very rarely or only during the night, but also to reproduce the perfume of

These delicate jasmine petals, wilting after being deprived of their odorous substance, have just sacrificed one of the most voluptuous and sensual essences in perfumery to the extractors. Nearly one ton of flowers is needed to make only two pounds of absolute (opposite).

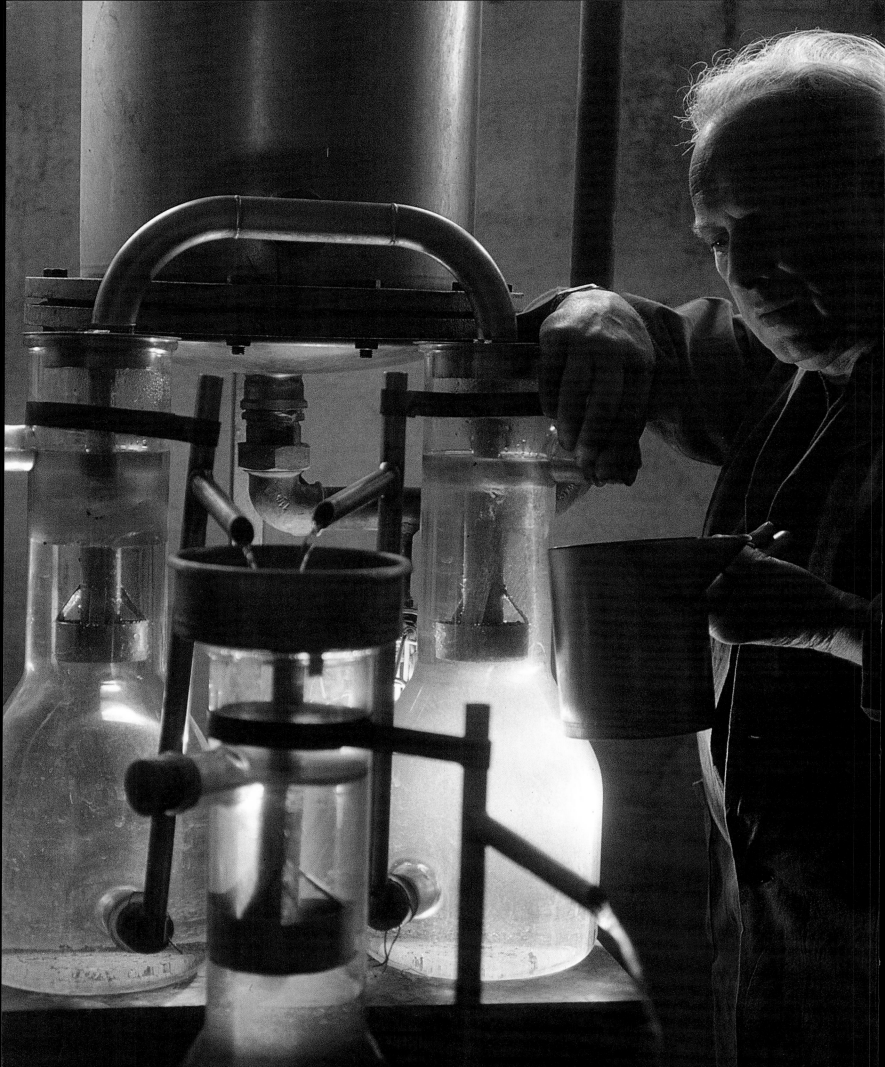

flowers, known as "the perfumer's despair," such as lilac, gardenia, violet and lily of the valley, from which it was impossible to extract their perfume by any of the previously existing methods.

THOUSANDS OF NEW ESSENCES

At the end of the last century, the perfume organ, with its wooden, fan-shaped form reminiscent of the musical instrument from which it takes its name, was the traditional worktable used by perfumers and it easily housed the majority of the products necessary for the creation of a perfume. Nowadays entire rooms are needed to accommodate the thousands of various odorous materials which creators have at their disposition.

In the space of a century, the perfumer's palette has expanded by more than two thousand new odorous products, all of which have been discovered through research. For many years these fragrances remained unknown to researchers. It was only in the 1880s, with the development of organic chemistry, that they started to produce new odorous molecules from natural raw materials. In actual fact, an essence extracted from a plant can contain several hundred odorous molecules; the rose, for example, contains more than three hundred. One of the techniques practiced by the research chemist consists of isolating one or more of these molecules and then recreating them synthetically. This is how linalol, an ingredient widely used by perfumers, is extracted from rosewood. Research carried out in the domain of organic products, such as petroleum or coal tar, has given rise to a considerable number of odorous molecules which do not exist in the plant universe, but have proved decisive in the development of modern-day perfumery.

The links between natural and synthetic products are very close. One of the greatest living perfume creators and theorists of our age, Edmond Roudnitska, has long been an

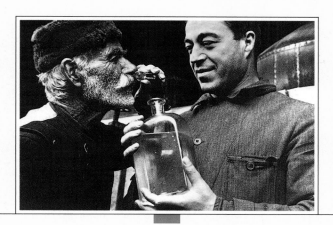

The art of perfumery resides in the subtle alchemy of intelligence, sensitivity and technique. Here a specialist controls the quality of a rose essence in the rose valley in Bulgaria (above). The distilled oils are collected in vessels which are known as Florence flasks (opposite). It was at this perfume organ that Jacques Guerlain (1874–1963) created the legendary fragrances Mitsouko, Shalimar and Vol de Nuit (overleaf).

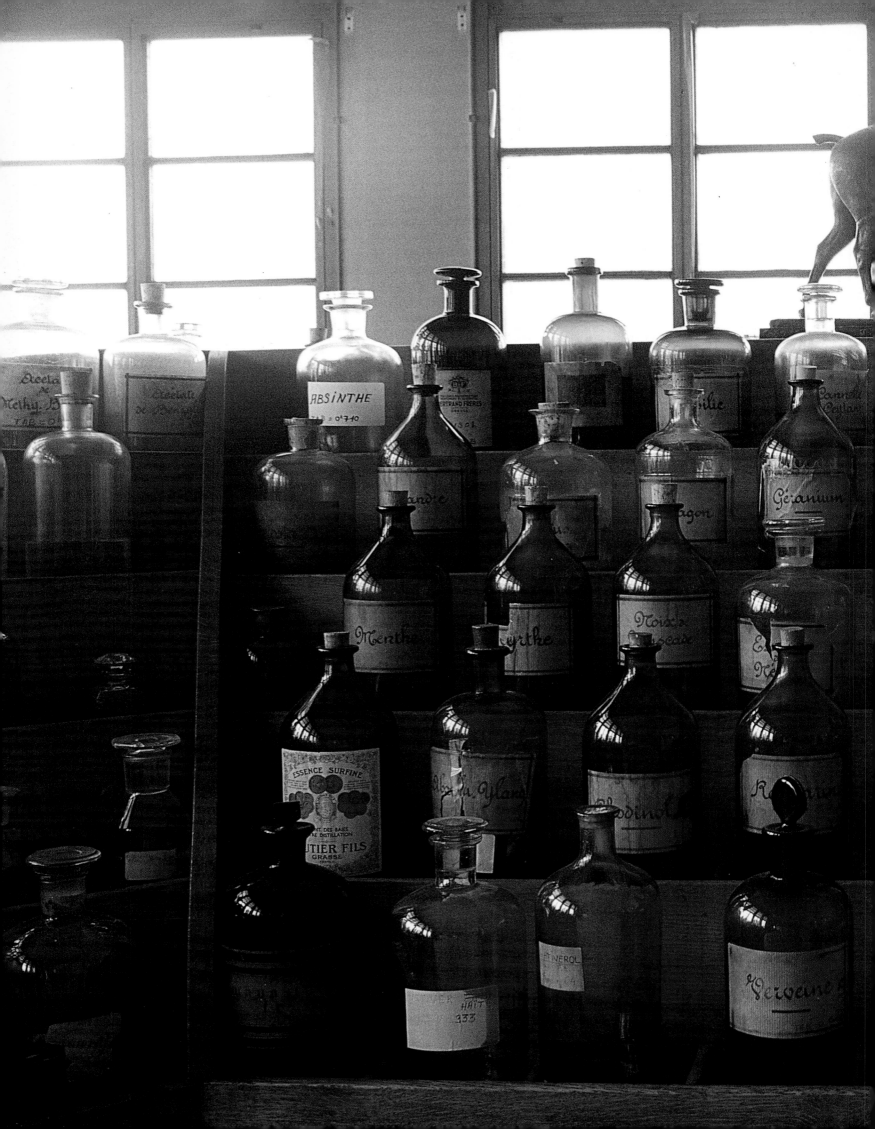

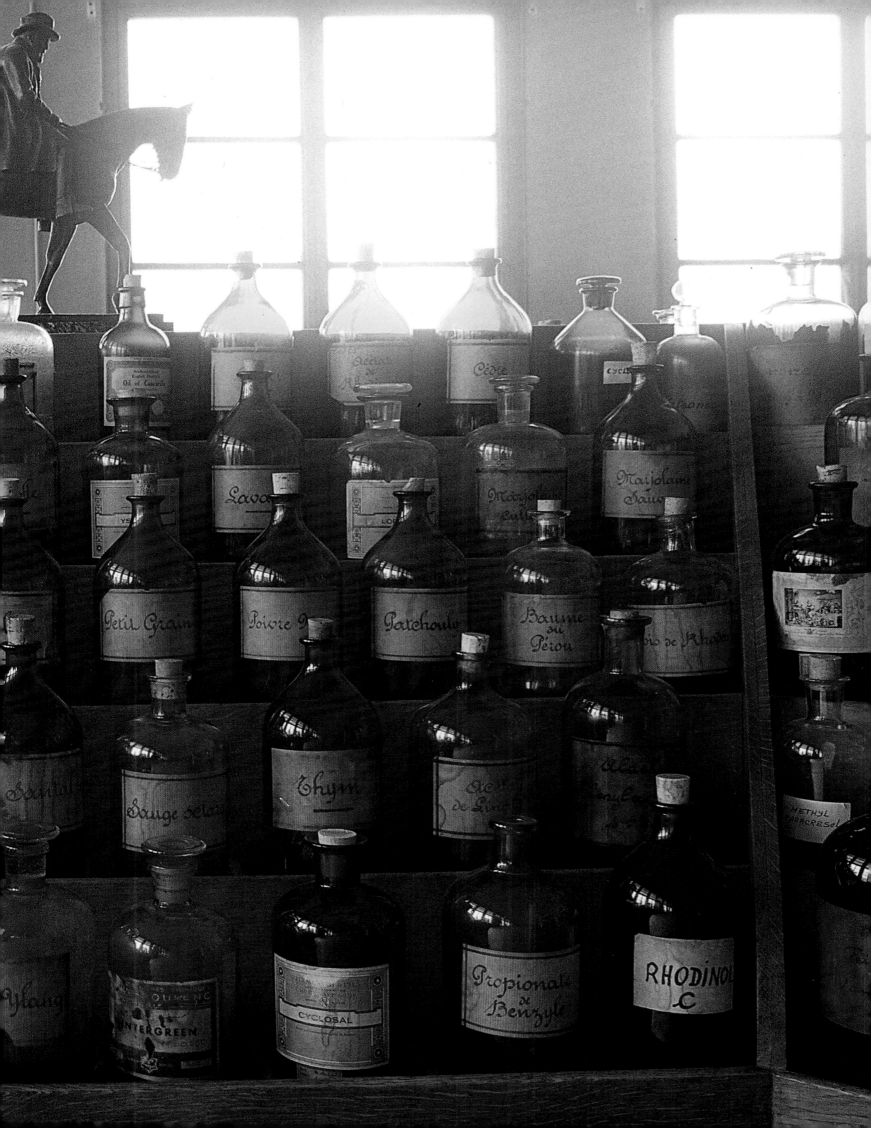

ardent champion of the latest perfumery techniques. It was Roudnitska who reproduced, with modern notes, the lily of the valley fragrance which haunts Christian Dior's Diorissimo. As far as he is concerned, natural products are "Nothing more than well-executed mixtures of chemical products provided by nature."

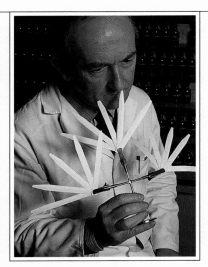

From the second half of the nineteenth century, new discoveries followed one another in rapid succession, thus enlarging the fragrance palette and developing our understanding of the world of odors. In 1882, for the first time, the perfumer François Houbigant used a synthetic molecule, coumarin, in a composition called Fougère Royale. Sometime later, Aimé Guerlain introduced vanillin into his perfume Jicky. Soon after, at the beginning of this century, the famous perfumer François Coty made wide use of this synthetic product in creations such as L'Origan or Le Chypre.

It was, however, the perfumer Ernest Beaux who established these little-known raw materials in the 1920s. By switching the roles and introducing very large proportions of certain aldehydes into his formula, he made Chanel N° 5 the leader of modern perfumes. These curious molecules, which have an odor which is like that of a hot iron placed on a damp cloth, have the effect of galvanizing the natural raw materials with which they come in contact. In this way, the magnificent Grasse

jasmine, which is used in the preparation of Chanel N° 5, acquired a hitherto unsuspected beauty and an incomparably more powerful impact. Ernest Beaux stated, "Henceforth it will be the responsibility of research chemists to discover new molecules to permit original notes to see the light of day. The future of perfume lies in the hands of Science," and with these words the celebrated perfumer succinctly summarized the decisive new direction he had given to perfumery.

Synthetic products, far from constituting an opposition to natural raw materials, complement them. Jean Guichard, a perfumer with Givaudan-Roure, maintains that he makes no distinction, when creating a perfume, between natural and synthetic notes, both of which have their specific properties and their own olfactory character.

Nothing, however, can replace natural essences. Their wonderfully rich, smooth impact is quite inimitable. Yet the evolution of the perfume industry is such that a return to entirely natural compositions is out of the question, since consumers are now used to the power and impact, the tenacity and trail of the synthetic products. It is these products which give contemporary creations their olfactory characteristics. Hedion, with its jasmine fragrance, contributed to the success of Christian Dior's extraordinary Eau Sauvage (1966), one of Roudnitska's creations. The

The "Nose," with his finely tuned senses and rich imagination, is the sole judge of a perfume. Jean Kerléo, perfumer for Jean Patou, smells a selection of perfumed blotter strips to check the quality of the essences (above). The rose concrete, after being filtered to eliminate waxes, yields what is known as the absolute (opposite).

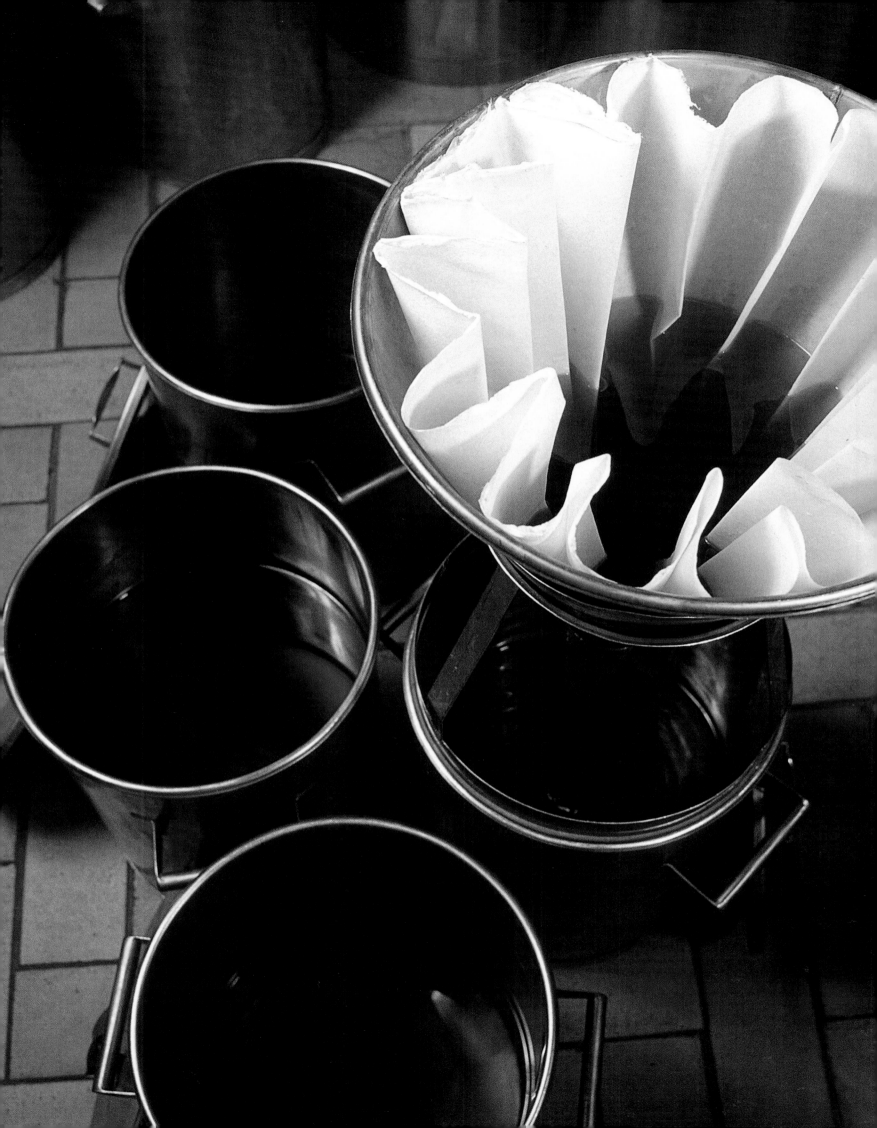

rose-like perfume of damascone gives that special touch to Guerlain's Nahéma (1979) and to Yves Saint Laurent's Paris (1983). The oceanic notes contained in calone and helional—found in New-West for Her by Aramis (1988), Escape by Calvin Klein (1991), L'Eau d'Issey by Issey Miyake (1992) and Kenzo for Men (1991)—are reminiscent of sea air blowing across the shore. These molecules can also substitute natural essences which have become too expensive, or too difficult to obtain for climatic or political reasons, as in the case of animal products.

The quality and interest of modern creations is linked to the extreme diversity of the odorous products which they contain. The discovery of new molecules represents a source of enrichment for perfumers. Jacques-Marie Decazes, the research director for Givaudan-Roure, sees the role played by the researcher as vital, since by offering unusual notes and new accords and techniques to the creator, he opens up whole new fields of creation for him.

THE ART OF COMPOSITION

Vast sunny beaches by the ocean, golden dunes caressed by the wind, the sky moving in rhythm with the sea—these ever-changing shores inspired Jean-Louis Sieuzac to create the new perfume Dune for Christian Dior. He thus imagined an olfactory landscape, a garden blossoming in the shelter of the sand dunes, full of lilies, gillyflowers, and peonies, and bathed in the scents of sea-spray and citrus.

On the table in his office, however, the only clues to his profession are a few perfume bottles containing the creations he is currently working on, a pencil, paper and a fan-shaped arrangement of blotter strips. Comfortably seated in his armchair, the creator conceives of the predominant features of his perfume assisted by his memory alone. As Edmond Roudnitska points out, it is with "recollections of sensations" that the perfumer begins his work, not by smelling essences, blending them, or carrying out tests. The perfumer exercises his olfactory sense daily and is able to

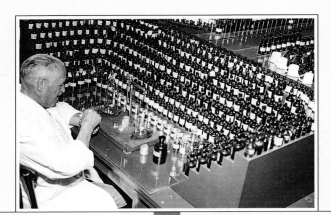

Like all creators, the perfumer needs to work in a calm atmosphere. Jean Carles, a perfumer with Givaudan-Roure and author of a revolutionary method used in perfumery training, sits at his perfume organ (above). Every year, the perfumer Annick Goutal returns to this monastic cell in Certosa di Pontignano, an artists' residence in Tuscany, in order to seek inspiration (opposite).

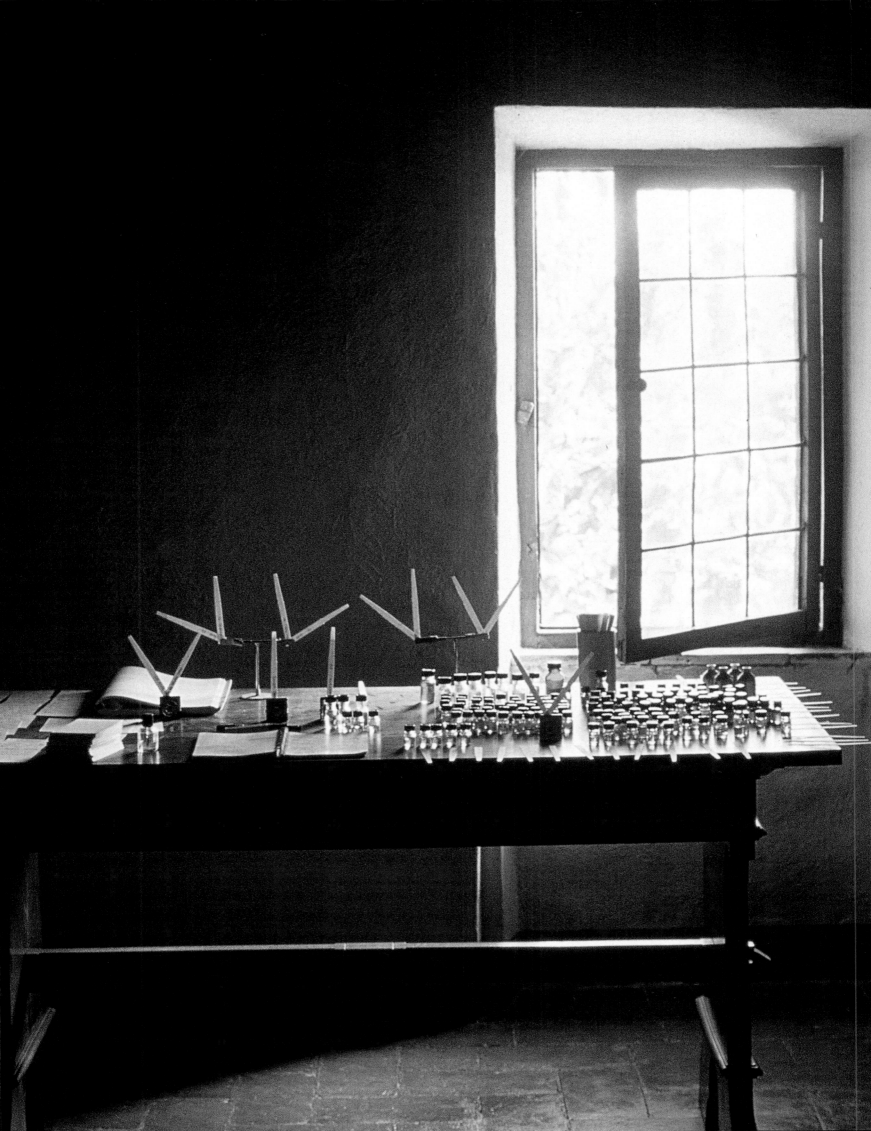

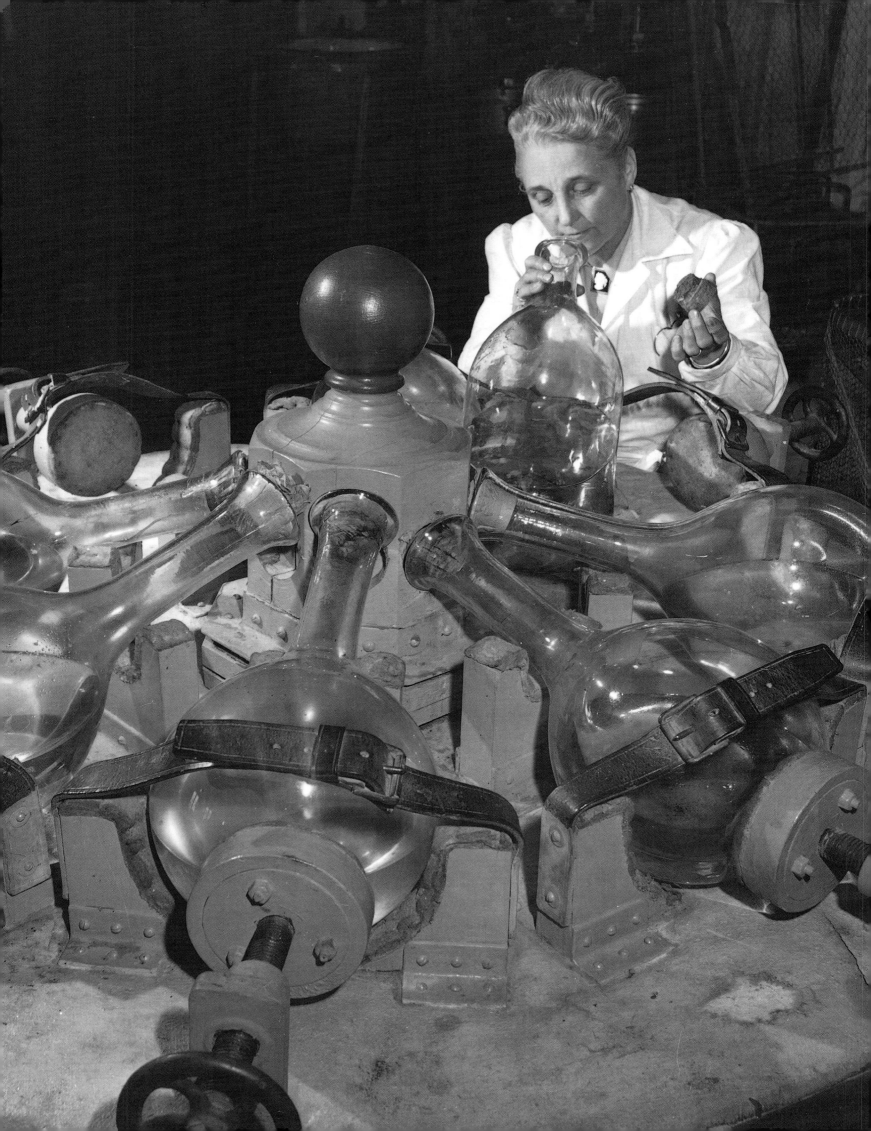

commit from two to four thousand odors to memory. Beside the raw materials which compose his palette, there are the odors which he comes across in his everyday life—the smell of a crowd, the aroma of a cedar tree in Marrakech, the perfumed shadow of a magnolia tree, or the exotic scents of a tropical forest. Moreover, his memory is so powerful that if he lost his sense of smell, he would still be able to invent and compose perfumes.

Equipped with this vast range of odorous materials, the perfumer sets to work. He still has to find the main idea, the olfactory theme around which he will work. This might take form either through a simple association of ideas, or intuitively—emerging suddenly when

he smells an odor for the first time, or when noticing a detail of a smell which had previously escaped his attention.

With his idea in mind—whether it be figurative, like a garden in the rain, or of a purely abstract nature—the perfumer starts by making a list of the odorous products which seem to correspond best to what he has imagined, opposite which he notes the requisite proportions of each ingredient.

Merely bringing together a certain number of odors is not, however, sufficient to compose a perfume. As Jean-François Blayn, the great critic and perfume historian, so accurately points out, "A perfume is composed not of a sum of fragrances, but of the rela-

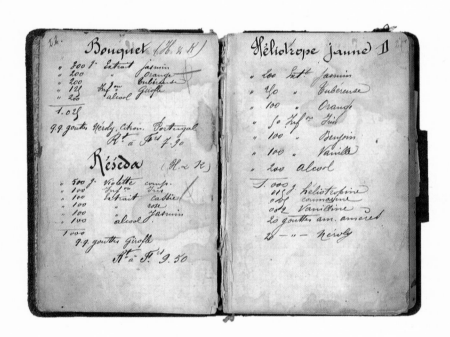

Perfumers work in the strictest secrecy, jealously guarding the mysteries of their art. Since the beginning of perfume, formulas have been kept hidden from prying eyes, like this one in a private notebook belonging to Molinard, dating from about 1905 (above). Extreme care is taken in the treatment of odorous raw materials, which, over a period of three months, are subject to constant tests and kept in constant motion in enormous vats known as *valseuses*, after which tinctures, originating from animal substances such as ambergris, are obtained (opposite).

tionship between them." Odors are alive. When mixed they produce chemical reactions; whether they harmonize, complement or smother one another depends on the delicate character of each ingredient. As a result, the perfumer requires not only a perfect memory of each odor he uses, but must also be capable of imagining how each raw material will react when in contact with another. Mixing ingredients can bring its surprises, however, and it is not uncommon to discover new, quite unexpected harmonies. To optimize these discoveries is the whole art of the perfume creator.

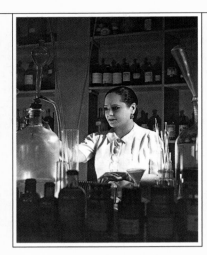

Jean-Louis Sieuzac has small quantities of the perfume he is creating made up at every stage so he can then put the results to the judgment of his nose. Smelling the product is in fact an essential part of the whole process. Edmond Roudnitska recommends "Three seconds of olfaction at intervals of at least fifteen seconds" so as to avoid saturation of the olfactory sense (which is known as odor fatigue). The perfume formula usually undergoes various modifications, perhaps adding a little freshness to the top note, making the perfume smoother, or developing the "green" notes (as in the case of Dune). Each test refines the perfume by accentuating the interesting effects and reducing any others.

While creating his fragrance, the perfumer works in the strictest secrecy. The formula he develops is confidential, known only to himself and the company he works for. The preparation of the perfume is entrusted to various laboratory assistants who only have access to one part of the formula. The mixture, in the form of a concentrate, is weighed then left to stand for several weeks in order to allow each ingredient to adjust itself to the others. After this it is diluted in 96° proof alcohol, then left for a maceration period of several weeks which gives the perfume time to find its equilibrium. The perfumer then smells the fragrance again to see if it is developing as expected and to see if any modifications are needed. The perfume is then "frozen" at a temperature somewhere between five and minus ten degrees centigrade and finally filtered in order to eliminate any insoluble residues.

This process of creating a perfume might appear uneventful, but in reality the situation is far more complicated. Apart from a few perfumers who work solely for the prestigious perfume houses and rare independent perfumers, like Annick Goutal, Edmond Roudnitska, Maurice Maurin, Monique Schlienger or Olivia Giacobetti, most composers work in teams employed by the large raw material and manufacturing companies, who in turn negotiate with the famous names. Gone are the days when perfumers were both creators and craftsmen, like François Houbigant, the Guerlains, François Coty, Paul Poiret, Ernest Beaux and Ernest Daltroff with Caron. Today

"By dint of seeking to penetrate fragrances, they themselves penetrate us. They inhabit us and become a part of us," wrote the great perfumer Edmond Roudnitska, photographed here in his garden by Edouard Boubat (opposite). As for Helena Rubinstein, a perfumer of Russian origin, it was from women, and women alone, that she drew her inspiration (above).

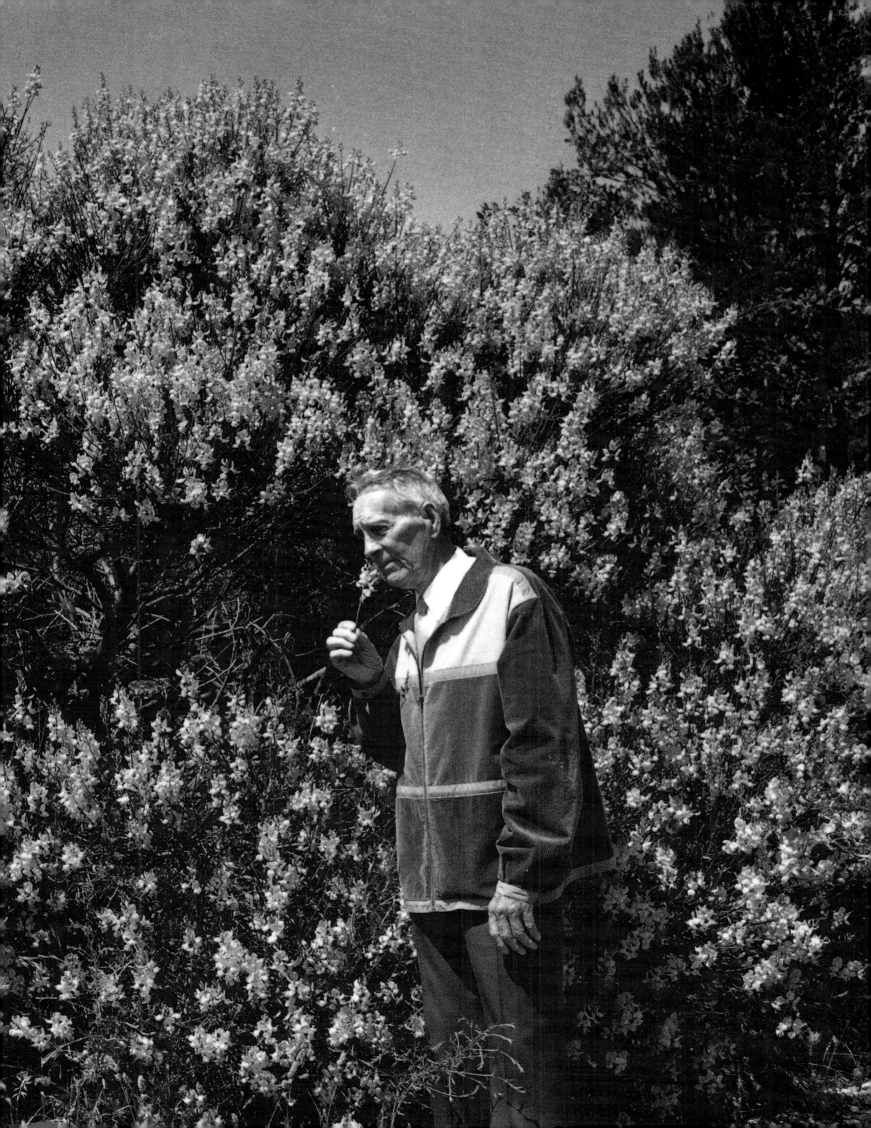

perfumers, whether they work in France, the United States, Switzerland, Germany or Japan, are obliged to compete with each other at the instigation of perfume houses such as Yves Saint Laurent, Laura Ashley or Escada, often only knowing the code name of the future perfume.

These men and women work under considerable pressure. Their job requires intuition, imagination and creativity. They work long hours in the office, have frequently to check the requirements of their clients and then spend long hours looking for inspiration outside their place of work.

One thing is certain, however, and that is the fact that only the perfumer possesses the secret of his art. He alone knows the magic of fragrances. Nothing, neither machines, nor analytical processes, no-one else can replace his experience, his savoir-faire and his refined talents. It is up to him to maximize his creativity despite restrictions imposed on him, to go beyond the generally accepted limits and to continue the search for perfumes which are beautiful, original and unique.

It is impossible not to aspire to creating the greatest, the most beautiful of all perfumes, impossible not to try to emulate the great perfumes, each of which, in its day, revolutionized perfumery and created new olfactory phenomena, in the same way as painters invent new forms of expression. There are numerous models to follow: François Houbigant with Quelques Fleurs, Ernest Beaux with Chanel N° 5, Coty's Chypre (no longer produced) or Germaine Cellier, one of the few female creators, who dreamt up Balmain's Vent Vert.

Yet, what use would the best raw materials and the purest odorous products be without the special art of blending them? Where the good perfumer is usually an excellent, imaginative technician, the great, the very great perfumer is an artist who intuitively makes the very most of the odorous materials at hand, transcending them even, to reveal that extra spirit which makes a real masterpiece, an incomparable source of emotion.

Edmond Roudnitska has spent his whole life striving to raise perfumery to the level of an art form. From his villa in Cabris, not far from Grasse, this very great perfumer—creator of Eau Sauvage for Christian Dior, Femme for Rochas and of the delightful Eau d'Hermès, to name just a few—maintains his passionate defence of an art which, according to him, requires the qualities of intelligence, imagination and intuition.

How does one recognize a truly great perfume? What distinguishes it from the others? Certain criteria such as character, vigor, power of diffusion, delicacy, volume and tenacity are essential. A great perfume must be technically perfect and develop harmoniously. This evolution depends on the evaporation rate of each raw material. Ideally, these should follow each other in a subtle pattern, without any gaps or sudden breaks in tone. The number of raw materials involved also determines the tone of the perfume. As Jean Kerléo explains, "Too many raw materials make a perfume heavy and confusing and hence difficult to appreciate, but at the same time, oversimplifying a perfume means it loses all its mystery." In the last twenty years or so, the number of ingredients used in perfume formulas has dropped, having reached a high

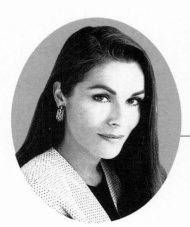

Working with perfume requires delicacy, passion and a constant open-mindedness and curiosity about the world around us. Annick Goutal (left) finds her inspiration in nature, of which she is a great lover, and her close friends, gathering together the impressions and sensations which form the very soul of her most exquisite creations, such as L'Eau du Ciel, or the magnificent Sables, inspired by the dunes on the Ile de Ré.

of several hundred. In response to a new demand for clarity, the preference is once more for compositions which contain only about fifty raw materials.

A truly great perfume, however, is one which provokes genuine emotion in the person who smells it for the first time. The heart misses a beat, emotion takes over and the person knows that for them this perfume expresses an essential truth. The best perfumes are ones which "give us a shock."

It is true that a perfume should possess a sort of excess, which could be considered to be a flaw, but which, as for a face, brings a beauty, a meaning and a personality which would otherwise be lacking. An excess of aldehydes, as in Chanel N° 5, or a slightly discordant note become appealing features which are sometimes capable of transforming a banal work into a masterpiece.

A beautiful perfume, however, always holds a promise of future happiness. The perfumer Constantin Wériguine (who worked for a long time with Ernest Beaux for Chanel) compares the pleasure we get from a perfume to the joy we feel in the presence of our children: "All the famous perfumes contain an element of happiness and the main reason for their success lies in this link with the very source of life."

GRASSE: A TOWN OF TRADITION AND MODERNITY

Grasse is the heart and soul of the perfumer. For several centuries now, successive generations of creators have followed each other there. Grasse, the cradle of perfumery, is now a place of pilgrimage for perfumers from all over the world. As soon as spring arrives, they can be seen wandering around this small town with its overpowering fragrances. "It was a tremendous pleasure for me to visit Grasse," admits Sophia Grosjman, a perfumer with IFF in New York, "I really had the impression of being at the very origins of perfumery's existence."

For more than three centuries now, Grasse

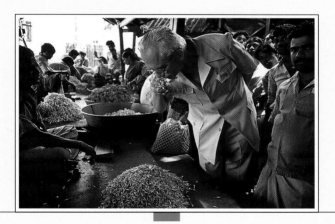

Traveling the world in search of the most precious flowers and plants, and selecting the most aromatic of them, those that will help to transform a simple perfume into a masterpiece—that is the dream of all perfumers. Every year, Jean-Paul Guerlain, the fourth representative of the Guerlain dynasty, goes to India to choose his jasmine (above).

has made people dream. In May, the smell of roses lingers in the dark alleys with their irregular paving stones and in the squares with their refreshing fountains, and although the fields of flowers have practically disappeared and the busy factories have been replaced by ultra-modern perfume laboratories, Grasse has lost none of its charm.

It was in the seventeenth century, here in this town situated in eastern Provence, nestling in a setting of mauve, pink and white hills, that—thanks to the energy and incredible faith of a handful of pioneers—perfumery was born. Until then Grasse had prospered thanks to its tanning industry, organized in to several guilds, including the glove and perfume-makers guild, created in 1582. Glove-making was in fact closely linked to the development of perfume, which was used to mask the unpleasant odors of the tanned skins. As the industry gradually shifted across to Nice and Italy, Grasse began to develop its production of essences which, from the seventeenth century,

became an industry in its own right. Thousands of orange trees were planted in the hills around Grasse; the Provence rose was introduced; jasmine, which was to make the town's reputation, was acclimatized and grafted; and carnations and violets tinted the hills. The distillation factories belonging to extremely powerful enterprises such as Chiris, Roure-Bertrand-Dupont, Cavallier, Lautier, Molinard, Méro-Boyveau, Sozio and Robertet, and which still exist today, were set up in the eighteenth and nineteenth centuries. The copper instruments continue to distill the best flowers; layers of fat still absorb the fragrant tuberose oils; bundles of moss still await treatment in the vast warehouses; at dawn, men, women and children still make their way to the fields and the scent of the lavender being distilled on site still wafts down from the hills.

At the end of the last century, increasing demand, combined with innovations and new standards of quality, led the more enterprising of the raw material companies, such as

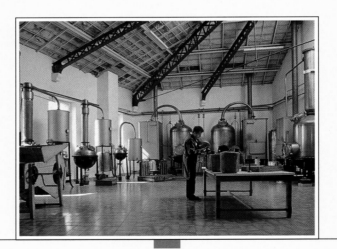

The Provençal writer Frédéric Mistral described Grasse as a "Valley of love, the promised land of perfume." The ample, tender fragrances of these fertile, sunny valleys have been enchanting travelers for several centuries (opposite, poster dating from 1930). Intoxicating perfumes escape from the distilleries. Here we can admire Molinard's distillation room in Grasse, with its metallic structure designed by Gustave Eiffel (above).

the Etablissements Chiris, to set up trading posts abroad in order to produce and process the numerous varieties of plants which could not be transplanted or acclimatized. The Etablissements Roure began to develop new techniques, such as extraction by volatile solvents, and to explore the possibilities of synthetic products. For a while, Grasse enjoyed a period of expansion and the excellent quality of its techniques, essences and raw materials gained worldwide authority, but after the Second World War the town went into decline. The younger generations, disadvantaged by the new political and economic situation, gradually sold off their family-run businesses to international pharmaceutical and chemical groups. The perfume town was no longer the epicenter of the industry, but its spirit traveled all over the world.

Grasse lives on in the hearts of perfumers. Those who were born there remain deeply attached to the town: the history of their ancestors is in the town records; their vocation began on trips to the fields at dawn in the company of their fathers and in the intoxicating atmosphere of the distillation factories. Jacques Polge decided on his destiny one sum-

mer, when, as a child, he went down to Cannes with his family to go swimming. On the way a pump attendant, in the midst of the petrol fumes, gave him a bunch of jasmine. As for Jean Guichard, he was marked for life by the smell of fresh petals mingled with that of jute sacks and machine grease that lingered in a small hut situated next to a rose plantation belonging to his father.

Grasse is not a nostalgic town. On the contrary, even if it is no longer the vibrant center of the perfume industry, it is very much alive. Despite the passage of time, its traditional craftsmanship remains unrivalled. Numerous raw material companies, such as Robertet, Mane, Chauvet, Camilli and Charabot, continue their culture and tradition with energy and enthusiasm, assisted now by the very latest modern techniques.

Few essences are produced in Grasse nowadays, but those that are produced there are the best in the world. The most demanding perfumers, people like Jean Kerléo, Jean-Paul Guerlain or Jacques Polge, still buy their supplies of Provence rose and Grasse jasmine in Grasse—proof indeed that tradition is still alive and well in the town.

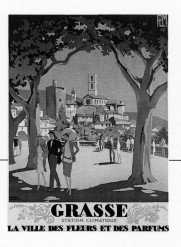

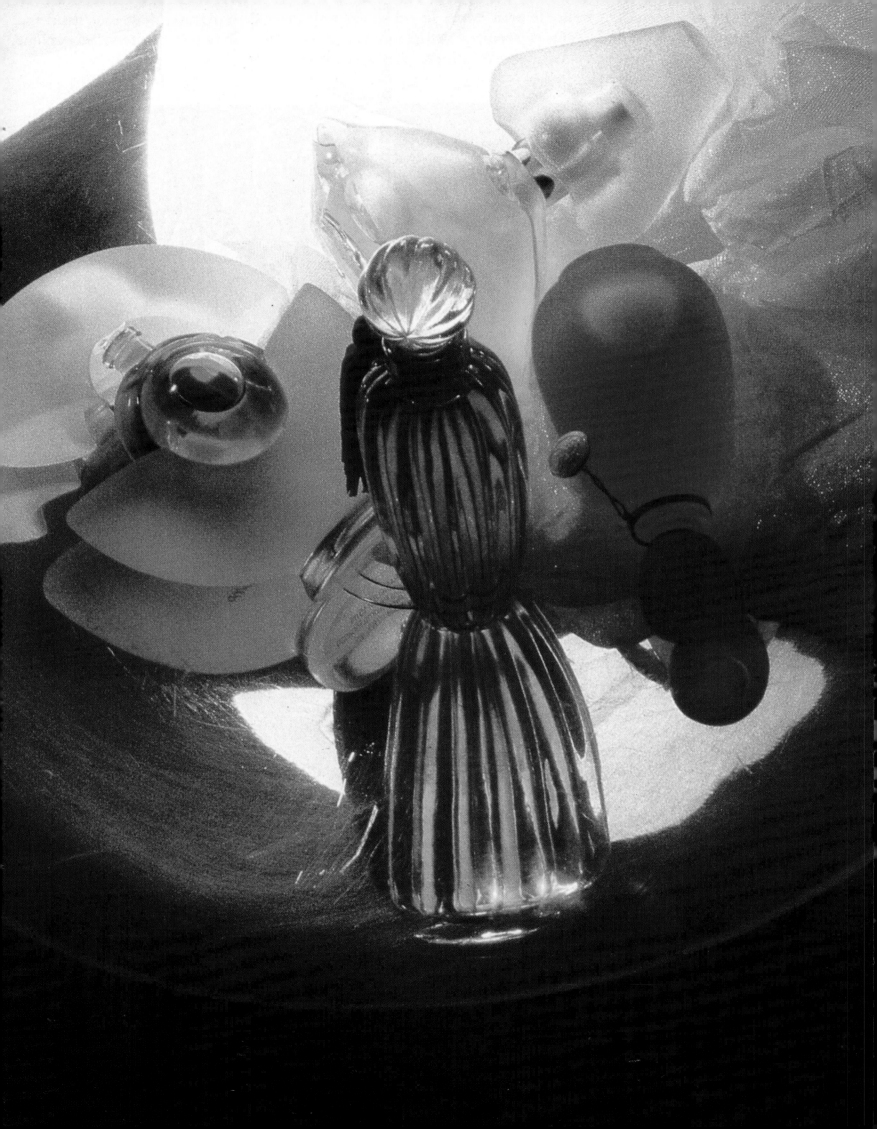

· THE ·
GREAT
PERFUMERS

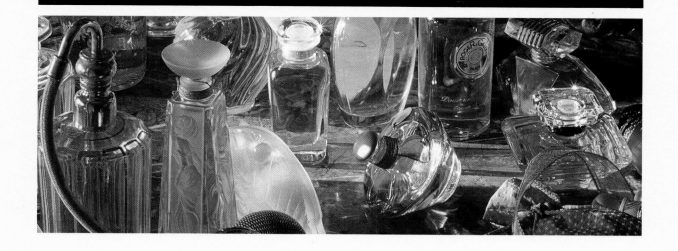

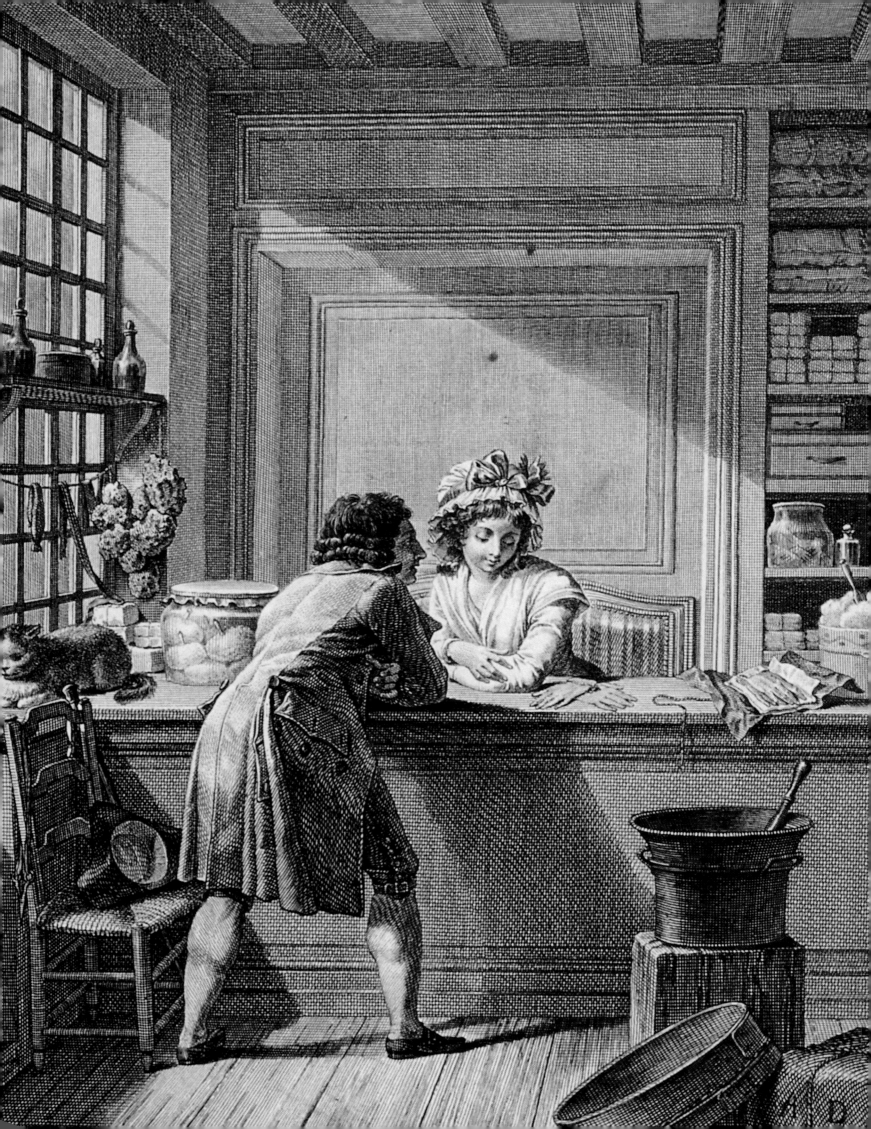

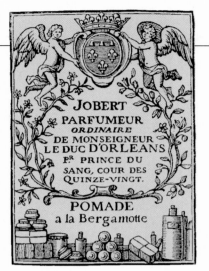

It was only at the beginning of this century that the perfumer really came into his own and gained recognition as a creator. Before the French Revolution, perfumers belonged to the glove and perfume-makers guild, governed by an edict issued by Philippe Auguste dating from 1190, which prevented them from developing their own trade. In those days, apart from a few personalities such as René Le Florentin, Catherine de' Medici's personal perfumer, who is said to have concocted beautiful fragrances as well as poisons in his boutique on the Pont au Change in Paris, or the celebrated Martial who officiated at the court of Louis XIV, perfumers worked anonymously in their dispensaries, endlessly repeating the same processes, making up perfumes following a handful of formulas.

After 1789, French perfumers were finally able to set up their own businesses, which began to spring up in great numbers, reaching their zenith in the nineteenth century. The perfumers of that period, motivated by a bourgeois population hungry for innovation and by the increase in raw materials which opened up hitherto unknown horizons, became genuine creators, on a par with painters or sculptors, who found ever-increasing possibilities for expressing their talent in their fragrances. At the dawn of the the twentieth century, Jacques Guerlain, François Coty and Ernest Daltroff, founders of the Caron perfume house, brought a new dynamism to the perfume industry with modernizing, state-of-the-art olfactory ideas which continue to inspire perfumers today.

In the space of a century, the trade of perfumer has changed from being a small-scale local family craft into big business on a global scale with a considerable social and economic impact. The companies that modern-day perfumers work for are varied. There are, of course, the traditional houses, such as Floris in England or Guerlain in France, who have remained indifferent to the vagaries of fashion since their foundation over two centuries ago. Then there are the men and women who, with intuition, and often with a touch of genius, created revolutionary accords, such as Gabrielle Chanel's N° 5 and Estée Lauder's Youth Dew. Finally, there are the more recent perfume houses who have become famous through the creation of a single perfume, such as Yves Saint Laurent with Opium.

One could name a great many more. We have chosen the most symbolic, those who have given perfumery a legendary fragrance, those who, through their original ideas, creativity and audacity, have influenced and continue to influence the evolution of the history of perfume.

During the reign of Louis XV, someone close to the king, as was the case becoming the official perfumer of for the perfumer Jobert, enabled one to start up a business (top). At the time, eau de Cologne (above) had yet to achieve widespread popularity and perfumers sold gloves as well as unguents in their boutiques (opposite). The amber transparency of perfume bottles encloses vibrant fragrances such as Valentino by Paloma Picasso, Private Collection by Estée Lauder and the surprising Salvador Dali (page 52), and Lalique and Trésor by Lancôme (page 53).

EAU DE COLOGNE

Everyone knows this exhilarating blend of lemon, orange, bergamot, rosemary and neroli. Of all the perfume accords, eau de Cologne is the oldest and most famous. The formula is said to have been discovered in the seventeenth century in Santa Maria Maggiore to the north of Milan, by a young man called Giovanni Paolo Feminis, a commercial traveler by trade. He

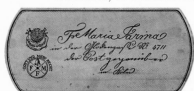

peddled delicate fragrances which were given the name of *aqua mirabilis* (miracle water) because of the therapeutic properties they were alleged to contain. If inhaled several times a day, they were said to cure headaches and palpitations of the heart. It was to their invigorating powers, however, that they owed their success: sixty drops of *aqua mirabilis* in a glass of water ensured health and longevity.

In 1693, Giovanni Paolo Feminis moved to Cologne in Germany to sell an *aqua mirabilis* which he claimed to be of his own invention. It was an immediate success. Was he really its creator? Several conflicting versions exist. Some people maintained that a soldier recently returned from India entrusted Feminis with the formula for an antiseptic which he subsequently modified. Others said that he obtained the secret from a nun in a convent in Santa Maria

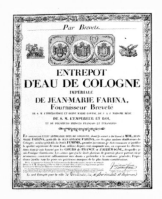

Maggiore. When Giovanni Paolo Feminis died in 1763, he bequeathed the secret to his son, Giovanni Maria Farina, thanks to whom the enterprise prospered. At the end of the eighteenth century, during the Seven Years War between the armies of the Rhine and the French, the latter were garrisoned in Cologne. There they became infatuated with the scent and exported it to France, where it soon gained the favor of none other than Napoleon himself, who, it is said, used to have sixty bottles a day delivered to him!

Giovanni Maria Farina's original formula soon inspired numerous variations. One of them was destined for fame and is today the most popular eau de Cologne in the world: the Eau de Cologne Originale 4711, by Mülhens. It all started with a wedding in Cologne in October 1792. Wilhelm Mülhens, the son of a lawyer from that town, was given a formula for *aqua mirabilis* as a wedding present from a monk, on the condition that the formula would receive the treatment it deserved. The young husband hastened to have a factory built in the rue des Cailles. In 1796 the houses in the town were numbered and Wilhelm Mülhens' factory was given the number 4711;

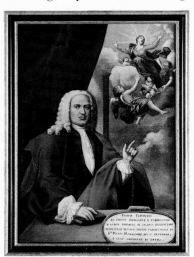

The inscription on the label of this eighteenth-century painting from the German town of Cologne translates: "Paolo Feminis, merchant and manufacturer of miracle water" (above). Feminis is considered to be the father of eau de Cologne, but it was his nephew, Giovanni Maria Farina, whose name is written in its German form on this label from 1874 (top left), who was responsible for the product's commercial success.

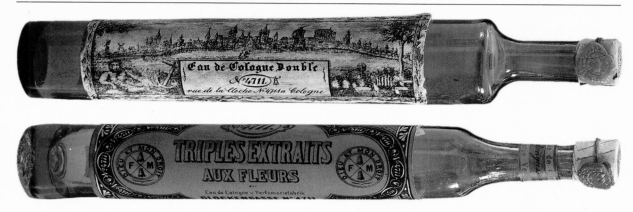

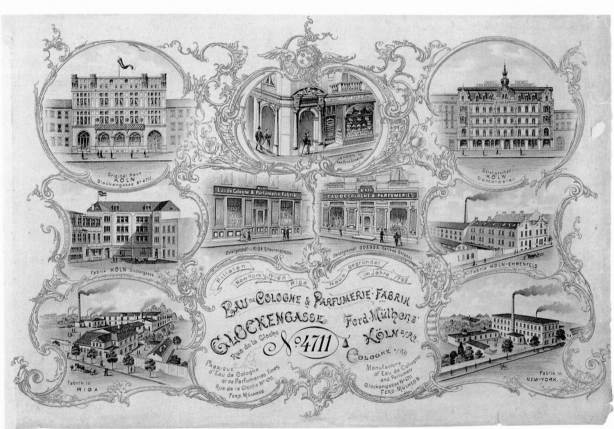

In the space of a century, the Mülhens family established the international reputation of their eau de Cologne and other perfumed products, which can be seen here in their original vessels, known as *Rosoli* (above). This document, dating from the turn of the century (above), shows the Glockengasse head office (top left), the elegant window displays in the London, Riga and Odessa boutiques, as well as the five factories where the products were manufactured. The New York boutique alone confirmed Mülhens' undisputed success (bottom right).

Kölnisch Wasser 4711 was registered as a trademark in 1875, by which time it had become popular throughout Europe. It was the composer Richard Wagner's favorite toilet water. In 1879, he wrote to the Mülhens establishment requesting them to send him three quarts of eau de Cologne in large bottles at a "reasonable price," taking into account his rate of consumption of a quart a month. Tourism, which started to develop at the beginning of the twentieth century, was good for business and it became fashionable to take the bottle with its blue and gold label back home from Germany as a souvenir. Nowadays, it

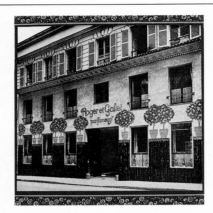

is no longer necessary to go to Cologne to purchase it. Eau de Cologne Originale 4711 is exported to sixty different countries and is currently set to conquer the Chinese market.

In Tuscany, meanwhile, there are toilet waters which are as ancient as eau de Cologne, but known only to the privileged few. They can be found in the shadow of the Florentine monastery Santa Maria Novella, in the pharmacy built on the site of the monastery's former Gothic chapel. It was in around 1200 that Dominican monks, recently settled on the banks of the river Arno, began to grow and distill medicinal plants.

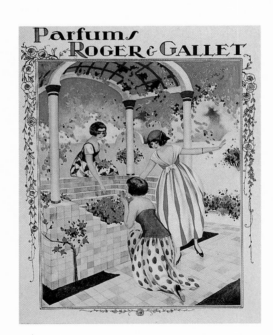

When they took over Giovanni Maria Farina's business, Roger & Gallet, named after its founders Charles-Armand Roger and Charles Gallet, inherited the celebrated eau de Cologne, which they began to sell in 1884. Their boutique in Paris, the façade of which can be seen here in 1925 (top), also developed fragrances of its own, using the newly discovered synthetic products, as illustrated by a poster advertisement dating from 1913 (below).

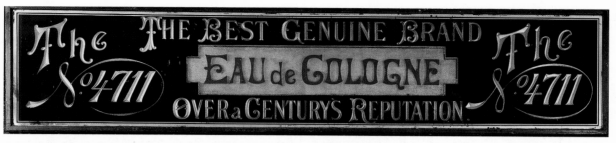

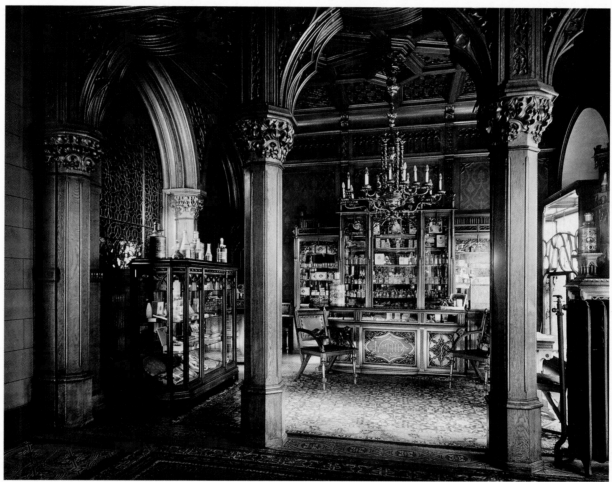

Although the Mülhens' eau de Cologne could be procured in the Bond Street boutique in London, whose shop sign can be seen here (above), real aficionados made the journey to Cologne to the main Glockengasse premises. Customers came to buy their favorite product in these Neo-Gothic surroundings (above). They might also have been tempted by such novelties as this case containing a selection of violet-perfumed products (opposite). The firm still has a boutique at this address in a building renovated in 1964.

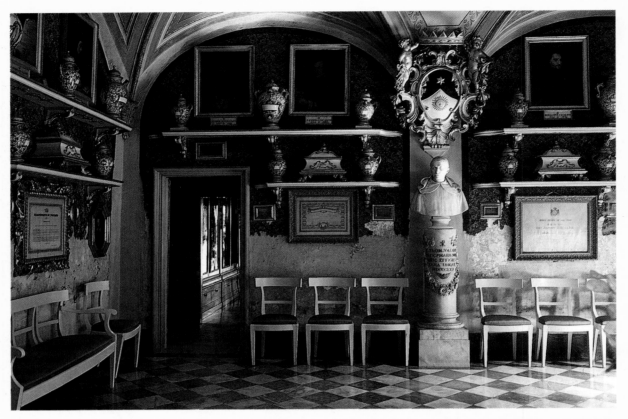

To begin with their use was private, but they soon became known around the town for their quality. News of their popularity eventually reached Catherine de' Medici, who made them famous throughout the courts of Europe. Today a stop-off at the Officina di Santa Maria Novella, which still lies off the beaten tourist track, is recommended on two accounts: for the beauty of the location and for its "old-style" fragrances, beautifully displayed on mahogany shelves— extract of heliotrope for handkerchiefs, rosewater, marzipan, essence of hay or lilac and potpourris gathered on the Tuscan hillsides.

GREAT ENGLISH PERFUME HOUSES

In England, the court of Elizabeth I went crazy over the spices, balms and animal essences which Venetian ships brought back from the Orient and Arabia. They were worn around the neck or on the belt, in pomanders (carved silver spheres) which diffused their heady accords at every step. Certain wealthy houses even had a stillroom, where people tried their hand at distilling essences. Small shops started to trade in fragrances but it was the barbers who gave English perfumery its noble reputation. They created dis-

This could be the private study of a Tuscan prince, but it is in fact one of the oldest perfume houses in the world, the Officina Profumo Farmaceutica di Santa Maria Novella. It is an enchanting, timeless place, open to the public. The green salon (above) contains precious historical objects—Medici parchments, portraits of former directors and porcelain jars which originally contained floral and plant essences. The salesroom, bathed in a milky light, is located in the former chapel, its dome decorated with frescoes representing the four quarters of the world (opposite).

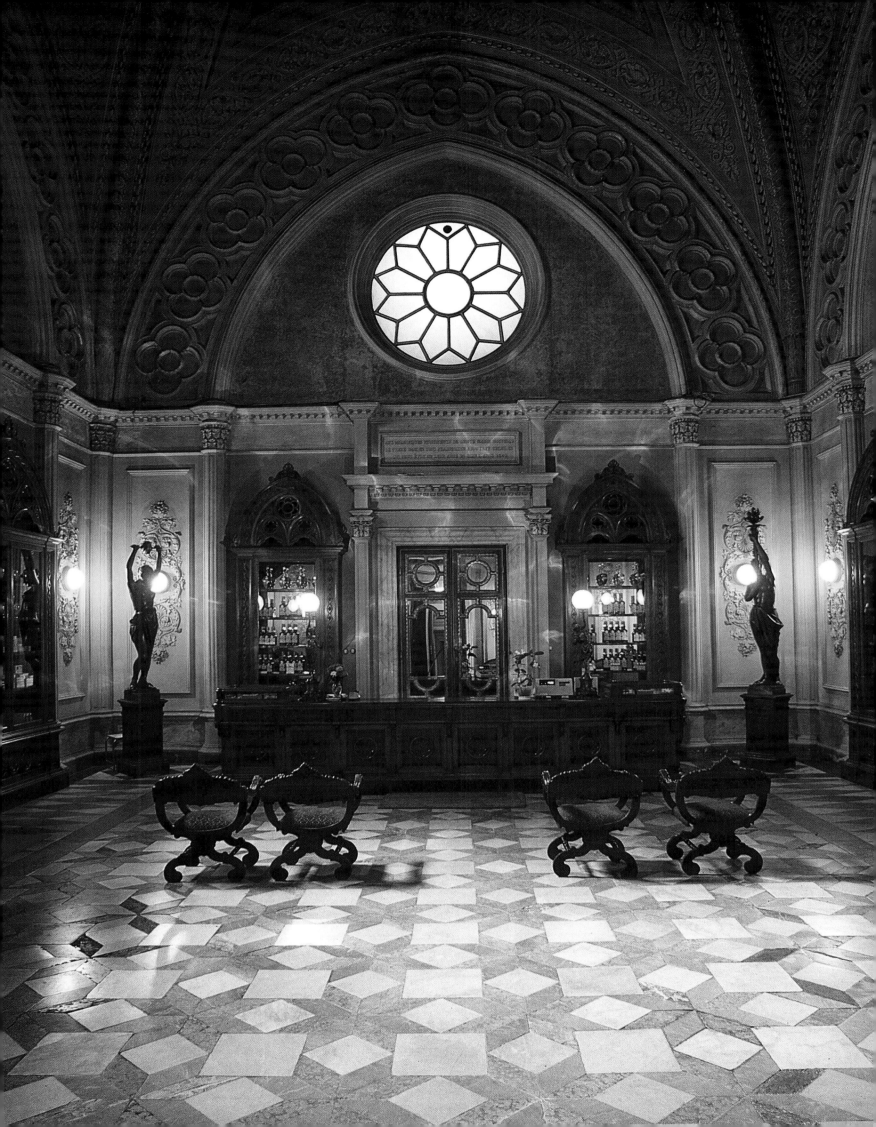

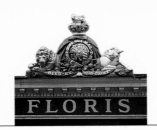

creet yet sustained perfumes which were highly distinctive and well suited to tweeds and flannels.

The first of these perfumer-barbers arrived in London in 1730. He was a young Spaniard from Minorca called Juan Famenias Floris, whose ambition was to open a perfumery in the upper-class district of St. James. At the back of a barber's shop, at number 89 Jermyn Street, he found what he had been dreaming of. The fragrances he created were nostalgic flights of fancy back to his native country, such as jasmine and sweet orange blossom waters, and the celebrated Lavender, which was to bring him his fame. Soon all fashionable London society patronized the Floris perfumery. In the eighteenth century, during the reign of Edward IV, this establish-

ment, which offered no less than one hundred and seventy-five fragrances, received a royal warrant. The "By appointment" certificate issued by the reigning monarch is every manufacturer's dream, as it enables them to exhibit the royal coat of arms on their products, giving them a distinct advantage over the competition. The warrant is reviewed every six years and today can only be granted by four members of the royal family: the Queen, the Queen Mother, the Duke of Edinburgh and the Prince of Wales. The two royal warrants awarded to Floris bear the coat of arms of the Queen and of her son, Charles, who, it is said, is very fond of the rose-sandalwood note of toilet water Number 89. With its original mahogany paneling, setting off

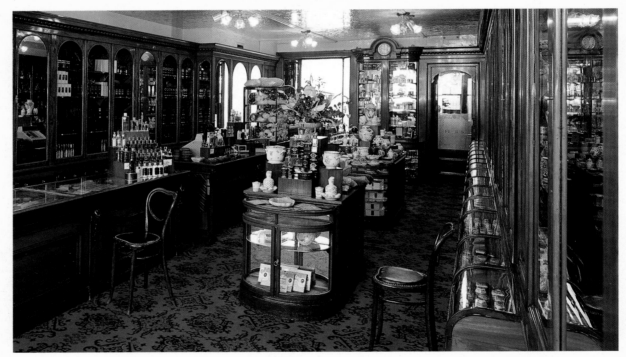

This Floris shop sign (top), graced with the arms of the British royal family, from whom it received its royal warrant, hangs above the London boutique at 89 Jermyn Street. Opened in 1730, this nostalgic place, sparkling with its highly polished woodwork and precious perfume bottles, is the only Floris shop in Europe (above). Two other boutiques in the same style have been opened in New York and in Kobe, Japan. Luxury and elegance characterize the perfume hall of the London department store Harrods, here photographed in 1944 (following double page). Floriss, one of the oldest lines, revives its old fashioned spelling for three timeless fragrances: lavender, wild hyacinth and moss rose (opposite).

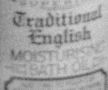

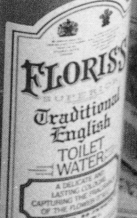

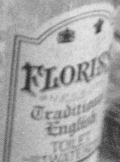

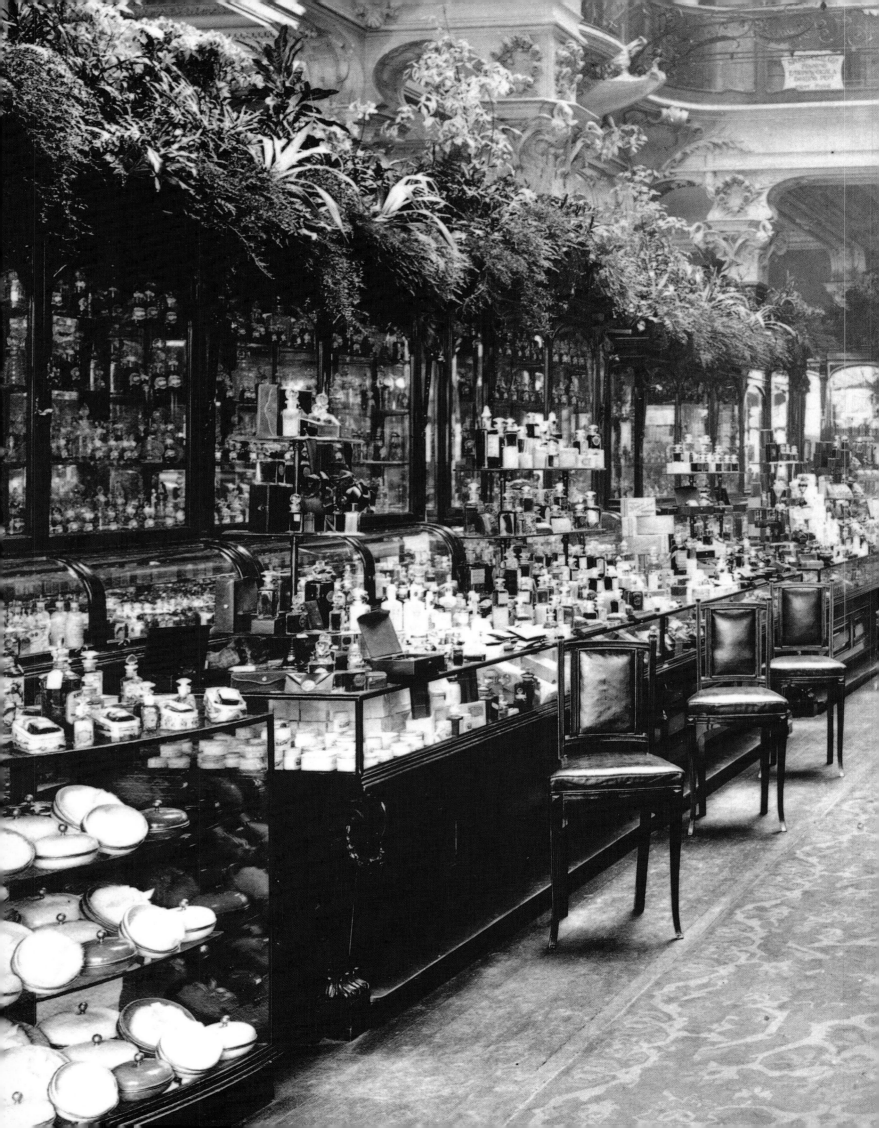

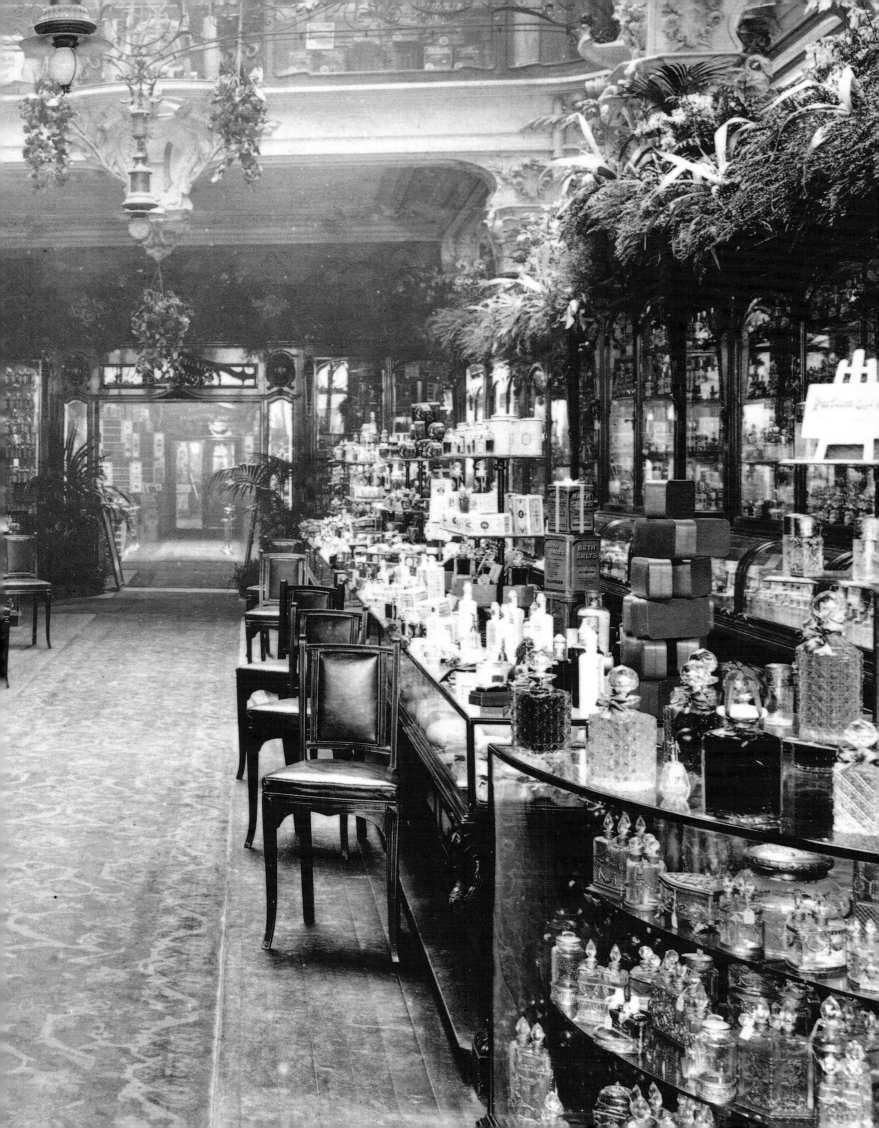

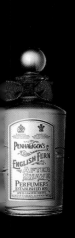
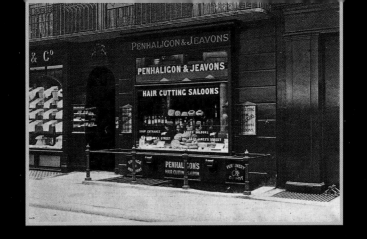
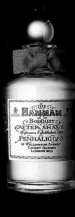
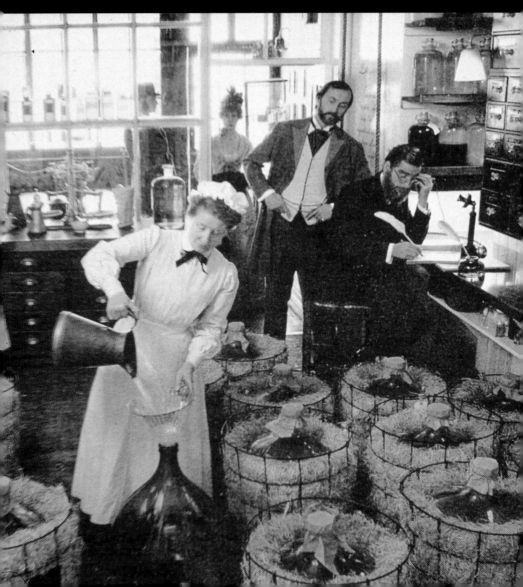

the famous blue and gold boxes, the boutique can still be found at its original address.

Another perfumer practicing in England who succeeded in passing his name down to posterity is William Henry Penhaligon. A barber by trade, in 1870 he opened a barber's shop in St. James, just a stone's throw from the fashionable Hammam Turkish Baths. Emerging from the purifying vapors, the gentlemen of London headed off to Penhaligon's shop to have their sideburns trimmed and their freshly shaved cheeks splashed with his wonderful fragrances. Penhaligon was devoted to his clientele and offered them only the most refined products. In 1872, he created Hammam Bouquet, a subtle accord of jasmine with a touch of sandalwood, which brought him wide renown. From then on, Penhaligon became the favorite supplier of the elite of London society, notably of the celebrated dynasty of bankers, the Rothschilds. In 1902, he created Blenheim Bouquet in honor of the politician Sir Winston Churchill, who was born at Blenheim Palace in Oxfordshire. Today, this discreet alliance of lime and pine is Penhaligon's most popular men's fragrance. After the Second World War the establishment sunk into oblivion. It remained almost forgotten until 1975, when Sheila Pickles, the manager of a perfume store located on the site of an old flower shop in London's former market, Covent Garden, decided to revive the original Penhaligon formulas. These had been mira-

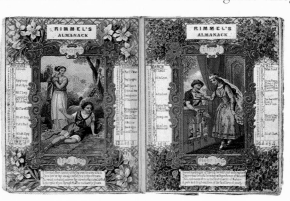

culously conserved in Sir William's diaries, where he recorded every detail of his daily activities as perfumer.

With access to archives such as these, it is understandable that Penhaligon remains a reference today. The new establishment made a point of respecting the original formulas, even though the requisite raw materials were often exorbitant. Hammam Bouquet, for example, requires a large quantity of Bulgarian rose absolute, which means the cost of producing it is high. But to replace its suave note would be tantamount to treason: Hamman Bouquet is the favorite perfume of the Duke of Edinburgh, to whom Penhaligon owes its royal warrant!

THE FIRST PARISIAN PERFUMERIES

It was in the second half of the eighteenth century, between the Tuileries gardens and the Palais Royal—the heart of Parisian fashion and chivalry—that boutiques selling perfume began to appear, their decorative shop windows gaily displaying all the secrets of feminine beauty, such as fragrant vinegars and smelling salts, complexion lotions, perfumed powders and delicate flower waters. The heady scents so highly prized by the courtesans of Louis XIV, powerful animal and spicy fragrances which were intended to mask any less hygienic smells, were no longer in vogue. The floral

In the nineteenth century, the Parisian perfumer Eugène Rimmel, like all the best European perfumers, opened new premises in London. His refined fragrances and perfumed objects, like this richly illustrated almanac (above), attracted a wealthy clientele, whose patronage he vied for with his rival, Penhaligon. Called Penhaligon & Jeavons until 1902 (opposite, top), Penhaligon's offered refined perfumes such as English Fern, an accord of moss and woody notes, and the first environmental fragrance, Hammam Bouquet. Here, Penhaligon is supervising the blending of fragrances (opposite).

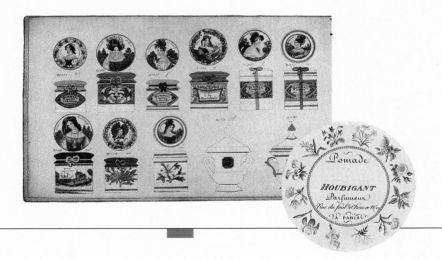

bouquets which appeared during Louis XV's reign were *de rigueur* at the court of Marie-Antoinette, who was particularly fond of rose and violet essences. In his novel *Perfume*, Patrick Süskind brilliantly conjures up this atmosphere in the description of his hero Grenouille's arrival in Paris: "It was here as well that Grenouille first smelled perfume in the literal sense of the word: a simple lavender or rose-water, with which the fountains of the gardens were filled on gala occasions; but also the more complex, more costly scents of tincture of musk mixed with oils of neroli and tuberose, jonquil, jasmine or cinnamon, that floated behind the carriages like rich ribbons on the evening breeze."

When, in 1775, Jean-François Houbigant opened his store, À la Corbeille de Fleurs, in the rue du Faubourg-Saint-Honoré, he was, of course, unaware that he had just inaugurated what was destined to become the oldest perfumery in France. His wig powders, perfumed pomades and flower essences were the delight of Madame du Barry, the late King Louis XV's mistress, and were especially prized by Marie-Antoinette who, on the day before her flight from Paris at the height of the French Revolution, hurried to the boutique to have all her perfume bottles refilled! The store, which happily suffered no damage during the revolution, became the regular rendezvous of the forerunners of the dandies, the Muscadins, so named because of their infatuation for musk. During Napoleon's reign, Houbigant's boutique was patronized by the Empress Josephine, for whom he concocted heady perfumes which flattered her Creole skin, but which met with the disapproval of her husband, Napoleon, who, we now know, only liked eau de Cologne! It is said that the empress's wardrobe was so strongly impregnated with fragrances, that the scent of musk and civet floated in her apartments long after her departure from Malmaison.

"Certain fragrances seem to have been composed to magnify the enchantment of loving embraces," remarked Edmond de Goncourt. During the nineteenth century, respectable women were expected to wear suave, discreet fragrances. As a result, perfume developed an extremely romantic image, as illustrated by this perfume sachet from the reign of Napoleon III (top), these ointment pots and labels from the 1820s (above) and this magnificent label for Eau d'Téou, a delicate fragrance by Dissey & Piver (opposite).

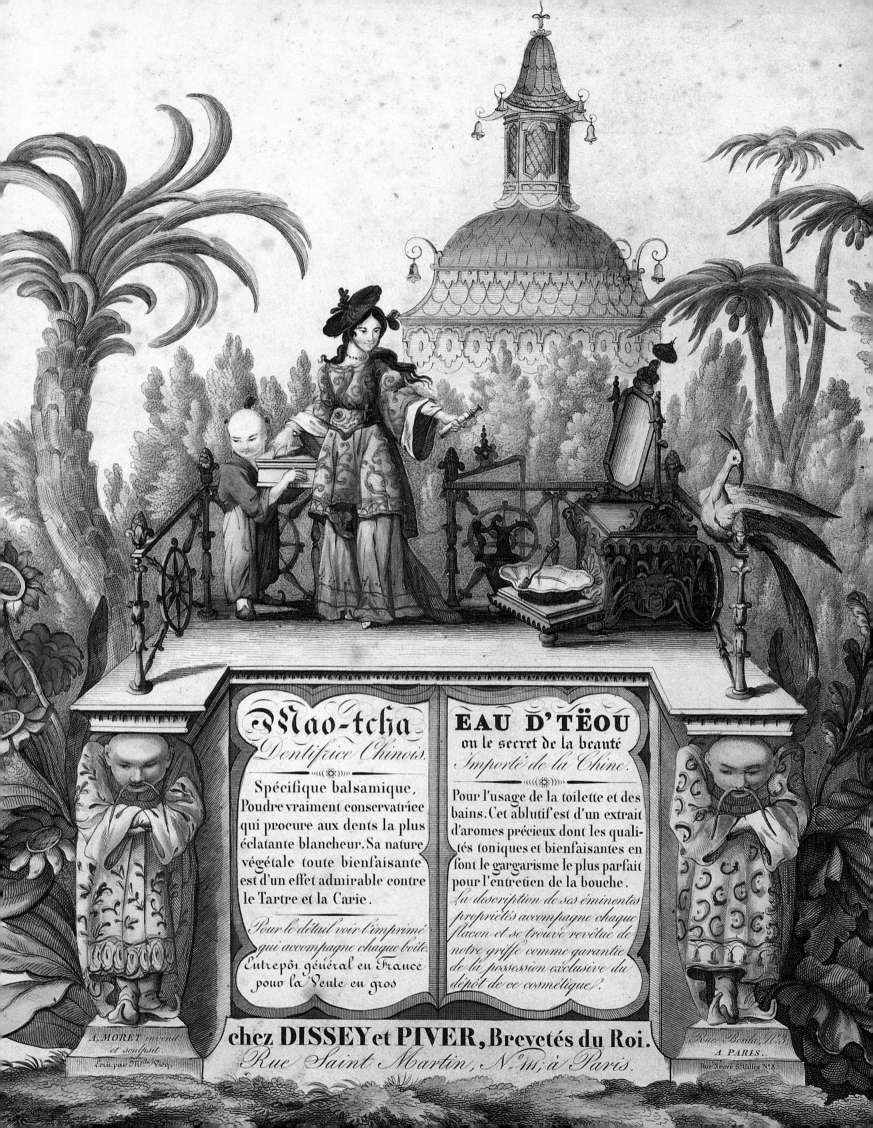

In the nineteenth century, the company exported its talents to the courts of Europe, creating Le Bouquet de la Tsarine for the Russian empress, Maria Feodorovna, wife of Alexander III, and, in 1882, Fougère Royale, which was to become the favorite perfume of the author Guy de Maupassant. In 1912, Quelques Fleurs, created by Monsieur Bienaimé, Houbigant's perfumer at the time, was a triumph. With its amber bouquet, reminiscent of the femininity of *La Belle Époque* and the effervescence of the Roaring Twenties, it is a powerfully evocative fragrance, given a new lease of life in 1985 under the name of Quelques Fleurs l'Original.

In 1798, Parisian women began flocking to a boutique called Aux Armes de France, recently opened by a certain Jean-François Lubin. There they found the myriad secrets of feminine seduction, which until then had been hidden away in haberdasher's or in stores selling trinkets. There were powders, smelling salts, lotions and perfumed milks, along with toilet accessories so tempting that even a saint would have been unable to resist them. Aux Armes de France, with its wealthy clientele, can be considered as the ancestor of Paris's modern perfumeries. Pauline Bonaparte, Napoleon's sister, later to become the Princess Borghese, favored Lubin with her custom and one of their perfumes, Pauline, was named after her. Eau de Lubin, said "to refresh and soften the skin," was composed in the first years of the nineteenth century and was extremely popular at the imperial court. Its formula far outlived the century, for its citronella, lavender and civet trilogy inspired Eau Neuve, a fragrance which only came into being in the spring of 1968!

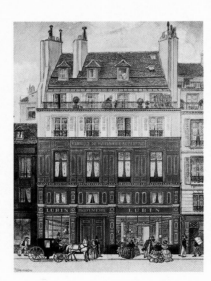

Lubin, whose Paris boutique can be seen here as it was in 1860 (above), was the first French perfume house to seduce the Americans, thanks to the protection of the duke of Angoulême. Four years before, Thomas Jones had opened a shop in Paris. His perfumes were presented in small boxes made of painted glass whose stylishness is reflected in this label in which the perfumer is depicted surrounded by flowers (vignette). The L.T. Piver perfume house also appeared at this time and soon had no less than five shops in Paris. This series of labels illustrates Piver's marvelous creativity: Eau de Ninon, Eau de Vénus and Trèfle Incarnat, which were quick to win favor with women of fashion (opposite).

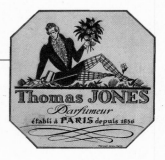

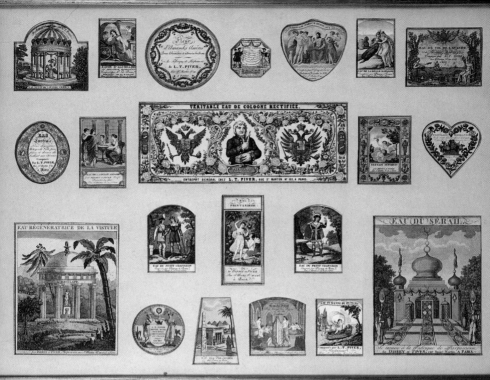

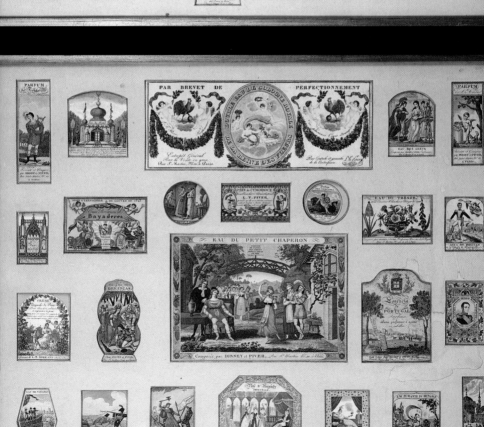

THE GUERLAIN DYNASTY

During the first decades of the nineteenth century, with the emergence of an ambitious upper-middle class population hungry for material wealth and power, perfumery experienced a boom. No longer considered a mere accessory to seduction, perfume became the accomplice of social ambitions in a society obsessed by social formalities and appearance. "If vanity is a cause of great torment to men," declares César Birotteau, the ambitious perfumer from Honoré de Balzac's *La Comédie Humaine*, "then good cosmetics are a blessing." Birotteau runs a boutique in Paris called La Reine des Roses and makes his fortune through his talent for business, his ability to pick up on the latest trends and by paying extremely careful attention to the design of the bottles and labels of his latest oils. As Balzac writes, "Newton did not put more mental effort into his famous binomial theorem than Birotteau into

his Comagenous Essence." The fashion at the time was for extremely discreet, modest perfumes, with soft fragrances, only perceptible to the practiced senses of men and women of "superior breeding." People were in the habit of perfuming linen, gloves, fans, mittens, slippers, the lace setting off the posy at the belt, and, above all, handkerchiefs, those indispensable articles of a woman's trousseau.

Only courtesans perfumed their skin. Charles Baudelaire caused a scandal in *Les Fleurs du Mal* by celebrating the disturbing sensual pleasure emanating from the body of a "daughter of darkness, slattern deity / rank with musk and nicotine." These are sinful fragrances because they are too provocative. Writing on this subject in a book of etiquette popular at the time, the Countess Bradi is quite clear: "I forbid you to use manufactured perfumes, however I consider those diffused by natural flowers to be perfectly permissible as long as they cause no inconvenience to those around you."

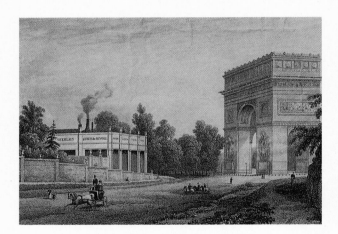

In was in this small workshop on the corner of the avenue Kléber, just a stone's throw from the Arc de Triomphe, that Pierre-François Guerlain, founder of the Guerlain dynasty, distilled his essences (above). His floral waters, like Fleurs de Serre, soon earned him a loyal clientele. In 1853, he introduced Eau de Cologne Impériale, presented here in its original perfume bottle and in a modern replica of the famous bottle adorned with bees, which brought him great renown. It is a harmonious blend of orange, lemon and bergamot, associated with lavender and rosemary, and was originally created for the Empress Eugénie (opposite).

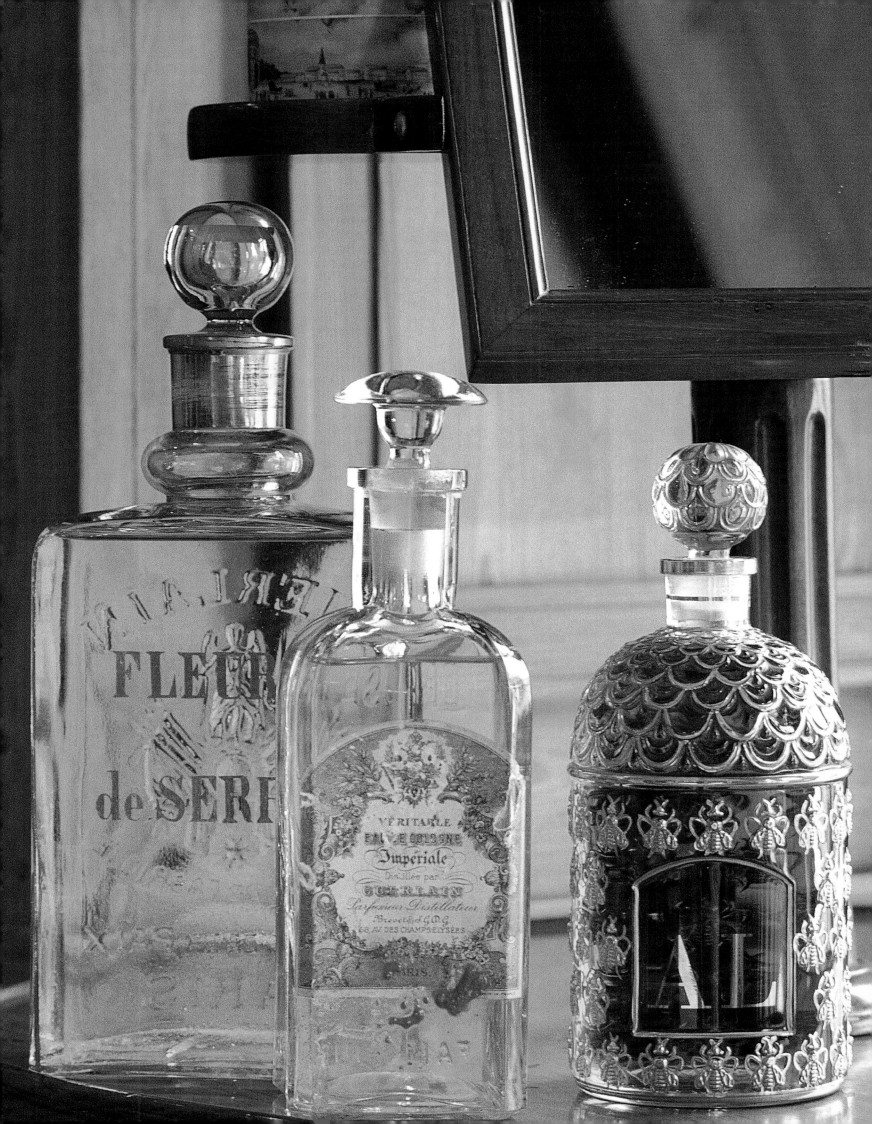

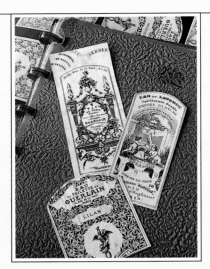

It was nevertheless in this climate, scarcely favorable to olfactory daring, that a prestigious dynasty of perfumers emerged, the Guerlains, considered by many as the veritable symbol of perfume. The Guerlain perfumes have an inimitable quality, a disturbing fascination. Pierre-François Guerlain, the first of the dynasty, opened his first boutique in 1828 on the ground floor of the Hôtel Meurice in the rue de Rivoli. It was not long before clients were flocking to the boutique; rumor had it that its fragrant waters were the subtlest in Paris. Their originality lay in the fact that they did not imitate a particular bouquet, but transcended the floral odors with a delicate harmony evoking a mood, a feeling or an atmosphere. In 1840 Guerlain moved to new premises at 15 rue de la Paix, home to the capital's most elegant boutiques. Clients included the Countess of Castiglione, the Princess of Metternich, the Prince of Wales, the Tsar Ferdinand of Bulgaria, for all of whom the perfumer composed "tailor-made" fragrances. In 1853, Eau de l'Impératrice, dedicated to Eugénie de Montijo, the wife of Napoleon III, earned him the much coveted "Royal Supplier" patent. The perfume bottle, decorated with bees, a royal emblem, highlighted in gold, is still manufactured today in traditional-style moulds.

On his death in 1864, Pierre-François Guerlain was succeeded by his two sons. Gabriel, the youngest, took over the management, while Aimé, the eldest, took charge of perfumery. In 1889, the year in which the Baron Eiffel erected his scandalous tower, Aimé created his first masterpiece, Jicky. This indefinable fragrance, with its eau de Cologne top note and civet base note, was as disconcerting as the metal tower and in fact the dandies, attracted by its ambiguous name, adopted it before the women did. Jicky, as it happens, was the nickname of Aimé Guerlain's favorite nephew, the highly talented Jacques, who was to succeed him in the family business. In 1912, Jacques Guerlain created L'Heure Bleue. This spray of roses softened by iris, musk and vanilla, evokes its creator's favorite time of day, the moment when, as he puts it, "The sun has set but the night hasn't yet fallen. A moment suspended in time. The hour when man is at last in harmony with the world and with light." The year 1919 saw the launch of Mitsouko, with its woody, chypre note, heightened by a touch of peach. It was the favorite perfume of Sergei Diaghilev, the exuberant founder of the Ballets Russes, whose performances were the delight of Paris in the 1920s. But Jacques Guerlain's greatest success proved to be Shalimar, launched in 1925, the year when the Exhibition of Decorative Arts introduced a new style inspired by African art. It was an entirely spontaneous but superb creation. It is said that Jacques Guerlain, enthused by a sample of synthetic vanilla he had just received, poured some into a bottle of Jicky . . . just to

Guerlain's floral waters (above), as delicate as their labels, were in vogue until the arrival of Jicky in 1889 (opposite). The latter was greatly admired by some, while others were scandalized by its audacious notes. "Jicky moves like hair blowing in the wind, releasing molecules of bergamot, like the legs of wild horses, galloping over vervain. Silky skin, saturated with sandalwood, can be immodest," affirms the author Denise Dubois-Jallais.

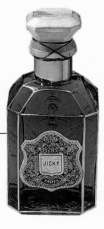

see what would happen. The result was rapturous, beyond his wildest dreams. Its name, Shalimar, is no less bewitching. It evokes the fabulous garden of Srinagar, which the Shah Jahan created in remembrance of his deceased wife, for whom he also built the Taj Mahal marble palace. If Shalimar alone, seventy years after its creation, represents sixteen percent of all Guerlain sales, it is because its breathtakingly luscious note is the most accomplished example of "Guerlinade," that indefinable touch which makes Guerlain perfumes so unique.

A Guerlain perfume is unmistakable. What is it that gives them their magic? What accords and in what proportions? The secret remains closely guarded. We do know, however, that vanilla and jasmine are involved, with underlying rose and tonka bean notes . . . but that is as much as Jean-Paul Guerlain will let on. Since the 1950s, Jacques Guerlain's

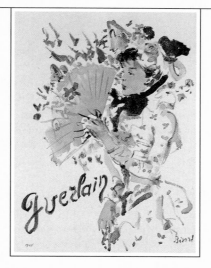

grandson is responsible for the creation of new perfumes, including the latest arrival, Samsara, a vibrant duo of sandalwood and jasmine conceived in 1989, which acts as the charming ambassador of an establishment determined to promote its products beyond Europe—an objective which has been attained, since today Samsara jauntily heads Guerlain's worldwide sales.

TRADITIONAL PERFUME HOUSES

In the traditional houses, perfumes are created with patience and respect for the profession, independent of fashion and the dictates of the market. Here the quest is for nostalgic trails, the powdered memories of *La Belle Époque*, or the wilder scents of the Roaring Twenties. Here the search is, above all, for the unusual, for secret accords and meaningful revivals.

For those who are fascinated by fragrances and

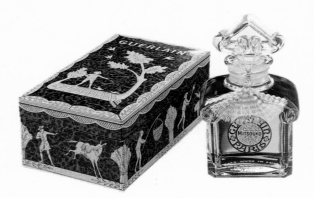

Each of the perfumes created by Guerlain, for whom the painter Christian Bérard designed this poster in 1945, incarnate the same ideal: emotion and sensuality. Mitsouko, launched in 1919, opened up this voluptuous avenue in bewitching notes of jasmine, patchouli and peach, conjuring up this fruit in all its ripeness. Offering femininity without vapidity, it was immediately adopted by the *garçonnes*.

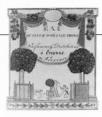

make the pilgrimage to Grasse, a visit to Molinard is not to be missed. Created in 1849, this perfume house has been in the same family for four generations and has chosen to remain in the birthplace of perfumery. It continues to make both its current perfumes and traditional formulas, notably the dazzling Habanita, to the same high standards of the past. The history of Habanita is an unusual one. The accord of vetiver and vanilla, created in 1921, was not intended to embellish the body, but to perfume the cigarettes which were the favorite props of the *garçonnes*, the sophisticated independent women of the 1920s. The publicity contained the following instructions for use: "A glass rod dipped in this fragrance and drawn along a lighted cigarette will perfume the smoke with a delicious, lasting aroma." It was also produced in a powder version in a sachet which could be slipped into the cigarette pack. In November 1926, the perfume was presented in a crystal spray bottle designed by René Lalique. The career of "The most lasting perfume in the world," according to the publicity slogan, was launched. It is still Molinard's star perfume, along with their delightful concretes which were brought out at the same time. These solid perfumes containing no alcohol, which perfume the skin with remarkable intensity, are manufactured from natural flower waxes according to an original technique developed by Molinard. Many attempts have been made to copy them, but to no avail. These charming momentos of old-style perfumery, with their little round hand-painted boxes, are quite inimitable.

The history of the Caron establishment began in 1903, when Ernest Daltroff, its founder, opened a perfumery at 10 rue de la Paix. His love of perfumes dated back to his childhood, when his mother, sitting at her dressing table getting ready for a party, dabbed a touch of heady scent behind his ear. This intoxicating memory was at the origin of Narcisse Noir, which he created in 1911. This provocative yet elegant, fervent,

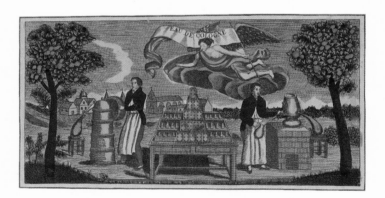

Molinard originally specialized in floral waters, those delicate masterpieces of Grasse perfumery, like the triple extract of orange blossom with its soothing properties (top), and the eau de Colognes with acidulous citrus accents represented on this label dating from the middle of the nineteenth century (above). From the 1920s, however, Molinard, whose atelier can be seen here, began to create heady perfumes like Fleurettes, launched in 1923, and Le Baiser du Faune, in its magnificent bottle designed by René Lalique, although Mimosa remained faithful to the traditional Provençal fragrances (opposite).

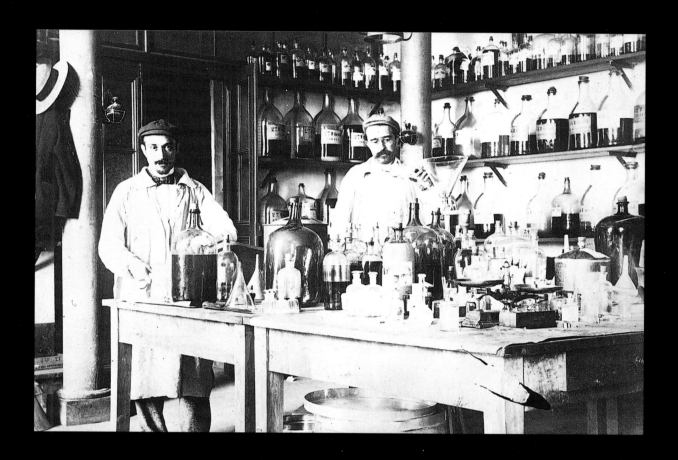

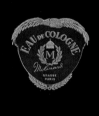

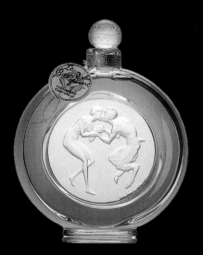

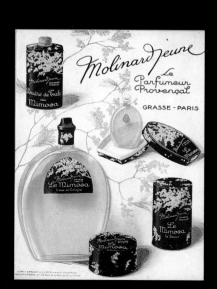

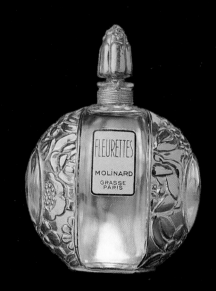

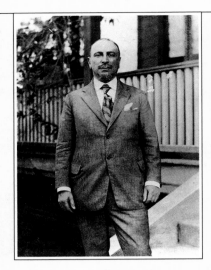

woody alliance of sandalwood and vetiver was immediately hailed as a masterpiece of perfumery and became one of the gems of Caron's collection. It even seduced the Hollywood stars; in the film *Sunset Boulevard*, Gloria Swanson turns the round perfume bottle in her hands. This first success established the Caron house style, that of heady perfumes with spicy accords, perfumes for furs and crepe de Chine. There is Bellodgia, for example, with its warm fragrance of carnation, jasmine and Bulgarian rose; Nuit de Noël, an oriental perfume with notes of ylang-ylang, tuberose and sandalwood, which was a great success in the United States right from its creation in 1927; and Royal Bain de Champagne, composed for an American millionaire who had a penchant for this particular beverage. It is also Caron who created Tabac Blond, the first perfume to contain a leather note. Designed for women smokers, this lightly opium-scented fragrance, reminiscent of the rich aroma of the tobacco of the time, heralded the magnificent olfactory family which was to generate Chanel's Cuir de Russie and, more recently, Bel Ami by Hermès, sold exclusively in their boudoir-style boutique which opened in the avenue Montaigne in 1982. Bel Ami figures among the series of twelve perfumes revived and luxuriously presented in foun-

tain-like Baccarat crystal bottles in a Louis XVI style. This collection also includes the romantic N'aimez que Moi, created in 1916, Narcisse Blanc, which for a long time was reserved exclusively for the American market, Farnesiana, with its powdery, mimosa fragrance, and the delicate En Avion, the actress Isabelle Adjani's favorite perfume, which was created in 1930 in the pioneer days of air mail.

Armand Petitjean, the founder of Lancôme, decided to set up his own company in 1935 and immediately began looking for a suitable name. He decided it should sound French, but be pronounceable in all languages. The name of a château in the center of France was suggested, that of Lancosme, like the royal-sounding names of Brantôme and Vendôme. The suggestion met with his approval, the only change made was the replacement of the letter *s* by a circumflex accent. In February 1936, only two months after the foundation of Lancôme, the company launched a range of lipsticks, a face powder, two eau de Colognes and no less than five perfumes—Conquête, an intense rose fragrance, Kypre, in tones of jasmine and amber, Tendres Nuits, haunted by magnolia, Bocages, with its delicate trace of lily of the valley and the languorous

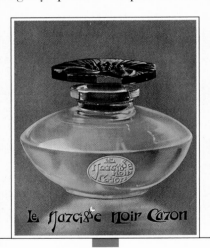

Le Narcisse Noir Caron

Narcisse Noir (above), launched in 1911, was the first great success of Ernest Daltroff (top), owner of the Caron perfume house. He lost no time in exporting it to the United States, where this sensual association of bergamot and sandalwood created a sensation in its magnificent Baccarat crystal bottle. Baccarat also produced the twelve dazzling perfume fountains which can be admired in the Paris boutique in avenue Montaigne. Despite only being opened in 1982, the store has all the refinement of a turn of the century perfume salon (opposite).

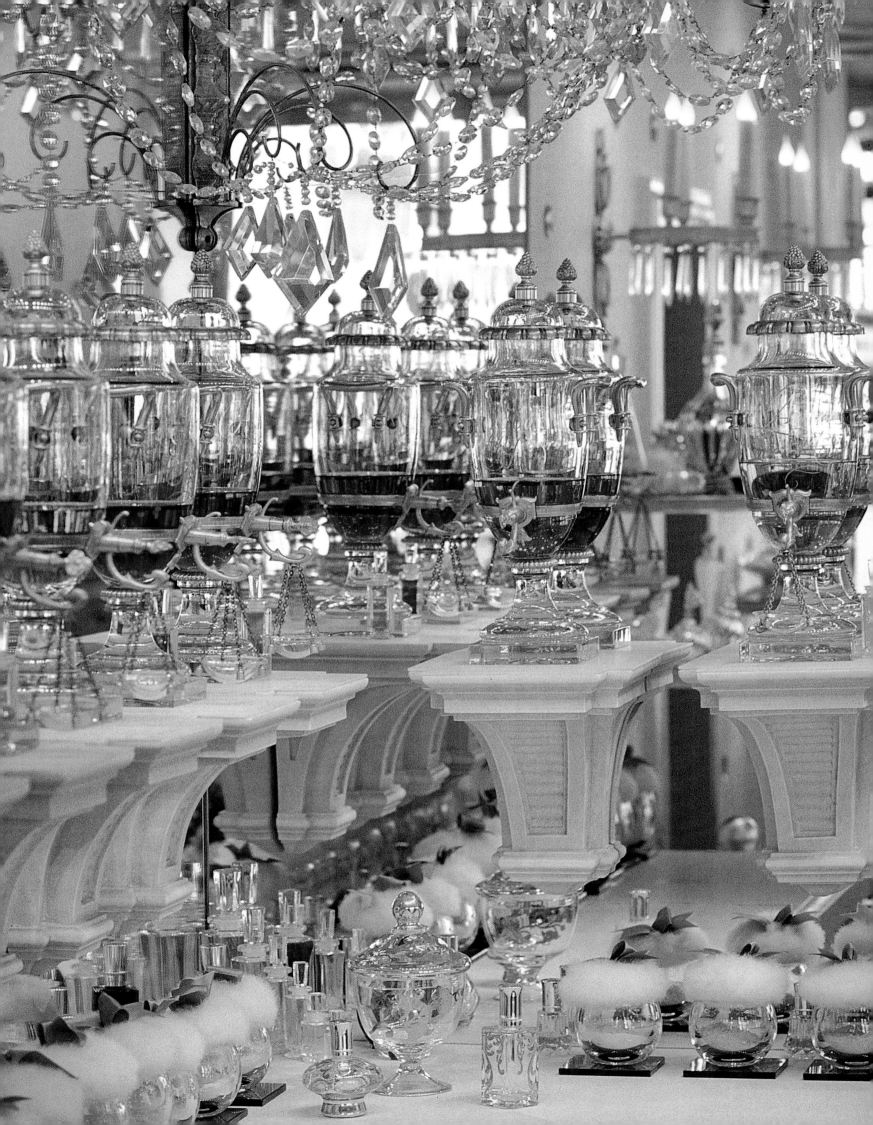

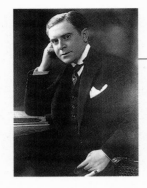

Tropiques, with its heady aromatic spice notes—all of which met with success at the Brussels World Fair. Tropiques was Petitjean's favorite and he had a text specially written for it: "Imagine a man strolling along a waterfront in the late afternoon. He finds himself at the corner of the landing stage where bananas, molasses, spices, exotic woods, rum and leather are being unloaded. These odors, accentuated by the sun, combine with the musty aroma of hemp and the acrid smells wafting in on the tide. A little later, the man returns to the residential district of the town where the air is full of the balmy scent of the gardens. After the confusion of the port, he finds the splendor of rare flowers, the cool shade of trees, the unbelievable luxury of serenity."

The great master perfumer, François Coty, used to maintain: "A perfume is seen as much as it is smelled," a lesson Armand Petitjean clearly never forgot. Magie made its debut in 1950, in a magnificent coiled-shaped crystal bottle packed in a prism-shaped presentation case sprinkled with multicolored sequins in the form of stars. Limited deluxe bottles are brought out for each new Lancôme perfume, the launch of which is always a memorable occasion. The celebrations for the launch of Trésor in 1952, for example, were held in the Palais de Chaillot in Paris on the occasion of the ball for the Petits Lits Blancs,

which Lancôme sponsors every year. Each debutante received a bottle of Trésor in the shape of an enormous cut diamond and the choreographer, Serge Lifar, created a ballet to music by Henri Sauguet.

Some perfume houses discontinue certain perfumes as and when fashions change, but this is not the case with Lancôme, who still produce their star perfumes, such as Magie, Climats, Sikkim and O Intense. In 1990, Lancôme went one better with a floral-fruity perfume named Trésor, today a member of the exclusive circle of the world's ten best-selling perfumes—proof that a beautiful fragrance, or a beautiful name never dies.

THE FIRST PERFUMES BY FASHION DESIGNERS

In 1911, when the fashion designer Paul Poiret founded his perfume company Les Parfums de Rosine, he was unaware that he had just sealed the strongest partnership in the world of elegance: that of fashion and perfume. These two sectors, both of which pursue their quest for beauty, quality and style whatever the risks, were bound to meet. In about 1930, the writer Colette affirmed, "The fashion designer is better placed that anyone else to know what women need and what suits them . . . Thanks to the designer-perfumer, perfume becomes more than a beauty

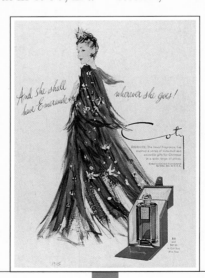

"Offer women the best fragrance you can produce, present it in a perfect perfume bottle of great simplicity, but of impeccable taste, charge a reasonable price and you have all the ingredients for the development of a trade more successful than the world has ever seen." It was by following this creed that François Coty, photographed here in the 1920s during the height of his career (top), made the reputation of his perfumes, evoked here by a poster (above) and by this graceful drawing by Helleu, an artist working at the turn of the century (opposite).

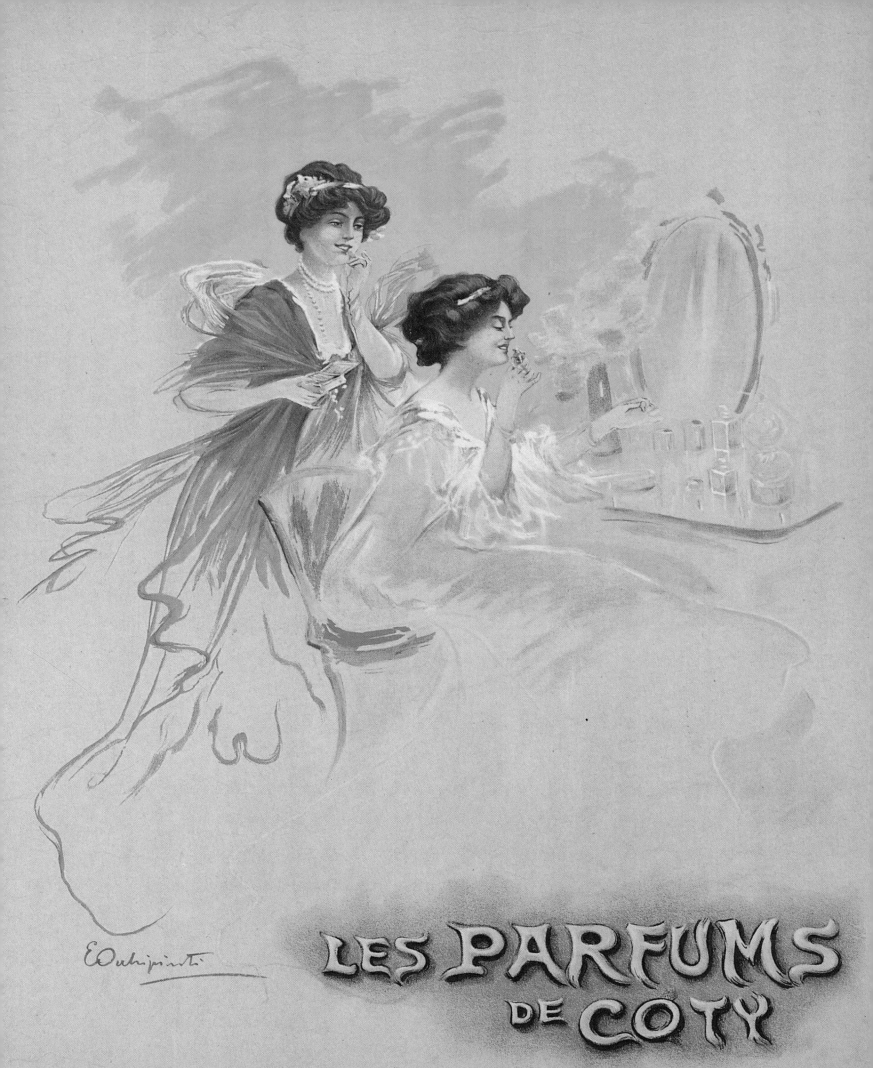

LES PARFUMS DE COTY

ESTAMPES D'ART
P. VERCASSON. 43 Rue de Lancry, PARIS

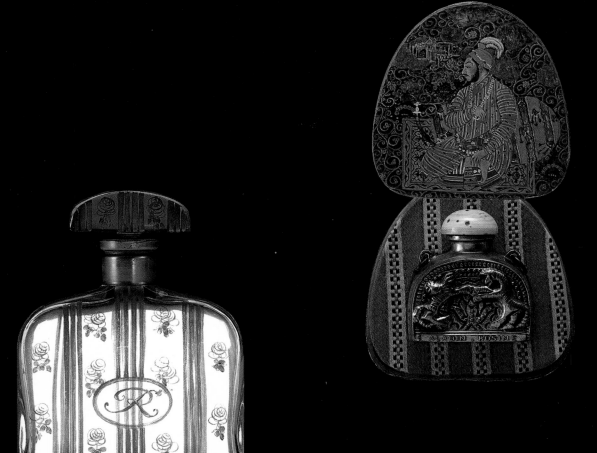

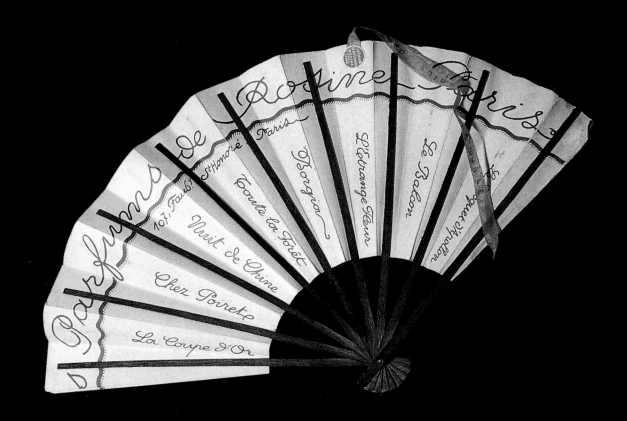

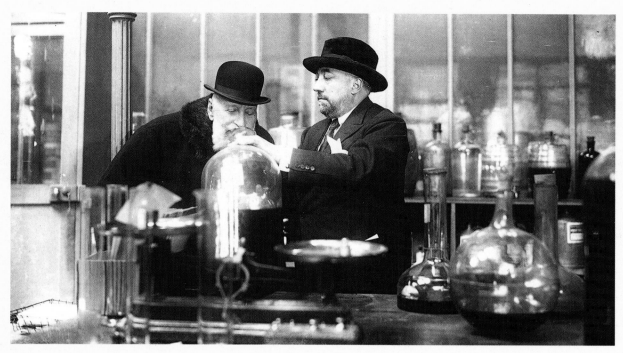

treatment in the orchestration of elegance: it can, it must, represent the direct expression of the tendencies and tastes of our era."

A dress is too frivolous? Perfume gives it soul, a certain *je ne sais quoi*, which is not bothered with outward appearance, transcends it in fact, because it is created for eternity. According to Jean Cocteau, "Fashion is what goes out of fashion," it is a "raging epidemic." And of course fashion does reflect the whim of the moment. Perfume, meanwhile, seems to withstand the test of time. The flared dresses of Christian Dior's "New Look" have long since gone out of style, whereas Miss Dior has lost none of its exhilarating charm.

Nowadays all the great fashion houses possess one or several perfumes, not only because they project the image of the make abroad, (perfumes represent 50 percent of all luxury goods exports), but also because the foreign currency they bring into France covers the colossal financial demands of the haute couture industry. If, in the 1920s, haute couture made possible the advent of the fashion designer's perfume, today it is perfume which ensures the survival of haute couture.

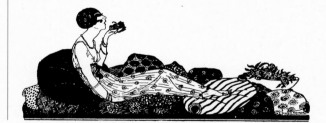

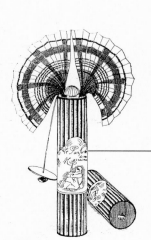

Paul Poiret, seen here in his bowler hat in the Parfums de Rosine factory in the suburbs of Paris with his perfumer Emmanuel Boulet (top), was the first to associate fashion and perfumes. Like this letterhead designed by Georges Lepape (above), Poiret's fragrances and perfume bottles were dazzlingly audacious and sophisticated: the dreamy Parfum de Ma Marraine, created as homage to soldiers' penfriends (opposite), the famous Rose de Rosine, in its bottle decorated with Lepape's rose—the company's logo—and Aladin, nestling in its delightful presentation case (opposite, top). This perfumed publicity fan was presented to clients as a gift (opposite, bottom).

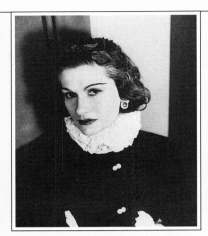

Gabrielle Chanel was the first to sense this new tendency. When this head-strong woman—she began her career as a hat designer—opened her perfume house in 1910 in the rue Cambon in Paris, Paul Poiret was still the reference in *La Gazette du Bon Ton*. People were beginning to tire, however, of his osprey plumes and harem-style garments. Women of leisure had had their day . . . it was time to make way for those with a more active lifestyle—business women, women who drove their Hispano Suzas with their hair flying in the wind. Time to make way for Chanel! She designed a wardrobe based on her own tastes and on what she herself wore—close-fitting sweaters, dark reefer jackets, wide trousers and the famous little black dress, said to be a souvenir of her boarding school years. Here was the new silhouette of the liberated woman. All that was missing was a perfume. None of those available really attracted her—they were all either to sweet or too insipid. Her friend the Grand Duke Dmitri of Russia had given her a taste for powerful fragrances, poles apart from the dainty floral scents then in fashion. In Grasse she met Ernest Beaux and a bond of trust was immediately established between the research chemist, who had spent his youth in Saint Petersburg, and the woman who inspired the love of the nephew of the late tsar.

On May 5, 1921, Chanel launched her first perfume, N° 5. It was forceful, polished and daring. For the first time in the history of perfume, here was a fragrance that did not imitate any bouquet or accord. It was unique, intoxicating in its originality. With its sharply defined bottle, a perfect example of Art Deco, N° 5 was to make Chanel's fortune. In 1924, she founded the Société des Parfums Chanel with horse-owning industrialists she had met in Deauville, the Wertheimer brothers. This was the first step down the road to success. In liberated Paris of 1945, crowds of GI's stood in line in front of the Chanel boutique in the rue Cambon, eager to buy this elixir of French elegance to take back home. Sometime later Marilyn Monroe was asked what she wore in bed. With her reply, "Chanel N° 5," the fragrance rocketed to the top of world sales and seventy years later it still holds its position. The rituals involved in its presentation have not changed. Sealing the fragrance in its famous bottle entails no less than nine operations, one of the most delicate being what is known as *baudruchage*. The *baudruche* is a fine natural membrane which is secured by a cotton thread knotted four times which seals the opening at the top of the bottle to ensure that it is perfectly airtight. Another delicate phase is the application of the logo of two interlaced letter *C*s, drawn by hand in black wax, that non-color so dear to Chanel. Other perfumes followed N° 5, and among the most popular today are N° 19, with its powdery, iris fragrance, the delightfully fresh Cristalle, and Coco, inspired by Ernest Beaux's magnificent Cuir de Russie, while for men there is Pour Monsieur, Égoïste and Égoïste Platinum. A Chanel perfume can be recognized by the quality of its raw mate-

"Women wear the perfumes which are given to them! You should wear a perfume you really like, your very own perfume. When I leave my jacket somewhere, I can recognize it straight away," affirmed Coco Chanel, pictured here in 1955 by the Hungarian photographer Hoyningen-Huene (above).

rials, for example the Grasse jasmine which the Chanel company still cultivates. It can also be distinguished by its spirited and powerful fragrance trail, which is quite remarkable on the skin of all women and just what Coco Chanel wanted: "I pity women who have to identify the perfume they are wearing," she used to say. "It should speak for itself. Perfume is utterly indiscreet."

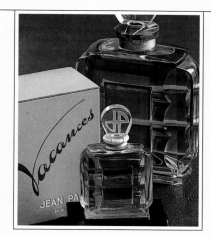

Jean Patou, renowned for his sweaters and tennis-style skirts, and who was Chanel's main rival at the time, also decided to turn his hand to perfumes. In 1925, he somewhat provocatively launched three fragrances simultaneously: Amour-Amour, Que Sais-Je? and Adieu Sagesse. For Jean Patou this was just the beginning. Perhaps he had sensed the changing trends, for in 1927 he invented the first sun oil, Chaldée, with its amber and floral fragrance and in 1931 the first unisex perfume, Le Sien, which, according to the publicity slogan, was intended "For modern men and women who play golf and drive at 75 miles an hour." These were followed by the first perfume bar, where, on request, a perfumer-barman concocted masterly olfactory cocktails. Not forgetting the small leather perfume cases in the form of cigarette lighters designed for elegant ladies to take on their travels. Then of course came Joy, to which Patou owes his reputation. It all began in 1929. With Europe suffering from the economic depression, Jean Patou dreamed of a sumptuous perfume as an antidote to the pes-

simism of the day. At his request, the perfumer Henri Almeras created a combination of Bulgarian rose and Grasse jasmine in unprecedented proportions which completely overthrew the norms of traditional perfumery. The accord was fantastic, so was the cost. "So what!" retaliated Jean Patou, "Let's be extravagant and aim for ultimate luxury!" Was it created for the lovely eyes of that fabulously wealthy client whose Christian name is said to have inspired Joy? The secret has never been divulged, but Joy soon figured among the legendary perfumes. Elsa Maxwell, the physically rather unattractive society woman with a sharp tongue which, in the 1940s, earned her the nickname "the Hollywood Busybody," declared, "It's the costliest perfume in the world!" This slogan has never changed, and, like Chanel N° 5, neither have the rituals involved in its manufacture. Each bottle of perfume is filled by hand, drop by drop, so as to lose none of the precious fragrance base, before being sealed and tied with a gold thread.

Arpège has been the pride of the Lanvin label ever since its creation in 1927. Jeanne Lanvin was then at the height of her fame. Nicknamed the "the Omnibus Kid" from the time when, as an apprentice milliner, she used to run behind the omnibus to save the price of the fare, she reigned over a fashion house which designed clothes for men and women. All Paris frequented her town house in the rue Barbet-de-Jouy, where they could admire

Hawthorn, the fragrance which stunned the young Marcel Proust, combined with lilac, mimosa and hyacinth makes up the joyous bouquet of Vacances (vacation) by Jean Patou, launched in France in 1936 in the euphoric atmosphere following the granting of the first annual paid leave (above).

paintings by Edouard Vuillard, who enjoyed her patronage. She had already launched fourteen fragrances, including the sulphurous Mon Péché/My Sin, which was graced with a double name since it was intended for the American market. But she wanted a perfume which would honor and epitomize her style, like Chanel N° 5. She approached the perfumer André Fraysse, then only twenty-seven years old, and asked Armand Rateau, her interior decorator, to design the bottle, which of course turned out to be the famous black sphere. The fragrance is intoxicating, a veritable floral symphony of more that sixty notes which subside into a trail of iris and vanilla. Jeanne Lanvin christened it Arpège (arpeggio) in honor of her daughter Marie-Blanche, an accomplished musician. As soon as it was launched, Arpège met with unanimous approval. Colette considered the perfume to be "thoroughly modern." In May 1927, on the strength of this success, Jeanne Lanvin founded the Société des Parfums Lanvin. From that moment on, André Fraysse never left his laboratory. L'Ame Perdue (Lost Soul for the export market) and Pétales Froissés were extremely popular, but even more successful was the leather note of Scandal, which in 1933 made furs so intoxicating. None of these perfumes, however, ever threatened the supremacy of Arpège among the Lanvin perfumes.

In 1931, Marcel Rochas, who had opened his fashion house at number 12 avenue Matignon, became the favorite designer of the Hollywood stars. Jean Harlow, Loretta Young, Carole Lombard and Marlene Dietrich snatched up his suits cut on the bias, his backless dresses, his divinely clinging sheath dresses and, above all, the wasp-waisted corset in black Chantilly lace, created for the most sensual of them all, Mae West. It is said that her silhouette also inspired the contours of the bottle for Femme. Many lines have been written about this perfectly named perfume, but the man who knows its history best is its creator, Edmond Roudnitska. "In 1944, Marcel Rochas came to see me and asked me to create a perfume for him. He wanted an opulent, feminine fragrance, evoking soft curves — according to him one should be able to smell a woman's perfume before seeing her. A year earlier I had composed a formula around a crystallized note, like a beautiful prune bronzed by the sun. It was my favorite and I suggested it to Marcel Rochas, never dreaming that he would immediately accept it." Accept it he did, and it is easy to see why. Femme exudes the generous sensuality which Rochas sought to give his dresses. A fruity note harmonizes with ylang-ylang, Grasse jasmine and a strange alliance of musk and amber. These, however, are luxury essences and the country was still at war. There was a shortage of raw materials and those needed for Femme were very costly, so Marcel Rochas decided to begin by bringing out a limited edition. Femme, in its Lalique bottle ensconced in a bed of black lace reminiscent of the provocative corset, was sold at first on a subscription basis to Parisian high society. The Duchess of Windsor, the Viscountess of Noailles, Madeleine Renaud, Arletty and Michèle Morgan all voiced their enthusiasm. In 1945, Femme was finally offered to the public at an exhibition entitled *Les Parfums à Travers la Mode*, a tribute to the recently deceased Paul Poiret.

Marcel Rochas launched Femme, with its black Chantilly lace packaging, a captivating echo of his notorious wasp-waisted corset, in 1945 to celebrate the end of the somber war years. It radiates femininity with its intoxicating fruity note. The suggestive curves of the perfume bottle were inspired by the figure of the American actress Mae West (opposite).

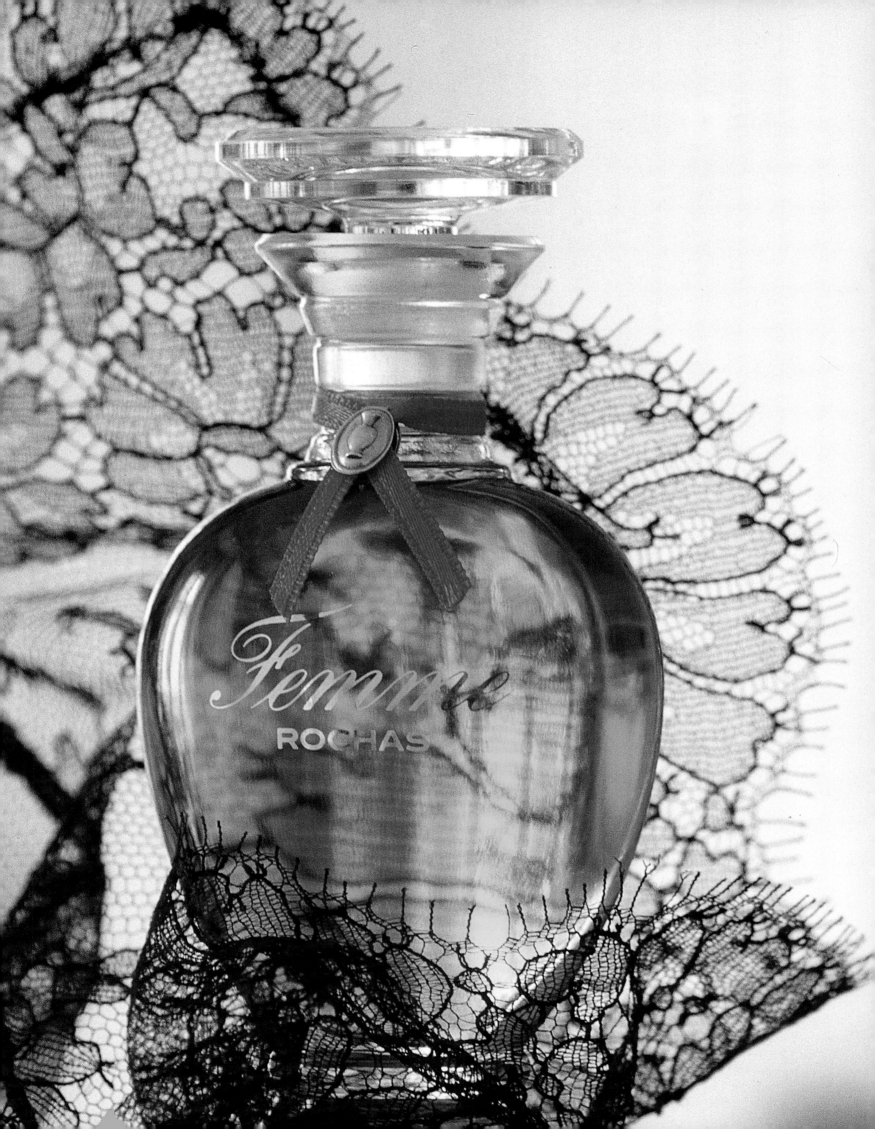

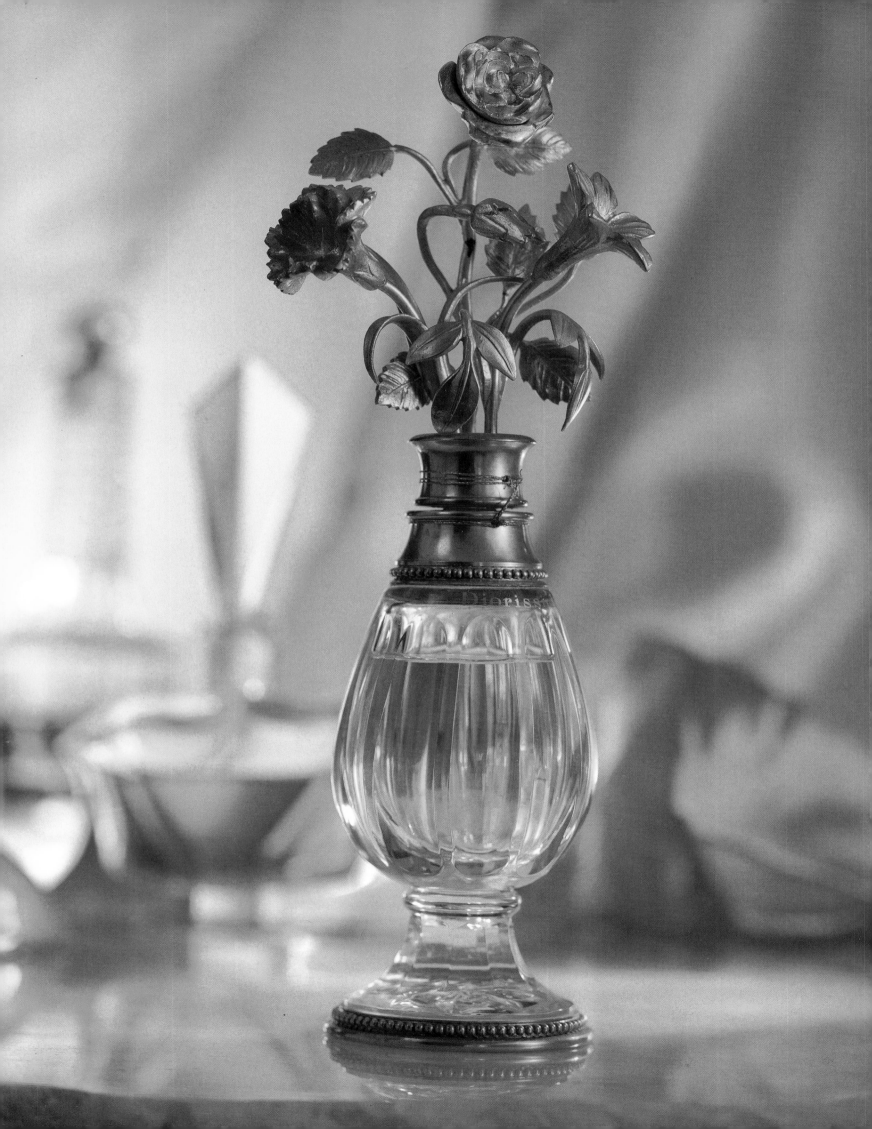

FROM BALMAIN TO DIOR, RICCI AND SAINT LAURENT

At the outset, perfumers were worried by the influx of fashion designers on the market. "The fashion designer is no more talented at making perfumes than perfumers are at making dresses," Marylène Delbourg-Delphis was quoted as saying in the *Excelsior*, one of the newspapers of the period. But a truce was rapidly signed. The perfumers soon realized that the fashion designers were looking for top-class perfumes, in keeping with their style. Perfume for the designers was no longer just a sideline, but an activity closely linked to fashion and of considerable economic importance for their image.

"As regards elegance, perfume is more important than accessories, jewels and shoes." So spoke Pierre Balmain in 1946. The young fashion designer, then just thirty-two years old, had just created the Balmain perfume company, only one year after founding his fashion house. His simple, uncoquettish style enthralled the American writer Gertrude Stein, who hailed it as the "New French Style." His perfumes were the best ambassadors of his talent, backed up, admittedly, by the presence of Germaine Cellier, creator of Vent Vert, and by his flair for publicity.

His most serious rival was Christian Dior, the inventor of the "New Look," whose first collection, in the spring of 1947, marked a return to opulence with clouds of chiffon and flared skirts made with yards and yards of material. His perfume company was founded in the same year, under the management of Serge Heftler-Louiche, formerly with Coty. What kind of perfume were women looking for, and what should it be called? "Miss Dior!" exclaimed Christian Dior, whose Anglomania was legendary. The hound's-tooth pattern of one of the materials in the "New Look" collection inspired the bottle's decoration. Created by the perfumer Paul Vacher, the green chypre fragrance with an animal base note did not meet with the company's unanimous approval, but Christian Dior, confident in his own judgment, held his ground and insisted that the perfume be sprayed in every room of the Dior fashion house. As he explained, "Perfume is the indispensable complement of a woman's personality, it is the finishing touch to an outfit, it is the rose by which one distinguishes a Lancret dress."

Robert Ricci, the son of Marie Nielli, an Italian fashion designer working in Paris, was in complete agreement with this statement, yet when he presented L'Air du Temps in 1948, he was far from imagining that he had just launched a legend! In 1932, he had persuaded his mother to open her fashion house under the name of Nina Ricci (Nina was the name she went by as a young girl). The serene femininity of her dresses soon propelled her into the limelight. The fortunes of the Ricci house suffered, however, because of the war and Robert Ricci decided it was time to branch out into perfumes. In 1945, A Cœur-Joie was created. "I wanted it to be noble and jaunty so as to reflect the joy of victory and the newly found optimism," recalls this youthful octogenarian. But it was L'Air du Temps which was to cause a stir. It is considered, and rightly so, as one of the five greatest perfumes in the world, along with Shalimar, N° 5, Arpège and Joy. It is, above all, the perfect symbol of a fashion house whose name is synonymous with romanticism. Robert Ricci is hardly

Diorissimo by Christian Dior made its debut in 1956, in a superb limited series Baccarat crystal perfume bottle in the form of a bouquet of bronze roses in an Etruscan-style vase. Its designer, Charles, is said to have been inspired by a baroque-style chandelier which illuminated the salons of the Dior fashion house in the avenue Montaigne (opposite).

the man to refute this. "I created L'Air du Temps for a woman, perhaps a famous one, or perhaps a woman one had merely caught a glimpse of, but above all for a woman you dream of and idealize. For me perfume is an act of love, real or imaginary love. I am a romantic, I cannot imagine life without dreams." This fragrance conceived by Monsieur Fauveron, a perfumer from Grasse, was very different to the heady accords in fashion at the time. Its fresh, floral, spicy notes enveloped the skin in a soft aura which can also be found in later creations. The poetry of the Lalique bottle and the beauty of the name which echoes like a promise, took care of the rest. In 1956, L'Air du Temps soared to the summits of the worldwide market and today a bottle is sold somewhere in the world every second!

These successful pioneers encouraged others to follow suit. Hubert de Givenchy dedicated L'Interdit to his muse, the actress Audrey Hepburn, whose clothes he designed both on and off the screen. Madame Grès, celebrated for her flowing, Greek goddess-style dresses, swept away two conventions: the reign of the floral aldehydes and the stilted belief that fashion must dictate what women ought to wear on an annual basis. Cabochard, a chypre with a leather note and an insolent name (*cabochard* means "headstrong"), at last suggested that to be elegant is to be oneself and nothing else.

Yves Saint Laurent bore this in mind when, in 1964, soon after taking premises in the rue Spontini, he created his first

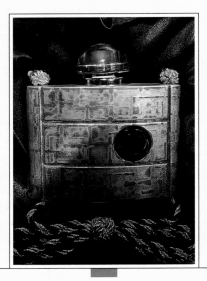

perfume, Y. The man whom Christian Dior presented as his heir broke away from the stilted elegance of his peers. Y plays on the paradox of freshness and suavity. In 1971, Rive Gauche underlined the joyful sensuality of emancipated women, and its spray bottle was as audacious as the transparent shirts and dinner suits they wore. In 1977 it was the turn of Opium to cause a stir. The financiers were reticent about the project, but Yves Saint Laurent stood firm. He had already chosen the name and the color of the bottle, inspired by a Chinese lacquer *inro* (a small, richly decorated, lacquer box) and he had in mind the notes of an oriental fragrance which avoided sliding towards vanilla. He did, however, allow blind tests—where the perfume is presented along with others, in identical plain, unlabeled bottles and customers are invited to state their preference—to be carried out in the United States, Germany and France. Opium won unanimous approval. From the first day it was launched, people went crazy about it and stocks quickly ran out. A turnover of half a million dollars had been projected for the first year, whereas a figure of seven and a half million was announced! Everybody wanted Opium. Men were enthralled by this perfume, which seemed to announce a return to sensuality, and they even went as far as going into perfume stores themselves to purchase the new fragrance (which Yves Saint Laurent, in his imagination, had created for the Empress of China) as a gift for the woman they loved!

The perfume bottle for Opium, which is as bewitching as the fragrance itself, was inspired by a Japanese *inro*. Although the perfume can be seen through a crescent-shaped window, it nevertheless remains mysterious, a mystery which is further accentuated in the deluxe bottle for the extract, by a worn, gold patina, reminiscent of certain pieces of jewellery by Yves Saint Laurent. This limited series perfume bottle is now much sought after (above). Kashâya, which Kenzo dedicated to women in love with the absolute, is a subtle, carnal, oriental perfume, presented in a plant-inspired bottle sculpted by Serge Mansau (opposite).

READY-TO-WEAR PERFUMES

"You look, you choose, you try it on and you take it with you!" So went the slogan for the publicity campaign conceived in 1954 by the French federation of ladies' wear to promote ready-to-wear clothes. The clothing revolution had been declared. The ready-to-wear industry's aim was to produce cheerful, practical clothes at reasonable prices. From now on, clothes were factory made and created by talented young designers. Two notable examples were Kenzo, the Japanese designer who, in 1970, created the "Jungle Jap" line of clothes, and the talented Sonia Rykiel, who four years later revolutionized knitwear with visible seams. Both of them rapidly became involved with perfume: Kenzo with King Kong and Sonia Rykiel, with 7ème Sens. Like their predecessors in the haute couture industry, the new designers used perfume to promote their style and draw in a wider clientele.

In 1975, the ready-to-wear clothing industry produced its first perfume, Chloé, the trademark of a make of clothes which were close to haute couture in their quality, but sold at more reasonable prices. Several designers have been associated with Chloé, but it is now in the hands of Karl Lagerfeld. The perfume owes much to Lagerfeld, not only its magnificent 1930s-style frosted glass bottle, but also the tuberose note which perfumery had long neglected and which gives the scent that haute couture touch.

In 1978, Cacharel's Anaïs Anaïs made the final break with tradition when Jean Bousquet, who had created the trademark in 1963, decided to launch the perfume in democratic fashion in the low-priced Monoprix chain stores. In the same year, a simple seersucker shirt on the front cover of the magazine *Elle* sent Cacharel soaring to the top of the ready-to-wear sales market. Then Liberty prints came into fashion, floral patterns which make women want to be young girls again—a trend which was instrumental in the creation of Anaïs Anaïs. Anaïs Anaïs is a tender fragrance, with a suave bouquet of orange blossom, jasmine and roses, presented in a white opaline bottle with a Liberty-print label. It captured the style of a generation and in 1985 topped worldwide sales. In terms of volume of fragrance, it is still the best-selling perfume in the world!

Another eloquent example of osmosis between a designer and his perfume is Claude Montana's Parfum de Peau, launched in 1986. Montana began his career designing leather jackets, establishing his structured, almost sculpted style from his first collection in 1977. He wanted to produce an equally powerful perfume which would lastingly impregnate the skin—a sort of olfactory tattoo. The result was a chypre fragrance, a daring combination of the blatant sensuality of musk, sandalwood and patchouli. The perfume bottle was equally remarkable, an impressive cabled column designed by Serge Mansau, presented in a box of Klein blue, the intense ultramarine tone created by the French artist, Yves Klein. In 1987 Parfum de Peau was awarded two Medici Prizes at the annual fair in Bologna, one for the perfume and another for the bottle.

Like Claude Montana, Thierry Mugler and Jean-Paul Gaultier belong to a generation of designers who, in the 1980s, played havoc with conventional elegance. They created per-

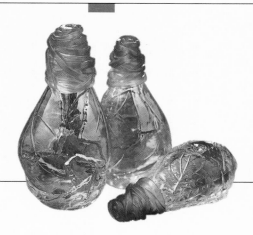

fumes to match their image. Angel, launched in 1992 by Thierry Mugler in a superb star-shaped perfume bottle, has a particularly surprising fragrance. One would have expected sinful intoxication in the style of his provocative clothes, yet the fragrance in fact evolves in tender notes of caramel, honey and chocolate. A sensational olfactory event which carried the so-called gourmand perfumes to extremes.

Although eccentric, Jean-Paul Gaultier's style is intended to be worn by all. He had to decide whether his first perfume was to reflect his corset-dresses, trouser skirts and tattooed T-shirts. Above all he wanted it to be traditional, to be taken seriously, even though Gaultier himself, in his own words, sometimes "looks like a clown." The perfume was launched in the spring of 1993 in an audacious bust-shaped bottle in a copper corset, presented in a metal case like a food can. The fragrance itself, however, was more restrained. It was inspired by rice powder, which Jean-Paul Gaultier had smelled for the first time as a child in the Châtelet theater. It is a successful balance between the desire to surprise and the desire to be lasting.

In Italy, ready-to-wear designers dominate contemporary perfume. The Italian market is dynamic, with the highest number of new perfumes each year. One name, however, stands out from this somewhat crowded sector, that of the fashion designer Giorgio Armani, who also

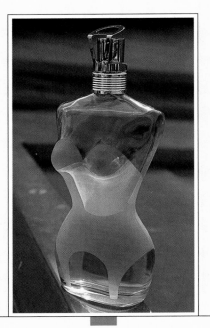

leads the Italian luxury ready-to-wear industry. Launched in 1984, Armani pour Homme—a light toilet water with a hint of pepper—still figures among the leading male fragrances, not only in Italy, but also in America. Giò, Armani's latest floral fruity perfume for women, created in 1992, bears the stylist's signature, Giò, traced in his hand, and the perfume bottle of his own design is reminiscent of his broad-shouldered yet softly contoured jackets.

In Germany, perfumes by the local ready-to-wear fashion industry are so popular they even eclipse the Italian, French or American ones. The fashion designer Jil Sander, known for the sophisticated sobriety of her clothes, has created three perfumes for men and four for women and leads the market alongside Hugo Boss perfumes and Joop!, a women's sportswear line. In 1973, Margaretha Ley, a designer of Swedish origin, chose to present her first luxury ready-to-wear collection in Germany and is now the country's leading creator in this sector. In 1990, she launched her first perfume under her fashion trademark, Escada. So far it is the only German perfume to have found favor with French women, who are not usually receptive to foreign fragrances. It owes its success to the red and gold heart-shaped bottle and its feminine fragrance produced by a note of hyacinth, Margaretha Ley's favorite flower.

A fashion designer's perfume reflects his style. "For those who like what I create, buying my perfume is a way of having a 'Gaultier' at a more accessible price than the clothes," remarked the designer Jean-Paul Gaultier on the subject of his first perfume for women (above). As for Issey Miyake's first women's fragrance, it reflects the pure lines which have always characterized the Japanese designer's style: a perfume bottle which might have been carved out of a glacier and a fragrance which is as pure and fresh as a dew-covered garden (opposite).

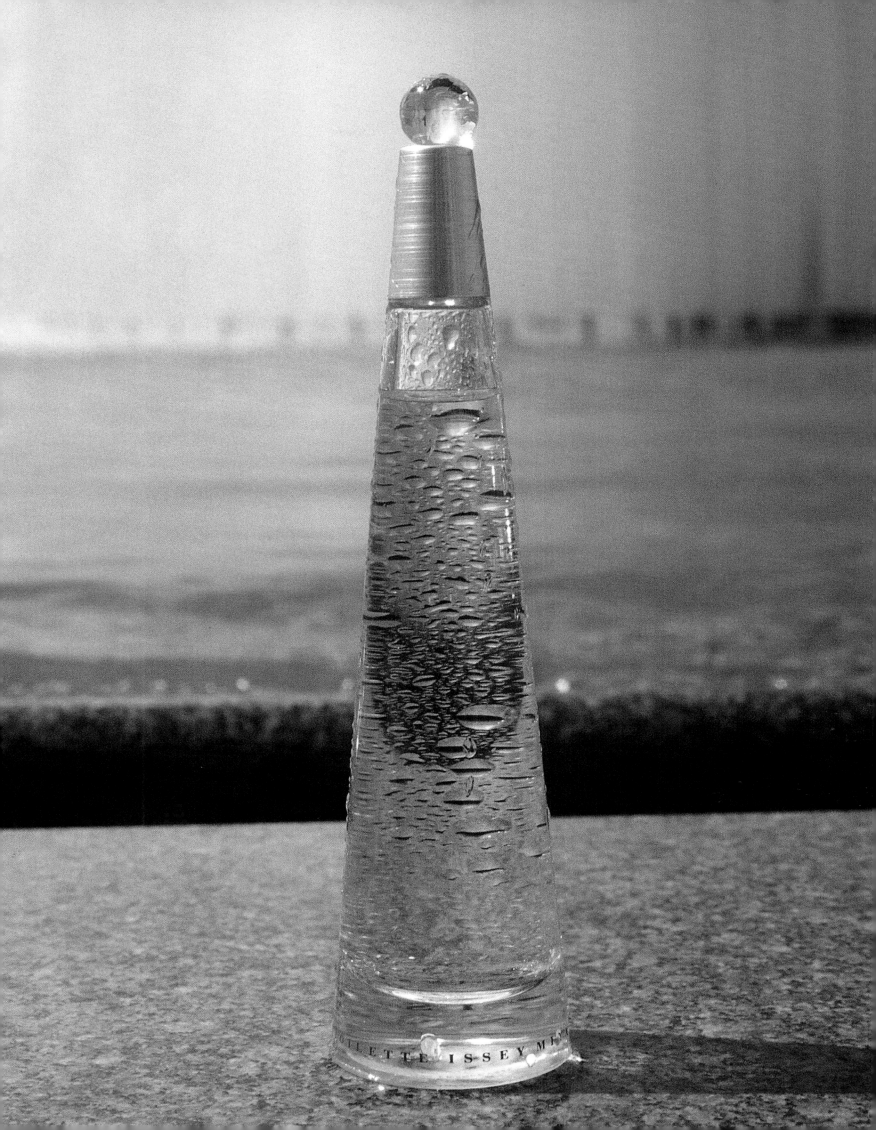

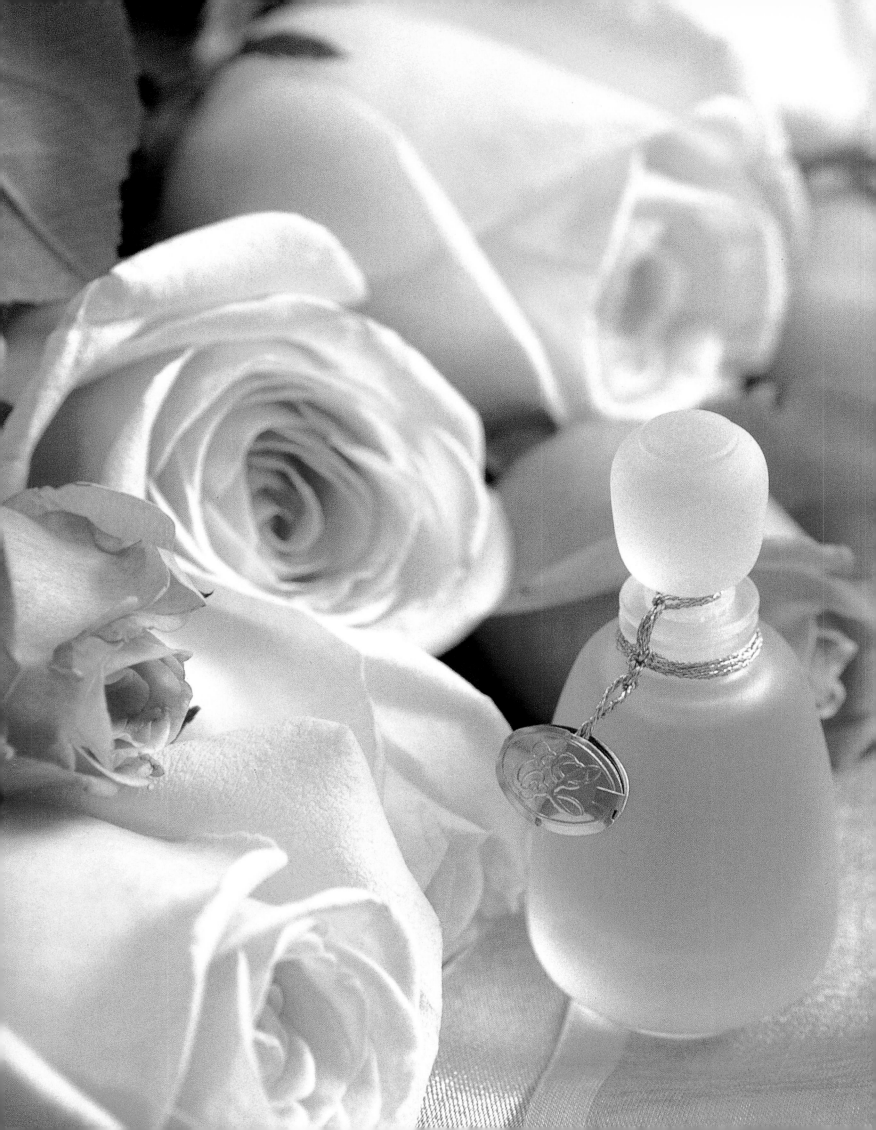

A GREAT AMERICAN LADY, ESTÉE LAUDER

The turnover figures for the American perfumery industry are the highest in the world. All the important European names set their sights on Saks Fifth Avenue and Bloomingdale's, New York's luxury department stores. The industry, however, is no more than fifty years old and owes its history to the imagination of one woman, Estée Lauder.

When this young woman of Hungarian origin founded her cosmetics company in 1946, 85 percent of fragrances sold in America carried the "Made in France" label. Women did not buy perfume for themselves, but were given it as a gift. In her autobiography, *Estée, a Success Story by Estée Lauder*, she explains how, at the time, perfume was considered as a love token. It was, as she says, "The perfect gift, and that was what was killing it." Very few women actually dared to buy their perfume themselves and it was conventional for the man to buy the perfume he liked, or that he thought his lady friend might like. One evening at a party at a friend's house, she found herself staring at a shelf where three unopened and dust-covered perfume bottles sat in solemn splendor. Suddenly she decided to persuade women to buy the perfume they really liked. How would she do it? Simply by producing a fragrance which was not in the form of a perfume. A perfumed bath oil, for example, that a woman could buy without risking her reputation. What could be more normal than taking a bath? And that is how Youth Dew came into being in 1953. Estée Lauder had the clever idea of leaving the stopper unsealed, so that the client could smell the fragrance, which is, in fact, much more heady than it's name might suggest. Its success was unbelievable.

Youth Dew, the first great national perfume, gave American women a taste for fragrances that hit "hard and long," which was to be the distinguishing style of American perfumery for several decades to come. Estée Lauder could have brought out a second perfume straight away, but the public had to wait fifteen years before being able to sample the white flowers which characterize Estée. The story behind another of Estée Lauder's perfumes, Private Collection, deserves a mention. Originally, it was reserved for Estée Lauder's exclusive use, and was not released on the market. When asked what perfume she was wearing, she used to reply "This is from my private collection." One day the Saks' sales manager called her to say that clients were constantly asking for a perfume called Private Collection. She wondered how and where they could have smelled it, and then she remembered that she had given a few samples to close friends who had lost no time in perfuming themselves with this unknown creation. Private Collection was launched in 1973 and became Princess Grace of Monaco's favorite perfume.

Teaching women to become more beautiful is something of a vocation for this great lady. In addition to providing American perfumery with its first masterpiece, Estée Lauder also succeeded in breaking down the very puritan American society's resistance to perfume. If nowadays Europe envies Estée Lauder's sales figures and creativity, and if, henceforth, the main olfactory breezes blow from American shores, it is thanks to an intrepid young woman who one day decided that "Perfume is like love, you can never get enough of it."

"A perfume is like a new dress. It makes you feel wonderful," affirms Estée Lauder. Private Collection, composed in a serene tempo of Bulgarian rose, orange blossom, mimosa and lime, blends languorous jasmine with heliotrope as light as chiffon (opposite).

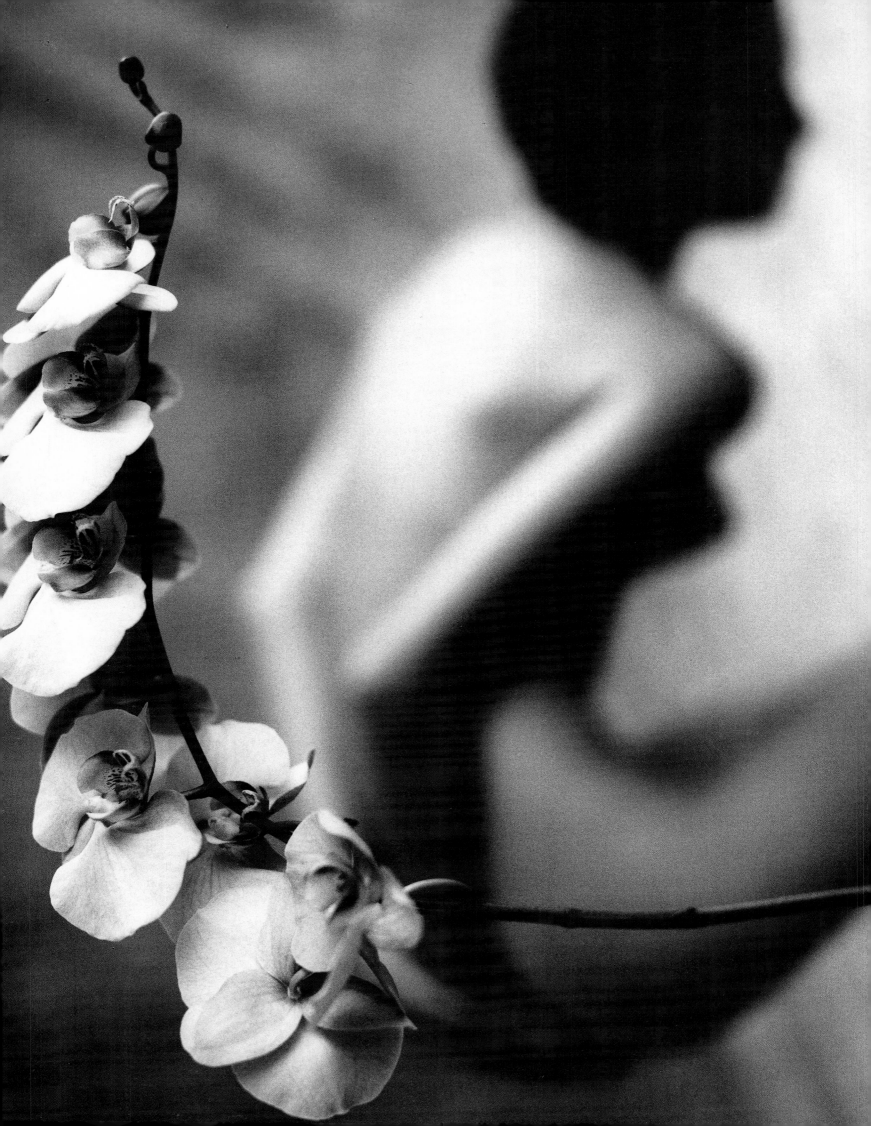

THE
POWER
OF
PERFUME

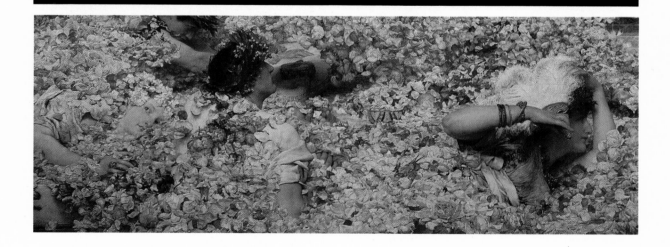

Perfumes, because they are linked with our sense of smell—the most uncontrollable and mysterious of all our senses—can be the source of intense emotions and extraordinary experiences. From the borders of sin to the frontiers of the sacred, perfumes stir up our desires and our passions, drawing us into unexplored regions of our emotions and the lost paradise of our memory.

Poets have always known that perfume is the faithful keeper of memory and each one of us has had occasion to experience it. Marcel Proust described this evocative power: "When from a long-distant past nothing subsists, after the people are dead, after the things are broken and scattered, taste and smell alone, more fragile but more enduring, more unsubstantial, more persistent, more faithful, remain poised a long time, like souls, remembering, waiting, hoping, amid the ruins of all the rest; and bear unflinchingly, in the tiny and almost impalpable drop of their essence, the vast structure of recollection."

When a face, an image, or a landscape has moved us, caused the skin to tingle and the heart to flutter, a fragrance is always there, intoxicating our memory. The smell of cut hay reminiscent of our first vacations, the aroma of the vanilla-scented apple tart we used to eat when we were children: so many sensual moments tinged with a nostalgic melancholy.

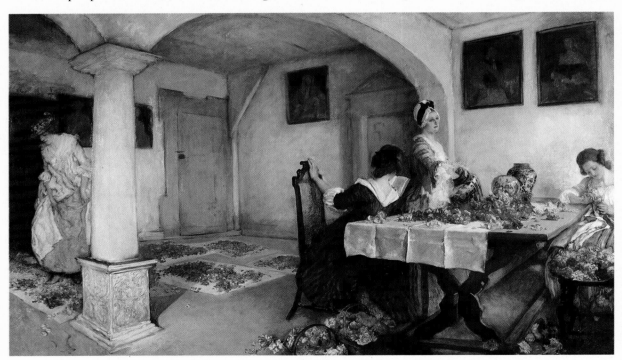

Perfumes divulge their secrets in an atmosphere of mutually shared emotion. The passions kindling in our hearts unveil the fragrant soul of roses, as illustrated in this work by John William Waterhouse (opposite). In this scene depicting the making of a potpourri, painted by E.A. Abbey (above), the rituals surrounding the preparation of the fragrances reveal the intimate thoughts of the flowers. Secret affinities exist between flowers and a woman's soul, a theme photographers (page 96), and painters such as Alma Tadema (page 97), never tire of portraying.

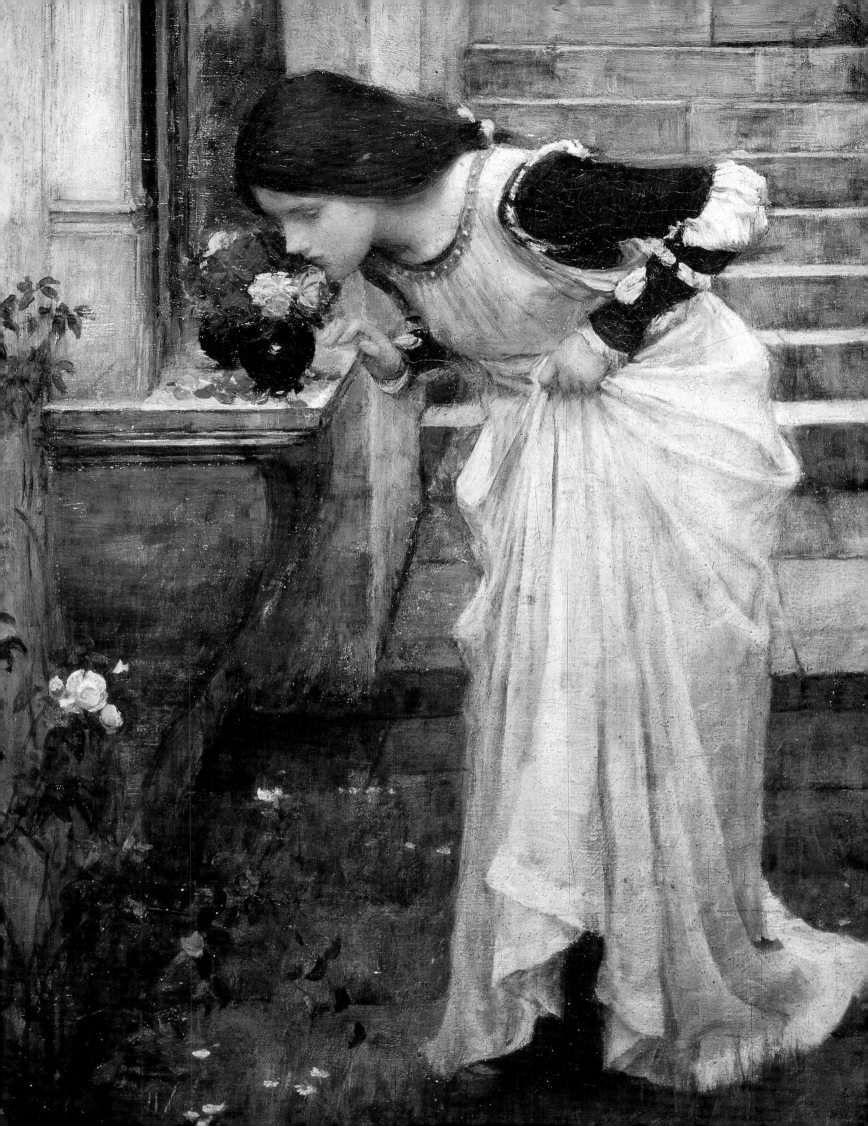

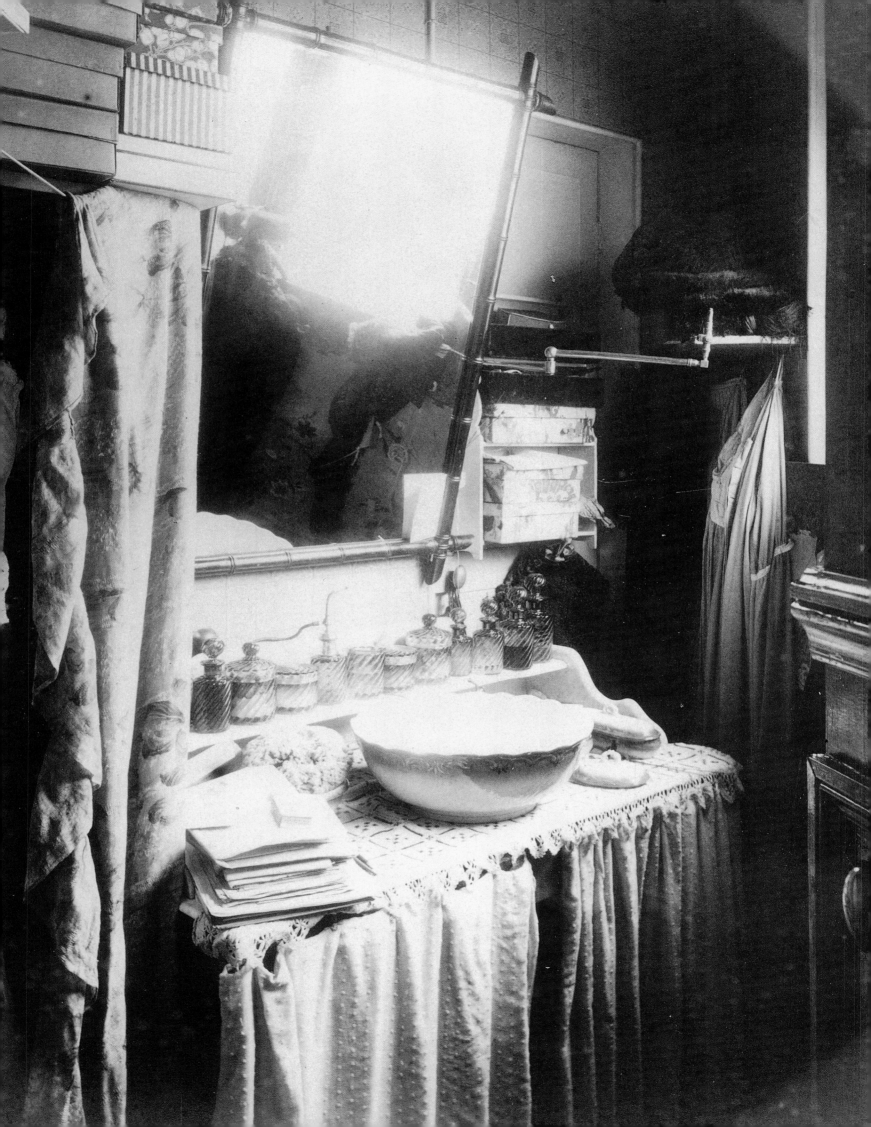

Many contemporary perfumes play on this nostalgia, with their fruity, or distinctly aromatic fragrances. Thierry Mugler's perfume Angel is as delectable as a Sacher torte in its combination of chocolate and cinnamon.

Sometimes, in moments of regret and sadness, we open the perfume bottles carefully hidden in the bottom of the cupboard. They tell the story of a lifetime. Ludmilla Mickaël remembers Carven's Vétiver, which her grandmother gave her when she was not quite twenty, and that other Vétiver by Guerlain, which she wore when she was at the Comédie Française theater, and finally Givenchy III, which she adopted after smelling it one evening in an actress friend's dressing room. The author Daniel Boulanger charmingly

describes perfumes as "Ferrets of recollection"! Perfumes are the liturgical objects of sentimental worship. There are women who keep the perfumes of old love affairs as the immutable proof of pleasures of the past, while others change their perfume with each new passion.

Perfumers draw inspiration from their innermost emotions and secret memories, embarking on intuitive journeys as explorers of their private experience of life, seeking themes which haunt them. The Japanese designer Issey Miyake's first perfume, L'Eau d'Issey, was inspired by a childhood memory. In Japan they celebrate boy's day on May 5 and traditionally iris leaves are put in the child's hot bath water, giving it a pleasant

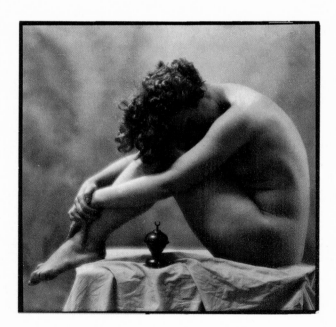

A woman is present body and soul in her perfume, which creates an aura of passion and emotion around her, as illustrated in this photograph (above) taken by the Catalan Josep Masana (1892–1979). Fragrances and flowers, perfume bottles abandoned on the dressing table and objects revealing the intimacy of an individual's existence leave a lasting reminder of a beloved person's presence, as in this photograph by Eugène Atget, taken in around 1910 (opposite).

plant odor. "On other days," Miyake recalls, "we used to put thick pieces of orange peel in the water and its perfume used to mingle with that of the wood of the bathtub." For his perfume Gardenia, the designer Tan Guidicelli wanted to capture the intoxicating scent of the white flowers which proliferate in the groves in Vietnam. "This fragrance is made all the more sensual by the fact that in my country it is synonymous with temptations of the flesh, for it is supposed to be the immaterial incarnation of the souls of courtesans."

In *Les Fleurs du Mal*, Baudelaire often describes the power of perfumes to evoke landscape:

When, with closed eyes, on some warm
autumn night,
I breathe your bosom's sultry fragrances,
Enchanted shores unfold their promontories
("Exotic Scent")

Baudelaire would certainly have liked Jean-François Laporte's perfumes, which are sublimated reflections of countries which this member of the French glove and perfume-makers guild has visited. "Datura evokes the sensuality of a Mediterranean garden into which I ventured at dusk when flowers give off their final scent. Geranium, a perfume to be worn indoors, was inspired by a visit to Egypt. I wanted it to be steeped in the heady fragrance of sun-drenched geraniums stacked on wooden carts."

Serge Lutens, who designs jewelry, make-up, images and objects, and composes perfumes for the Japanese firm Shiseido, has an equally personal approach. His perfumes could be described as interior journeys, for, although they are inspired by actual places (Feminité du Bois evokes the milky odor of the cedarwood sculpted by craftsmen in the quarter of Marrakech where he lives part of the year), they express, above all, the emotions the artist experiences in these places.

For Lalique, the first perfume produced by the famous establishment of the same name, Marie-Claude Lalique, the granddaughter of the celebrated glass artist, today the company's artistic director, was inspired by the immense magnolia tree which stands in her garden in Provence blending animal-like fragrances with the innocence of peonies. Ungaro's Ombre de Nuit began as the fashion designer's personal perfume, before taking its place next to Diva as his flagship perfume. "Having found nothing to my taste," relates Emmanuel Ungaro, "nothing which corresponded to my secret flights of fancy, I asked a perfumer friend to compose a fragrance. I wanted it to be somber and sun-beaten, like the city in Tuscany where I spent the most intense moments of my adolescence, and above all I wanted it to reflect the ambiguity of my status as an artist, at the same time masculine and feminine, fragile and tyrannical, steeped in contradictions."

THE SENSE OF SMELL

Take an old hunting jacket. Its strong odor of damp tanned leather assaults your nostrils, and yet the tender emotions it provokes can bring tears to your eyes. Odors conjure up a whole world of forgotten sensations and,

Perfumes have the power of revealing the passions and emotions which haunt us, a power Paul Morel, the hero of D.H. Lawrence's *Sons and Lovers*, discovers in a garden of flowers at night: "The air all round seemed to stir with scent, as if it were alive. He went across the bed of pinks, whose keen perfume came sharply across the rocking, heavy scent of the lilies . . . The scent made him drunk." It only takes the magic of a flower evoking Italy, like orange blossom for example (above), or the green, tender, penetrating fragrance of the peony, for one's life to change completely (opposite).

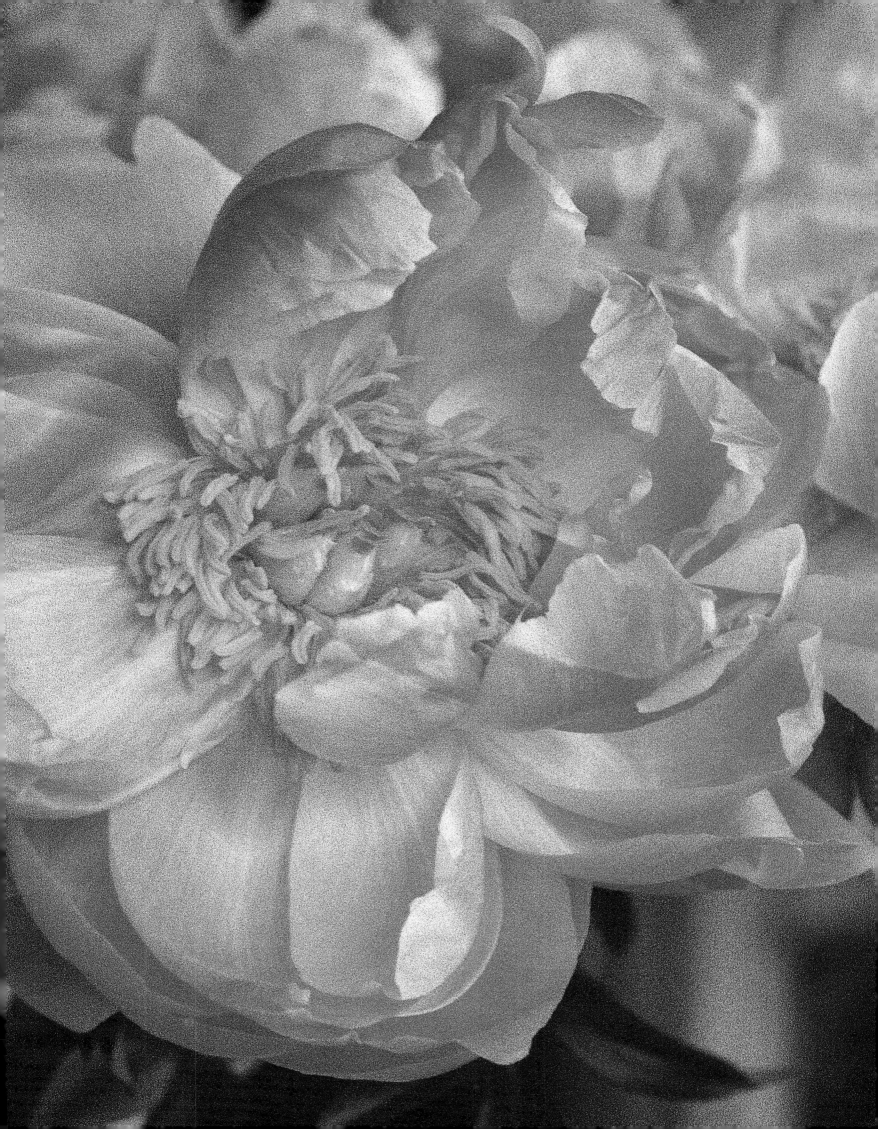

because of the particularly close links which unite them to our emotional life, they offer us one of the richest and most complex sensory experiences that exist.

Of all our senses, the sense of smell is the least known, despite the fact that very early on philosophers and doctors attempted to penetrate its mysteries. In the fourth century B.C., Aristotle first tried to describe the mechanisms of this organ, as did the Roman philosopher Lucretius in the first century B.C. The Middle Ages deliberately ignored the sense of smell, associating it with sinful, voluptuous pleasures, and it was not until the Renaissance period that Michel de Montaigne sang its praises, evoking its beneficial effects on the soul. On the subject of odors he wrote, "I have often noticed that they change me, affecting my spirit depending on what they are," while in the eighteenth century Jean-Jacques Rousseau, particularly attentive to the most subtle emotions, called our sense of smell "the sense of the imagination."

In the nineteenth century, scholars became passionately interested in the analysis of the human senses. Numerous works were devoted to the sense of smell, which was considered a fascinating faculty, but somewhat capricious and eccentric. It was not until the 1940s and the development of electro-physiological experiments examining the effects of electric signals on the brain, and later, in the 1980s, with the triumph of molecular biological research, that the sense of smell began to divulge some of its secrets.

One factor in particular which slows down the analysis of the sense of smell, is that we have no language which immediately corresponds to odors. We experience them only as sensory memories. When we look at a picture, for example, the words to describe its colors, forms and textures come spontaneously to mind, whereas if we smell a perfume, prior to any analysis, what comes to mind are memories of impressions associated with it. Smell is always the smell of something else.

In order to understand this phenomenon, one has to go back to the origins of mankind, when the sense of smell played a decisive role in man's survival. It was vital for looking for and choosing food, sensing danger, recognizing others and choosing a partner. It acted as a signal, it warned, informed and reassured. But with the development of civilization, man's olfactory perception became less acute and he relied increasingly on sight rather than smell in his perception of the world.

Although we use our sense of smell far less than in the past, it has not diminished but is simply lying fallow. In a newborn baby it constitutes one of the first means of communication with the outside world. The infant isolates the calm and reassuring odor of its mother. Between the ages of three and six, the child stores up numerous olfactory impressions. Studies have proved that at this early age there is no such thing as a "bad smell." Whereas our sense of hearing can be conditioned by listening to music and that of sight by looking at painting and sculpture, no specific education exists regarding our sense of smell, which is instead dictated by our immediate cultural and social environment. Diet, personal hygiene habits and exceptional geographical and climatic conditions, such as extreme heat, humidity or high altitude, all

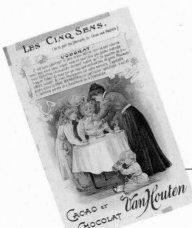

The odors of childhood constantly haunt us. For most people, the smell of chocolate (left) conjures up the cosy, familiar atmosphere of children's teatime. These aromas from carefree times in the past influence our adult preferences and desires. It is with great joy that we transmit these precious delights to our own children (mother and child, photographed by Gertrude Käsebier, opposite).

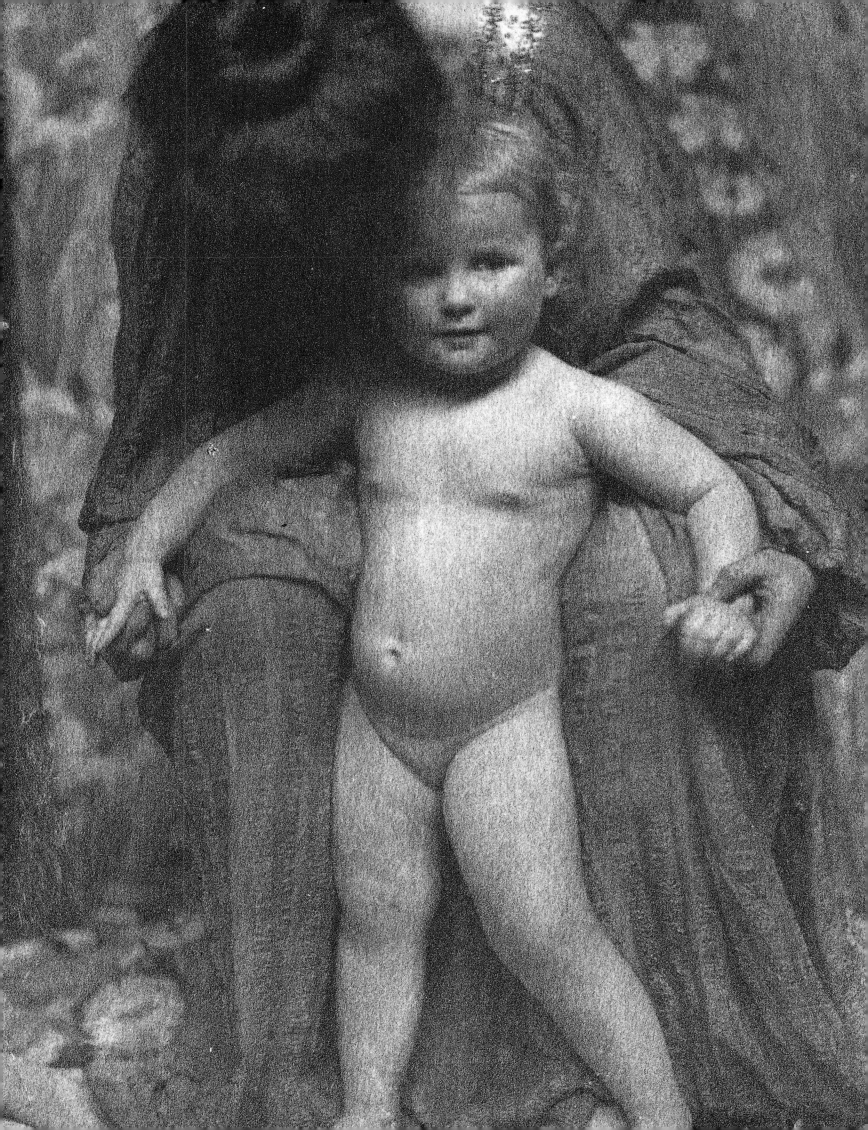

create fundamental differences in the olfactory preferences of different populations.

An individual's perception of odors is as unique as their fingerprints or as their genetic code.

Odors play a decisive role in how we perceive our environment and in the aesthetic and emotional pleasure we derive from it. Cases of anosmia—the total or partial loss of sense of smell—are fortunately fairly rare and mainly occur as a result of shock or illness. For people deprived of other senses, the sense of smell remains a vital means of perception. For Helen Keller, the blind, deaf-mute American girl, her sense of smell was a source of enrichment and pleasure which enabled her to transport herself into the past, to distant places, or, more practically, to find her way around. As she explained in her autobiography, *Midstream, My Later Life*: "I normally know what part of the city I am in by the odors. There are as many smells as there are philosophies . . . I find it quite natural to think of places by their characteristic smells."

LOVE POTIONS

According to Jean-Jacques Rousseau, "The soft fragrance of a boudoir is not as weak a trap as one might think, and I do not know if one should pity or congratulate the wise or somewhat insensitive man who has never trembled at the flowers his mistress wears at her bosom." Since time immemorial, odors and perfumes have played a decisive role in the art of seduction. In his work entitled *L'Empreinte des sens*, the biologist Jacques Ninio relates that in the past it was common practice for people to "sniff another person's hand or face" in order to know who they were dealing with! The odor of another person can become an intoxicating perfume. Alexander the Great smelled naturally of musk, which consequently made him very popular with women, while the powerful odors that Rasputin apparently exuded were said to be the reason for his magnetism and irresistible charm.

Flowers conceal considerable attractions behind their chaste appearance. Popular wisdom was well aware of this when it advised young girls not to walk in the tuberose fields after dark. The Romans passionately exploited the voluptuous fragrance of roses. During the course of a banquet, Nero drowned his guests in an odorous sea of fragrant petals. The iris was one of the favorite scents of the Renaissance period: gloves, clothes, fans, hair powders and sometimes the whole body were

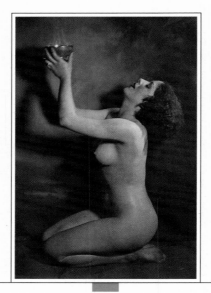

Perfume modifies a person's most intimate being, lending them, for an instant, a certain grace and passion which seems to come from deep within (photograph by Josep Masana, above). But perfume is also capable of weaving tender, lasting relationships between people; it is the messenger of love, a throbbing heart, a passionate and fervent soul which floats and lingers from skin to skin and imparts a magnetic power to every thought and gesture (opposite).

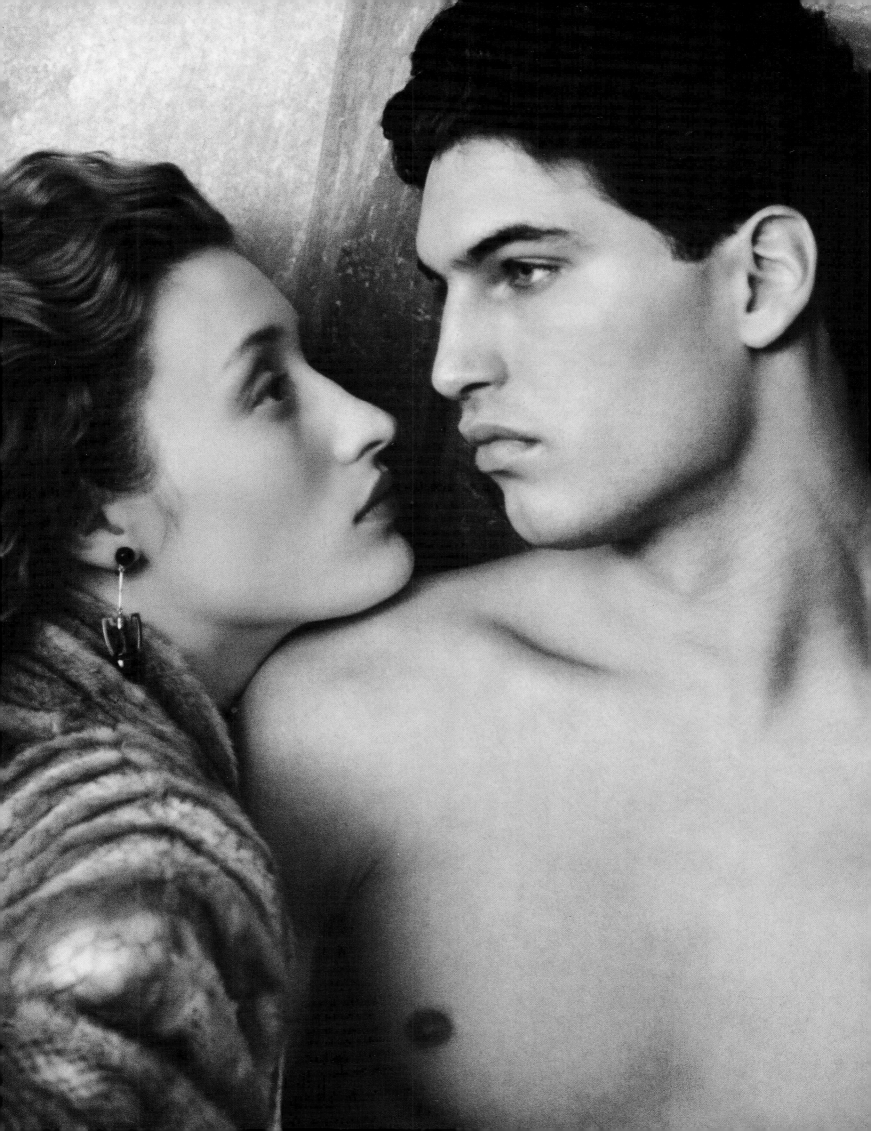

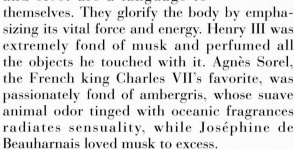

saturated with a powdery iris-scented perfume originating from Florence, which no doubt owed its success to the fact that it evoked the smell of fresh, smooth skin. During the seventeenth century, perfumes became highly fashionable. Every inch of the body, every article of clothing, every room in the house was perfumed with different fragrances. In the eighteenth century, love boudoirs were adorned with the most delicate flowers and suggestive perfumes. In *Félicia ou mes fredaines*, the poet Guillaume Apollinaire describes a labyrinth dedicated to Eros, planted with orange flowers, jasmine and honeysuckle, a discreet and odorous tribute to the sensual gardens of the Italian Renaissance. As for the velvety, herbaceous smell of the violet, it aroused such extreme passions in the women of the last century that the more

extravagant among them actually gave themselves subcutaneous injections of the essence.

Whereas flowers exalt feminine beauty by highlighting its delicacy, lightness and sweetness, the powerful animal essences such as musk, amber and civet are a language to themselves. They glorify the body by emphasizing its vital force and energy. Henry III was extremely fond of musk and perfumed all the objects he touched with it. Agnès Sorel, the French king Charles VII's favorite, was passionately fond of ambergris, whose suave animal odor tinged with oceanic fragrances radiates sensuality, while Joséphine de Beauharnais loved musk to excess.

Perfumes, whether tender or powerful, rapidly became a part of the paraphernalia of seduction. Balms, with enveloping sweet fragrances such as incense, myrrh and benzoin, transformed bodies into living censers. Cleopatra welcomed Mark Antony enveloped in clouds of incense. The Old Testament tells how Esther bathed in myrrh for six months before conquering the heart of Ahasuerus, king of Ancient Persia. But perfume can also be used as a weapon. At the request of Catherine de' Medici, René Le Florentin concocted such violent perfumes for her female rivals' gloves that they are said to have been deadly.

Perfumers are the modern-day wizards and alchemists. Formulas have changed: musk and amber, for example, those wonderful but excessively costly natural essences, are practically never used now. Perfume houses like Guerlain, which still uses ambergris

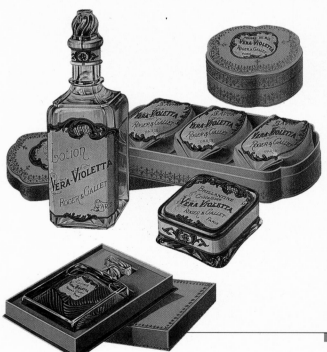

The same captivating, evocative scent of flowers, landscapes or moods can be captured not only in the sophistication of perfume, but also in more modest perfumed objects, such as powders and delicate, charming soaps (top and above).

(which radiates from their perfume Mitsouko), are rare nowadays. Modern musks can be found in Jovan's appropriately named Musk and in Lancôme's fragrant Trésor, where they are blended with a peach note. Reconstituted ambers vibrate in Tan Guidicelli's L'Ambre and Shiseido's L'Ambre Sultan and synthetic floral notes exude from the majority of perfumes.

Despite this move away from animal notes, perfumes have certainly not become any more restrained. They are more ardent and subtle than ever before and composed of bouquets which combine the delicate amplitude, richness and radiance of natural notes with the drive, audacity and immodesty of synthetic notes. Estée Lauder's Youth Dew, the perfume which defines itself as "The sexiest perfume in the world," arouses delicious sensations, intermingling sweetness and wild tenderness which intoxicate and liberate the senses.

"The love of pleasure is man's eldest-born," wrote the English poet Edward Young. Today, perfumes invite us to follow them to the borderline between the conscious and the subconscious. They are a far cry from those magnanimous elixirs, those aphrodisiac potions composed of mandrake or marjoram, perfumes which are too strong and irritate the senses. Nevertheless, the search for euphoric products, those molecules of pleasure, continues as ardently as ever, and when, in 1965, researchers discovered a new molecule which they called pheromone, it was seized upon as the miracle ingredient which would be able to transform the weakest of attractions into passionate love. The function of this molecule is to regulate the sexual and social relations of the insect in which it was first discovered. It did not take long for people to imagine that if introduced into human beings, it might make them irresistibly attractive by emitting forceful subliminal messages. The scientific community examined the question. Would we be

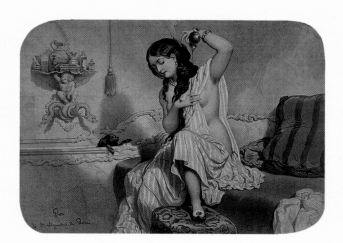

The author Italo Calvino exalted the mysteries of the perfumed aura: "For every woman there exists a perfume ideally matched to the perfume of her body, a note which gives color, taste, odor, gentleness, thus the pleasure of passing from one woman's body to another can never reach an end." Perfume is the art of creating harmonies, as evoked by this picture of a woman preparing to take a bath (above).

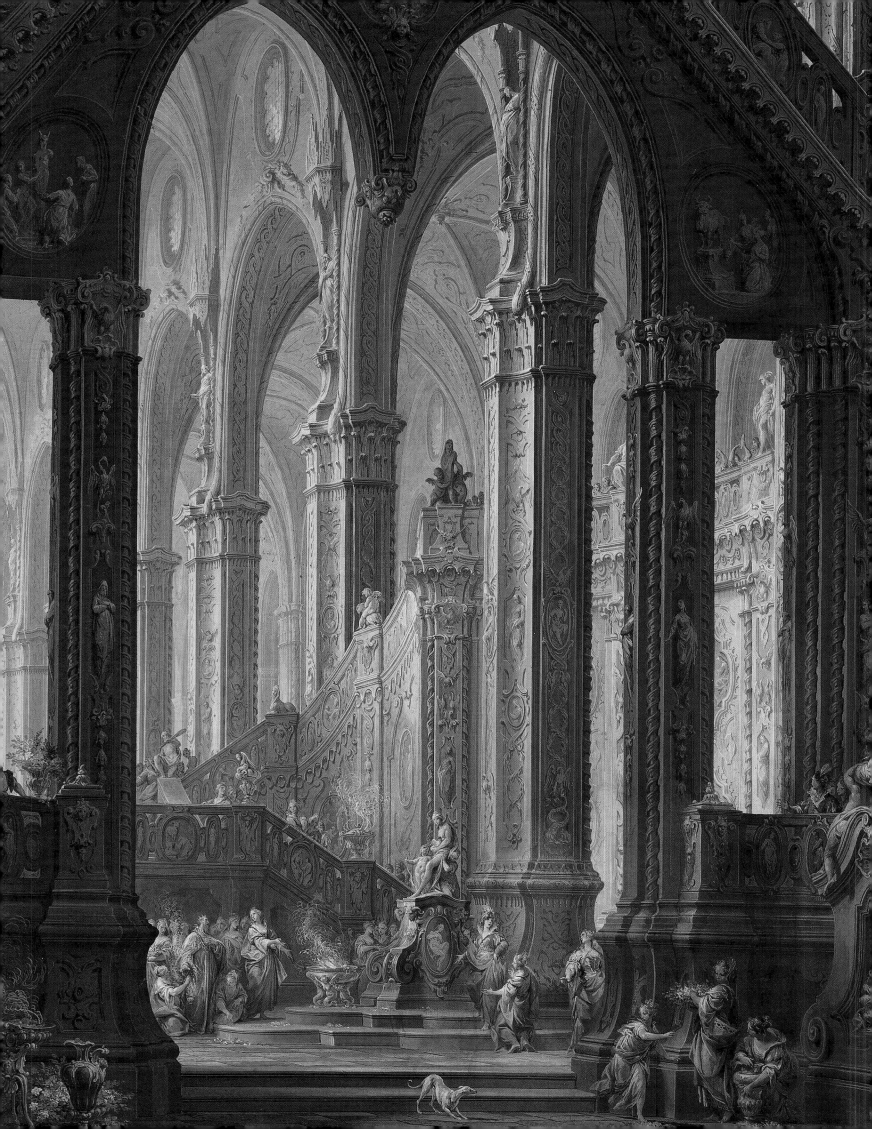

able to resist such impulses? With no proof to the contrary, several perfumers monopolized the "magic" properties of pheromones. These mysterious molecules caught the public imagination and became the source of much speculation. It was a return to the secretive and sulphurous atmosphere which surrounded the commonest of aphrodisiacs. In 1980, an American, Marilyn Miglin, created a perfume called Pheromone; the name speaks for itself. That the perfume smells nice comes as no surprise, as pheromones have no odor. From then on, a series of perfumes with evocative names followed each other in rapid succession, all of which expressed this idea of uncontrollable, devastating impulses born from the discovery of pheromones: there is Volcan d'Amour by Diane Von Furstenberg, Obsession by Calvin Klein, Animale by Suzanne de Lyon, Désirade by Aubusson, a perfume which is advertised as "The essence of desire," Hot by Bill Blass and finally Estée Lauder's latest perfume, Spellbound, all proof that passion sometimes prevails over impulse . . .

PERFUMED OFFERINGS

The ecstasy of love is not very far removed from religious ardor and the fragrant wreaths of smoke in sacred rituals often help us to bridge the gap between the two. Since the Dark Ages, places of worship have been infused with fragrances from odorous woods, balms and various essences intended to call upon the favor of the gods with their subtle fragrances. Cypress and cedarwood were burned in the temples of Mesopotamia, while the smell of incense and rancid butter hangs in Tibetan monasteries. In India, the air in sacred places is thick with the scent of the sandalwood from which the holy statues are carved, and the lotus flower unfolds its fragrant petals at Buddha's feet. Rose and musk essences are enshrined in the heart of mosques, while aromatic, peppery basil haunts Orthodox places of worship. Incense, whose purpose, according to Michel de Montaigne, was "To delight, arouse and purify the senses in order to make us

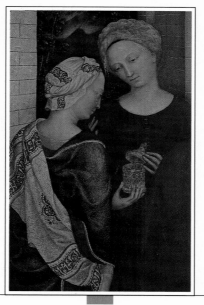

From time immemorial perfumes have been used to honor the gods. As Honoré de Balzac wrote, "What do we give to God? Perfumes, light and songs, the most refined expressions of our nature." Fragrances in the form of balms and odorous resins can be distinguished in this detail of *The Adoration of the Magi*, by Gentile da Fabriano (above). Sometimes perfume takes on a more carnal, profane form, like these petals scattered on sacred ground in *Solomon Burns Incense to the Idols*, by the artist V. Bigari (opposite).

more fit for contemplation," clouds the naves of cathedrals.

The lily and the rose, both sacred flowers, adorn altars dedicated to the Virgin Mary. The pure bodies of saints, having renounced earthly pleasures, join the mystic, floral procession, exhaling the pure and spiritual odors of sanctity. The odor of sanctity is not simply a figure of rhetoric: to combat the noxious emanations of the devil, the bodies of saints are transformed into divine censers. Saint Catherine of Ricci smells of violets, Saint Rose of Viterbus of roses and Saint Lydwine of Schiedam and Saint Thomas Aquinas of incense. Odors reflect the most intimate changes in our being and it is said that when a woman entered the confessional the pious priest of Ars knew whether she maintained an "odor of chastity."

"The twenty-first century will be religious or will not be," declared André Malraux. What will perfumes be like? Will they transform us into odorous cloisters or celestial bouquets? It is possible that perfumes help to uplift our souls. As for the perfumers, they amuse themselves by treading the borderline between the sacred and the profane. Jean-Paul Guerlain paved the way for the third millenium when he made Samsara into a heavenly garden planted with sandalwood and jasmine, or, as the publicity says, "A few

drops of Samsara, a few drops of eternity." Sacred perfumes conjure up mysterious, somber rituals, burnished gold and powerful divinities. The Caron perfumers, who were interested in scented rituals, introduced essence of *hood*, a sacred Indian tree venerated by Muslims, into their perfume Yatagan. For Parfum Sacré, they created a bouquet of rose macerated in musks and spices, like a vibrant offering in the cool shade of a crypt.

"Sacred the fragrance that enrobes her flesh," wrote Charles Baudelaire. Transparency, purity and eternity are themes which haunt many perfumes today. Eau du Ciel by Annick Goutal is a delicate balm made from essence of hay and beeswax. Eternity by Calvin Klein has a virginal transparency with the merest suggestion of a rose fragrance. Shiseido's Féminité du Bois, radiating dry, sparkling cedarwood, invokes an atmosphere of calm and serenity. Wandering along the frontiers of paradise lost, one dreams that its doors will be opened by Cacharel's Eden, whose fragrance conjures up a garden where the sacred lotus flower blooms.

On the path towards these odorous Elysian Fields, we may not gain in sanctity, but at least our appeased souls will imagine that they are finally acceding to the center of the mystic rose celebrated by Dante.

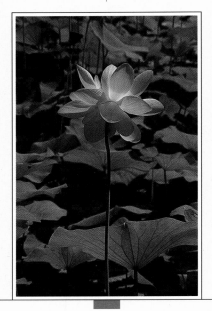

Flowers, by the beauty and perfection of their form and the softness of their scent, have been the privileged mediators between heaven and earth since time immemorial. In the Christian world, the rose, for example, symbolizes the Virgin Mary, the lily represents innocence and virginal purity, while in the Orient the perfume of the lotus flower (above), which for the early Egyptians evoked "a fragrance of divine life," is a symbol of universal harmony. This superb publicity document was created by the Rimmel perfumery (opposite).

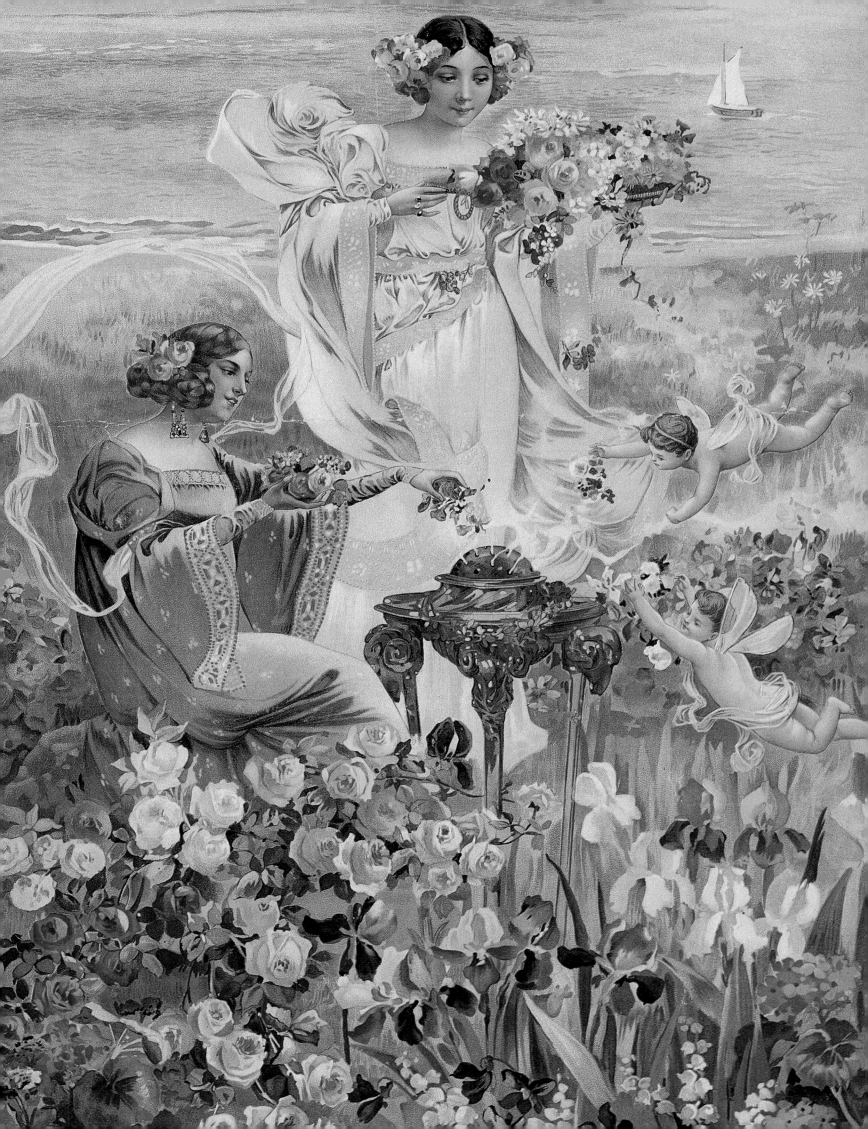

IN SEARCH OF WELL-BEING

"A sea fragrance arrives on the breath of the wind which salts the lips, refreshes the eyes and soothes the heart," wrote Jules Vallés in *L'Insurgé*. If fragrances excite the senses and elevate the soul, they also help us to find calm and serenity. Even in antiquity, Hippocrates, Aristotle and Pliny the Elder emphasized the beneficial properties of plants. Carolus Linnaeus, the renowned Swedish botanist of the eighteenth century, classified plant odors according to the effects they produced on the human organism. They were either aromatic, fragrant, ambrosial, alliaceous, hircine (like a goat), putrid or nauseating. Even nowadays we are aware of the power of plants and perfumers take good care not to use certain substances such as the essence of rue, a plant with a dry and penetrating perfume known for its abortive properties.

Man had to confront many catastrophes on his path to modern civilization, not least of which was the plague, which decimated populations in their millions. Until the eighteenth century, aromas were considered the principal antidote to the plague. Strong perfumes with purifying powers were dispersed using various methods to combat the putrid fumes: braziers of odorous wood were placed at town gates and doctors cov-

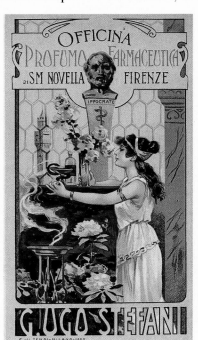

ered their heads with black masks adorned with long nose-pieces filled with cotton wool saturated with aromatic substances. Strong-scented materials were also used to fill the pomanders they hung from their clothing and the hollow knobs of their canes with which they whipped the air, as if in combat with the deadly vapors. But, as the perfumer Louis Peyron cautioned, "It is not sufficient to put up an odorous screen between oneself and the world, it is also advisable to consume light meats boiled and spiced with cloves, cinnamon, nutmeg, ginger, sorrel and vinegar." Failing this, the best method was to flee the city altogether. In 1348, with a great plague raging through Europe, Boccaccio took refuge in Fiesole, a small town in the hills outside Florence and it was there that he wrote his *Decameron*.

The research laboratories of the large raw material companies increasingly tend to favor fragrances associated with a sense of well-being and happiness. Experiments carried out in large firms have demonstrated the beneficial actions of certain odorous raw materials. Vaporizing mint or lemon, for example, significantly reduces stress and fatigue and increases staff productivity in offices and factories. Familiar smells give us a feeling of security, such as the soothing odor of a place we know well. In the absence of its mother, for

The celebrated Santa Maria Novella perfumery in Florence (above) has always invited women to exalt the senses. The delicate fragrances prepared from aromatic essences transport you to the beauty of the Tuscan countryside. In Morocco, the perfume ceremony is a purely feminine ritual, as illustrated in this picture by John Singer Sargent, *Smoke of Ambergris*, painted on a visit to Morocco around 1880, which portrays a woman perfuming her skin and clothes with delicate fragrances (opposite).

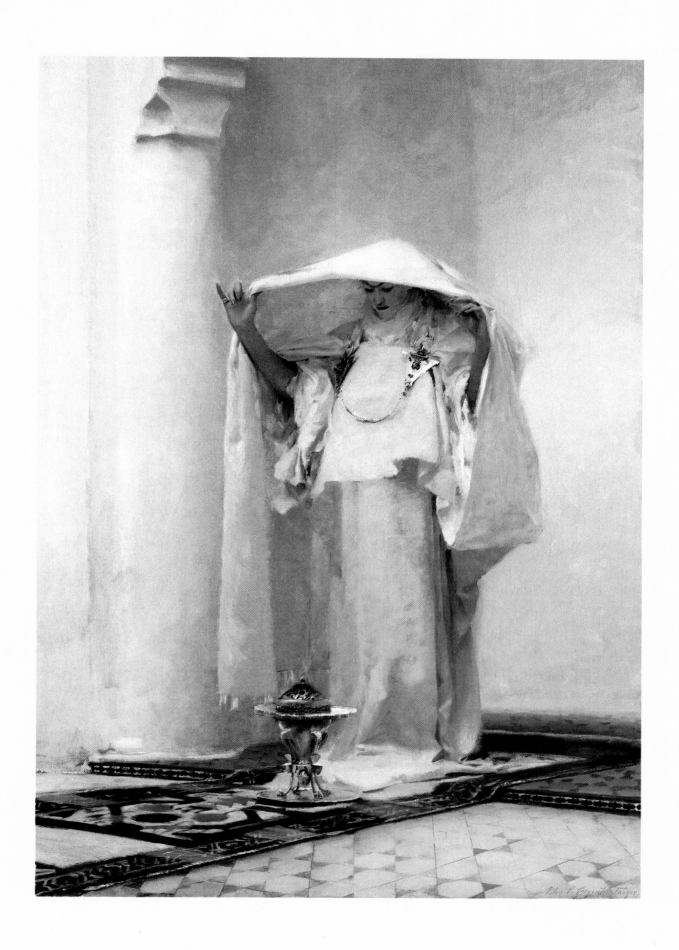

example, a child will go to sleep more easily if given a scarf or any other garment impregnated with her smell. The use of fragrances can have beneficial effects in places generally associated with anxiety, such as hospitals, subways, airports and planes . . . as good a way as any of making people more comfortable.

Aromatherapy has always been linked to perfumery. We have seen the success of *aqua mirabilis*, said to improve one's mental and physical condition. Basing her ideas on these empirical findings, Carol Phillips, the founder of the American cosmetics and perfumery company Clinique, created Aromatics Elixir, "The perfume that goes far beyond," which announced a new generation of perfumes promising both seduction and well-being. The innovative aspect of Aromatics Elixir lay in its subtle combination of stimulating and soothing essences and in the fact that it claims to have a beneficial effect on one's mood.

It has been noticed that certain odors tend to make us more extrovert, while others on the contrary seem to make us shrink away. The perfumer Paul Jellinek has classified odors according to their effects. According to him, lavender is restful, patchouli and vetiver exciting, incense and tonka bean exalting, rose, violet, magnolia and cyclamen intoxicating, and jasmine, tuberose and lily of the valley stimulating. You only have to take a walk in Provence, for example, to observe the beneficial tranquilizing and fortifying effects of powerful aromatic odors.

The new perfumes promise us internal harmony and equilibrium. The 1980s made us understand that charm is not simply a question of outward appearance. It is a feeling of personal stability and well-being that makes one attractive. Wearing a perfume you like makes you feel more beautiful, more in harmony with life and more sure of yourself.

Needless to say, the traditional codes of seduction have not disappeared. Languid looks, provocative poses, luxurious materials and shady alcoves still are, and always will be, the expression of a certain femininity. But whereas the 1970s brought us perfumes for active women, like Revlon's famous Charlie—lively, not too heady perfumes, which could be worn from morning to night—the 1990s offer us healthy, invigorating perfumes, perfumes of a new age based on creating or accentuating our sense of harmony with the world around us.

Following the paths of memory, perfumers reconstruct pleasant olfactory landscapes. New West for Her by Aramis conjures up the vitality of a Californian lifestyle, with oceanic notes evoking fresh air and the body and health cult practiced in that part of the world. The outdoor style also animates Escape by Calvin Klein, which, after Obsession, the name of his first perfume, offers an airy, light fragrance in keeping with a new state of mind.

These evocative perfumes bring us eternal images of happiness, like the beaches of our childhood and their dunes dotted with spicy-scented everlasting flowers. The sea breeze heated by the sun comes to life in Annick Goutal's perfume, Sables. Distant shores, skin salty from the sea, torrid heat and the light rustle of the palm trees casting their shade on the white sand rise up from Montana's Parfum d'Elle. The windswept Atlantic coast and

Perfumes are, first and foremost, an invitation to happiness, whether it be from the pharmacopoeial angle, as suggested by this vignette of the Parfumerie de la Société Hygiénique (left), which presents perfumes and odors as a healthy and salutary condition of well-being, or by suggestion and imagination, as expressed in this photograph entitled *Towards Happiness*, taken by a representative of European pictorialism, Robert Demachy (opposite).

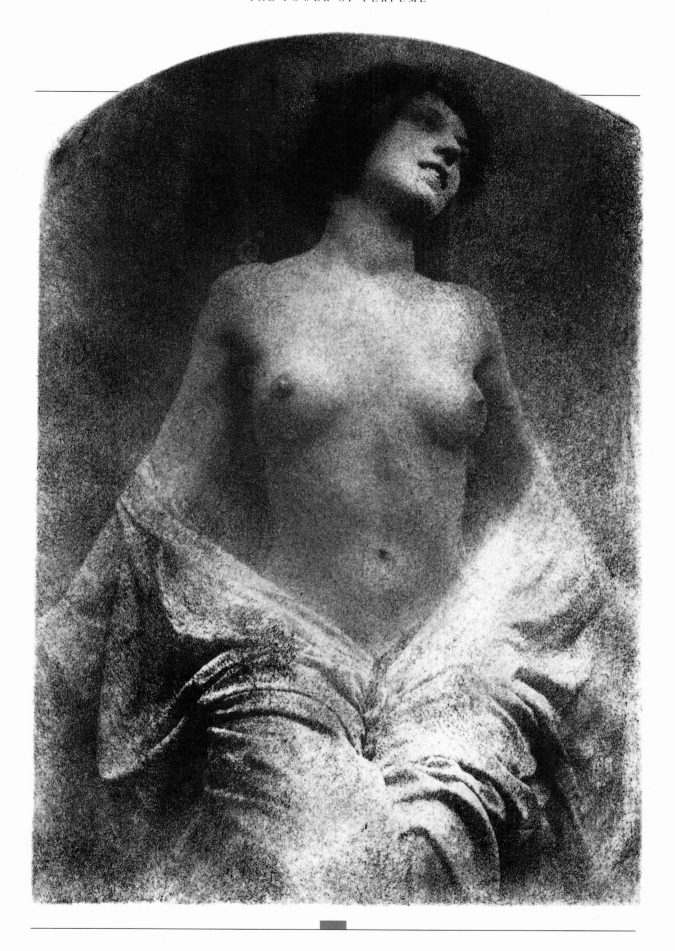

shores, caressed by a salty spray, echo in the strong oceanic notes of Kenzo Pour Homme, while tender impressions of June mornings, honey, languid flowers and the soft sun on one's skin vibrate gently in Kenzo's Parfum d'Eté, distilling fresh, floral sensations, enthusiasm and a sense of well-being in one's heart.

PERFUME AS A WORK OF ART

For Andy Warhol, capturing fragrances in bottles was a way of controlling his experience of life, a process which allowed him to smell the fragrance he wanted when he wanted, evoking memories to suit his mood. In this way he transformed perfume into an aesthetic experience, just like the aesthetes of the late nineteenth century, who considered perfume the ultimate stimulant of the senses. Des Esseintes, the hero of Joris Karl Huysmans' novel *À Rebours*, is the most accomplished of the olfactory dandies. Excessively nervous and weakened by life, Des Esseintes learns every-

thing there is to know about the mysterious art of perfume. To break the melancholia assailing him, he creates bouquets of scents which he sprays in his room, creating imaginary odorous landscapes: ". . . there rose piles of hay, bringing a new season with them, spreading summer about them in these delicate emanations." Another dandy, Oscar Wilde's hero Dorian Gray, took an interest in the effects of perfumes on the soul: "He saw that there was no mood of the mind that had not its counterpart in the sensuous life, and set himself to discover their true relation, wondering what there was in frankincense that made one mystical, and in ambergris that stirred one's passions, and in violets that woke the memory of dead romances, and in musk that troubled the brain and in champak that stained the imagination."

We have all played with the evocative power of odors. At one time or another, everyone has brought back from a journey a bunch of everlasting flowers, a sea shell, or a few sachets of spices which compose little odorous

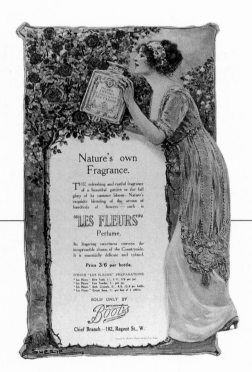

pictures. As a child, the writer Pierre Loti used to bring back from his much-loved family home, La Limoise, "an odor of wild and common thyme, sheepskin and some indefinable aroma which was particular to that corner of the land," which he used to like to inhale in expectation of the next vacation.

Odors, by recreating a familiar and reassuring universe, facilitate thought and inspiration, something writers know well. According to the critic Edouard Maynial, "Gustave Flaubert liked to work in a quiet, closed room which retained a familiar odor and where the perfume of amber rosaries and oriental tobacco lingered among the exotic idols," whereas Guy de Maupassant appreciated fragrances "For the mysterious shock they communicate to the imagination and for all their enriching secondary sensations."

Whereas the home is the privileged place for expressing the most intimate emotions, gardens and nature offer us the inexhaustible effusion of the world's energy. Odors invigorate the spirit and exalt the senses. Francis Bacon, the English Renaissance philosopher, advised carpeting garden paths with burnet, wild thyme and water mint to benefit from their fragrance when taking a walk. The scent of plants arouses special emotions, it awakens undying emotions in us, linked with our youth or with springtime. This is how Jean-Jacques Rousseau describes Julie's garden in *La Nouvelle Héloïse*: "The densely planted, closely cut, verdant lawn was interspersed with wild and common thyme, balsam, marjoram and other aromatic herbs." The combination of taste with the other senses creates a sensation of real symbiosis: "My senses are all fused/ by

subtle transformation," wrote Baudelaire. Great chefs have mastered the art of guiding us to unique moments of savory pleasure, experienced quite differently by every diner. The dishes they compose are perfumed landscapes, like the *garrigue* with its densely growing aromatic herbs, forest floors with odorous mushrooms, hillside paths in Provence lined with wild thyme and savory, mountain pastures with invigorating herbs, or the Orient with its mysteries and spices. Flowers accompany these odorous feasts with their familiar scents, such as smooth, peppery nasturtiums, delicate, tender pansies and begonia flowers with their crisp green leaves.

Perfumes are also a source of inspiration for artists. Marcel Duchamp created the imaginary perfume label *L'Eau de Voilette, Belle Haleine* (literally, "little veil water, beautiful breath"), a play on words evoking *eau de toilette, eau de violette* (violet water), and *belle Hélène* (beautiful Helen); the painter Titus-Carmel added fragrances from damp woods to his work *Forêt vierge, Amazone*, in order to emphasize the decomposing vegetation. Arte Povera artists, like the Italian Giuseppe Penone, incorporate various odorous materials into their work, such as sacks of grain and coffee beans. Pier Paolo Calzolari, for example, diffuses the aroma of coffee in his installations and works with dried and fresh moss. The American artists Kate Ericson and Eric Ziegler asked a perfumer to create a perfume reminiscent of the odor which pervades the Archives Nationales in Paris. The result was a work entitled *Êtes-vous servi?*, comprising a silver tray containing a perfume spray bottle and blotter strips in the form of bookmarks.

For the Belgian author Maurice Maeterlinck, "It is quite possible that this sense, the only one directed towards the future, immediately perceives the most striking manifestations of a form, captures the happy and salutary state of matter which holds many surprises in store." It is this almost divinatory intuition, source of happiness and exaltation, which this advertisement—created by Boots, the English chemists, for the perfume Les Fleurs—seeks to express (opposite).

Catherine Willis, a sculptor and something of a magician, creates mysterious relations between people, odorous plants and the world. "Our senses are complementary," she maintains. "It is therefore necessary to reintegrate odors into our perception." She has traced circles of mint in the heart of forests, planted clumps of fragrant sun-drenched lavender in the snow and caused salty sea vapors to rise up from the middle of a quiet river in the French countryside. She also pays odorous tributes to literature and has created several precious perfumes in limited editions, such as Le Parfum du Baron Perché, dedicated to Italo Calvino, Le Parfum du Sourire du Chat, dedicated to Lewis Carroll, and Le Vétyver de Dan Yack, in honor of Blaise Cendrars.

As far as images and, more particularly, the cinema are concerned, sometimes all that is missing to make the show complete are odors. Jacqueline Blanc-Mouchet, an archeologist by training, is fascinated by odors and in 1984 created the Odorama under the auspices of the Museum of Science and Technology at La Villette in Paris. This ingenious apparatus provides the corresponding odors to famous film sequences. A series of scenes from Volker Schlöndorff's film *Swann's Way*, for example, are accompanied by odorous atmospheres. Depending on the close-ups selected by the spectator, they can inhale the perfume of a cattleya, the orchid that Odette used to wear, or that of her lipstick, or the fresh smell of her clean, white linen. Jacqueline Blanc-Mouchet also organizes exhibitions of wood, wine, chocolate and, of course, perfume, in order to remind her public of this indispensable source of emotion, without which all substances would be lifeless.

Show business also takes an interest in perfume. Just as certain odors are inseparable from the circus—the thrilling reminder of the presence of live animals in the ring—it can be enriching to associate certain shows with a particular odor. The aromatician Michael Moisseeff, for example, composed a mysterious and, needless to say, sulphurous perfume to accompany a magic show.

Some populations have elevated odors to works of art, as is the case of the Japanese. The incense ceremony, known as *koh-do*, obeys rituals which are as complex as other traditional ceremonies, such as the art of tea or the art of the bouquet, known as *ikebana*. This game of *koh-do*, referred to as early as the eleventh century in the *Sayings of the Genji* by Murasaki Shikibu, was very popular at the imperial court and has recently made a comeback with modern-day aesthetes. It is closely linked to literature and consists of associating sequences from a poem with a bouquet of perfumed incenses.

The art of perfume is, above all, a pleasure. It is a pleasure which arouses subtle emotions and associations woven into the world by perfume. An attraction to a perfume is never neutral but rather expresses our deepest aspirations. To chose a perfume is to talk about oneself in veiled terms, but it is also to reveal one's true character, for, as Jean-Paul Guerlain charmingly put it, "What is left of a woman at night if it isn't her perfume?"

Charmingly decorated perfumed fans were used in the past as a refined form of publicity for newly created perfumes, like this one, inspired by the Ballets Russes, for L.T. Piver's perfume Gerbera (opposite, bottom). This astonishing image of a woman transformed into a powder puff, known as the "Powder Puff Number," appeared in a 1925 Hollywood-style commercial for Guerlain's Extase and L'Heure Bleue (opposite, top).

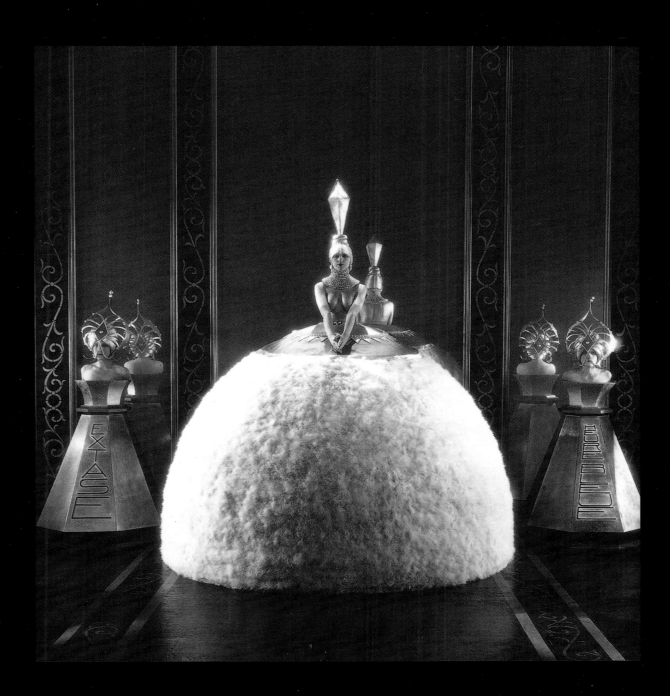

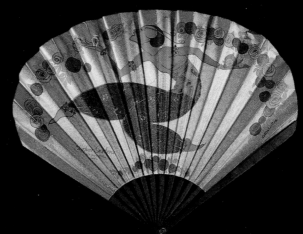

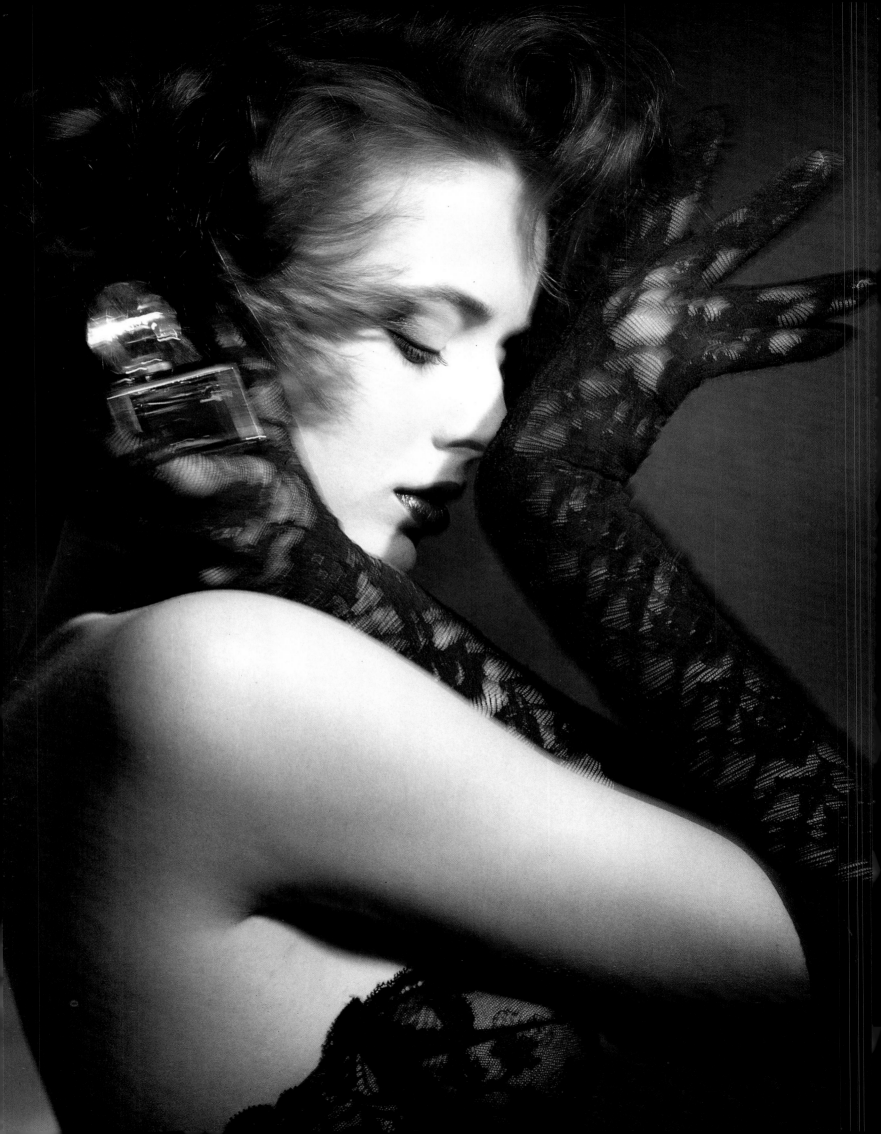

A
FRAGRANCE
OF
ONE'S OWN

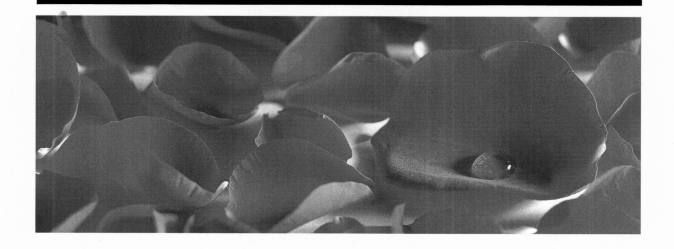

erfume is the most intimate, the most magical of all our finery. In the designer Sonia Rykiel's words, it is "Like a melting, merging extension of oneself, something one leaves behind, something strange which makes people turn round, once to look and then a second time to question what it is they have seen." What could be more wonderful than to feel oneself enveloped, exalted and transformed by a fragrance of one's own? Nowadays a multitude of beautiful perfumes exist. Recognizing their different accords and knowing exactly when and how to wear them are the first steps to finding the fragrance which is best suited to your needs.

Everyone has dreamed of possessing their own exclusive perfume, a perfume which follows their every mood, a perfect fragrance which makes them quite unique. This is what Grenouille, the hero of Patrick Süskind's *Perfume*, dreams of: "Yes, that was what he wanted—and they would love him as they stood under the spell of his scent, not just accept him as one of them, but love him to the point of insanity, of self-abandonment, they would quiver with delight, scream, weep for bliss, they would sink to their knees just as if under God's cold incense, merely to be able to smell *him*, Grenouille!"

For some people this dream becomes reality in the form of an exclusive "signature fragrance," custom-made especially for them. At the end of this century, where standardization is the rule and the rich variety of life is threatened by a leveling of tastes and desires, wearing a perfume designed exclusively for you is a way of creating a poetic, emotional refuge all of your own, of creating a world in which you resemble no-one but yourself. This haute couture version of perfumery remains a luxury, however, which only the happy few can afford—those who are willing to pay up to twenty thousand dollars in order to own a perfume to which they have exclusive rights.

The perfumer Nicolas Mamounas worked for various prestigious names, and in particular for Rochas, before trying his hand at the art of composing custom-made perfumes, an art which requires patience, an understanding of psychology and a keen sense of observation. "The slightest detail," he affirms, "can reveal a great deal about someone's personality. Décor is very important and a room's furniture, pictures and color scheme compose an intimate landscape to which the custom-made perfume is the sensual counterpart. I am very proud of the fragrance I created for a friend who, as the result of an accident, had became anosmic, that is to say, incapable of distinguishing the slightest odor, not even that of her own skin. To overcome this terrible handicap, she asked me to compose a perfume just for her, a perfume that expressed her whole self." Perfumers who are willing to spend hours in their laboratory making tests for a perfume which will always remain private are few and far between. "It is both a personal and financial investment which cannot be measured in terms of profitability," explains Patricia

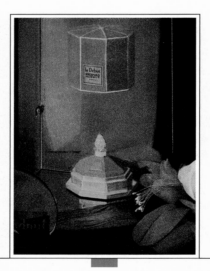

As suggested by this fashion photograph featured in a 1930s edition of *Harper's Bazaar* (opposite), perfume exacerbates the narcissistic trait which exists in all of us. "Perfume betrays our self-image while odor translates what we really are. It is the age-old question of being and appearing to be," affirms the philosopher Michel Onfray. The precious box, here that of Richard Hudnt's Le Début, adds to the seductiveness of the flacon. The ardent haze of an evening fragrance, a moving aria of dewy petals, a perfume wells up and captivates us (previous pages).

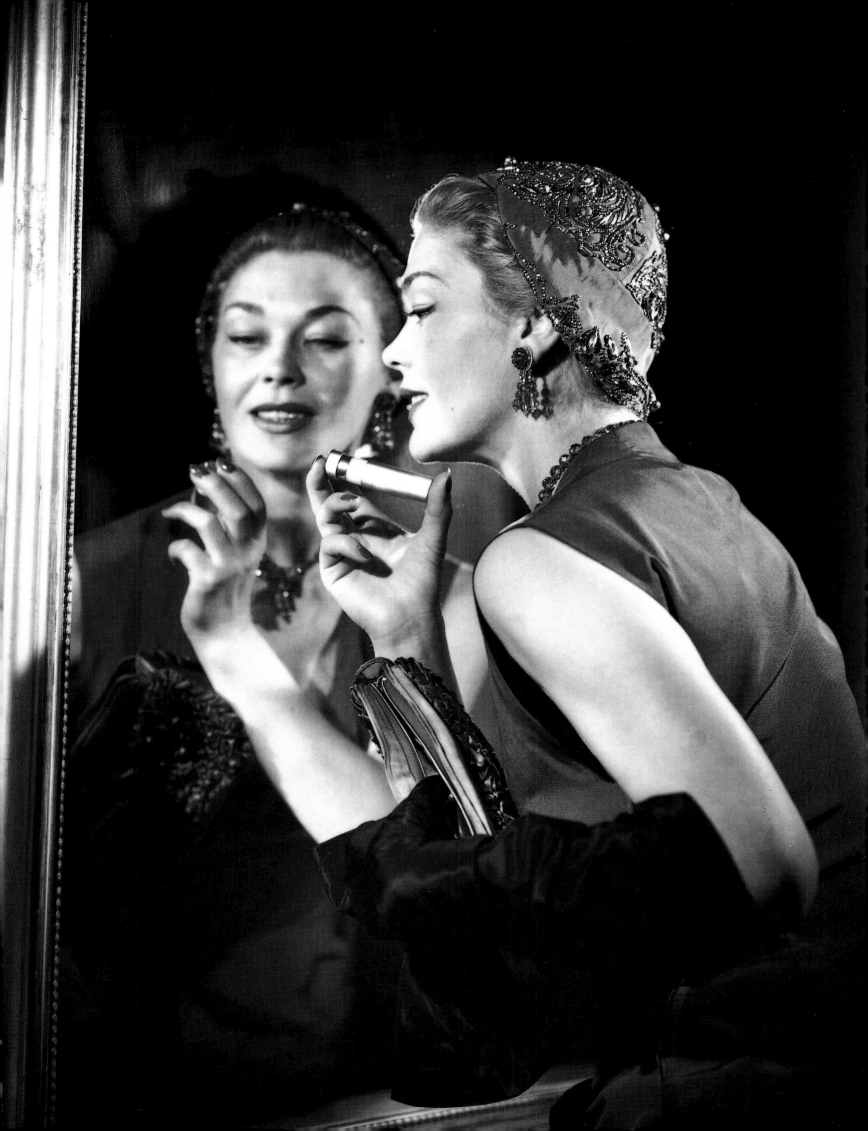

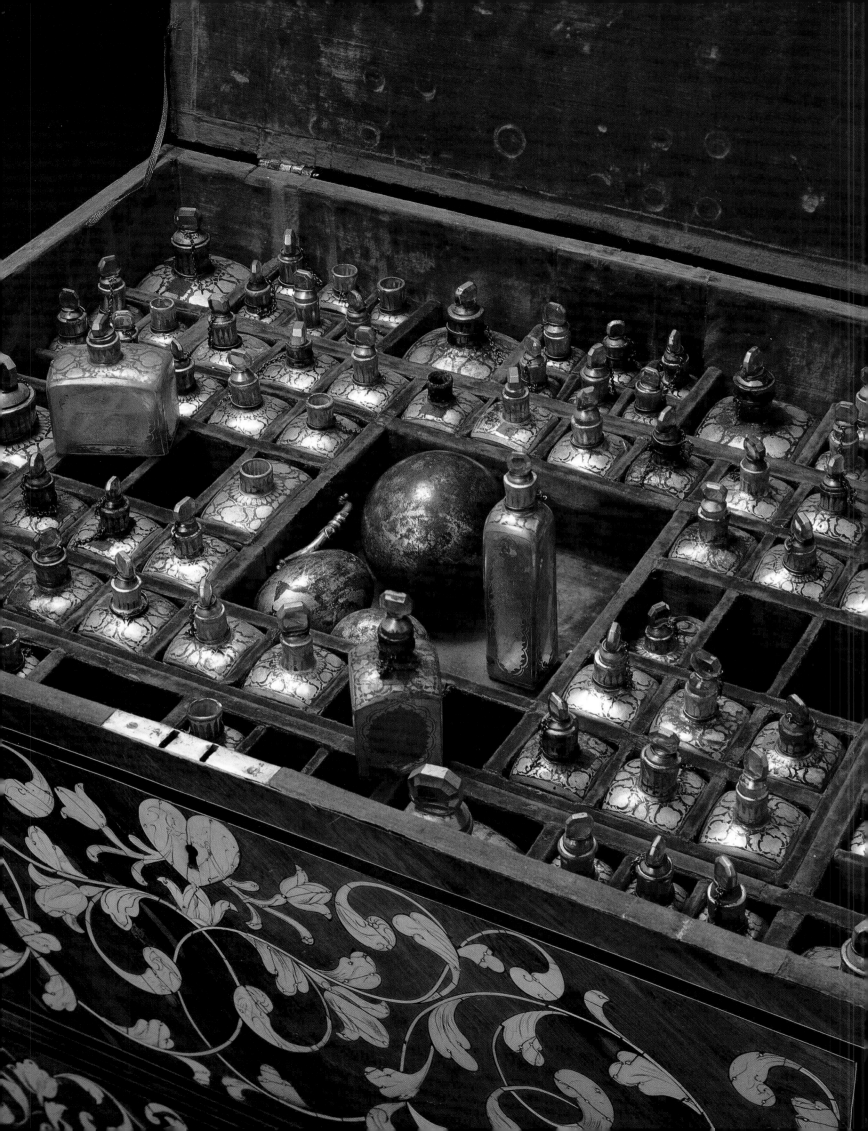

de Nicolaï, who launched a range of perfumery products under her own name in Paris. "The custom-made perfume represents a very small proportion of my turnover, but on the other hand it stimulates my creative capacities, especially when the client proposes an original idea which I am interested in developing." This enterprising young woman, a descendant of the Guerlain family and winner of the international award for the best perfumer in 1989, has some very demanding and eccentric clients, such as the fabulously rich Japanese woman who is known for her passion for roses. Patricia de Nicolaï created a rose-scented fragrance for her client, who promptly ordered three thousand bottles in Baccarat crystal to give as gifts to her friends!

Although creating custom-made perfumes remains an extremely marginal activity in the perfume industry, interest in the field is steadily growing. Perfumers are looking towards less costly ways of producing exclusive formulas—modifying the accords of existing perfumes to suit the taste of each client, for example. Creating

for this market, the perfume house Creed carries a selection of one thousand five hundred new, unused formulas to meet special orders. The most improbable requests can be satisfied, ranging from a perfume evoking the well-worn leather seats of an old Jaguar, to the fragrance given off by a forest floor after a rain shower (the particular favorite of a close friend of the Belgian royal family).

Lorenzo Villerosi's premises are situated in Via de' Bardi, in the Altrarno district in the heart of Florence, traditionally home to the city's craftsmen. This thirty-nine-year-old perfumer, a former doctor of philosophy, inherited a taste for flowers and a sense of style and elegance from his botanist father and his Hungarian grandmother. He only starts composing his custom-made perfumes after a fairly long interview with his clients, during which he tries to get to know their personality and understand exactly what it is they are looking for. "The majority of clients don't have much knowledge of raw materials. It is up to me to find out whether their dream per-

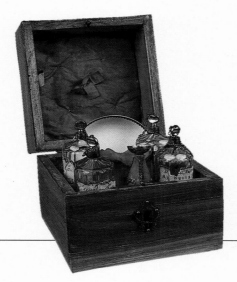

Concentrates of ambergris, musk and benzoin, tuberose, jasmine and citron, and essence of neroli and Turkish rose, are the fragrances which haunted the perfume boxes that accompanied ladies of the court on their travels. Only a few examples have survived to this day, like this marquetry casket dating from the time of the Marquise de Sévigné (above), or this superb eighteenth-century perfume cabinet in the Natural History Museum in Paris which contained 146 gilded glass perfume bottles (opposite).

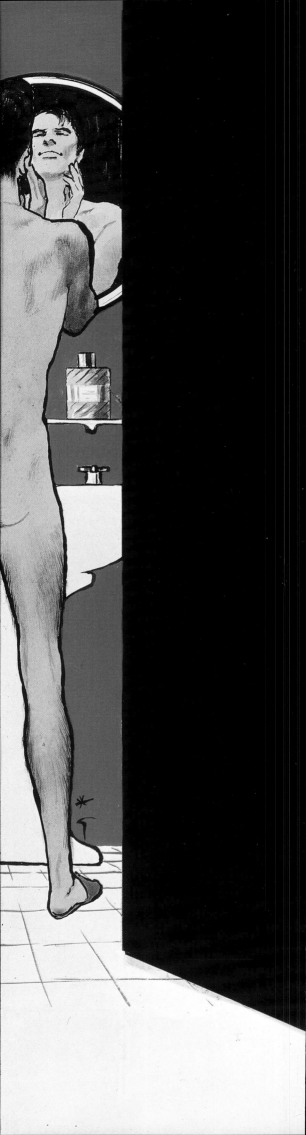

fume contains sandalwood or bergamot. Disappointing the people who make this sort of request is out of the question. It is essential that I satisfy their wishes, even the most bizarre, like those of a man who wanted a perfume for his mistress which evoked the odor of a horse after a race!" Lorenzo Villerosi is very proud of a perfume he composed for Jacqueline Kennedy, a citrus symphony with a spicy top note which, he feels, successfully matched the imperious character of his famous client.

CLASSIC FRAGRANCES FOR MEN

In the Song of Songs, Solomon's bride declares: "Your love is more delightful than wine; delicate is the fragrance of your perfume." Numerous literary works, such as *The Thousand and One Nights*, the memoirs of the Duke of Saint-Simon, a chronicler at the French court of Louis XIV, and the Shakespeare plays, which set the scene for civet-perfumed dandies, all testify to the occasionally immoderate use that, over the centuries, men, even the most virile among them, have made of perfume. We know of Nero's passion for roses and his banquets strewn with rose petals, and King David's habit of saturating his clothes with aloe and cassia (a kind of cinnamon). All that changed with Napoleon at the beginning of the nineteenth century. The emperor, who would only tolerate the invigorating fragrance of eau de Cologne, considered the more heady per-

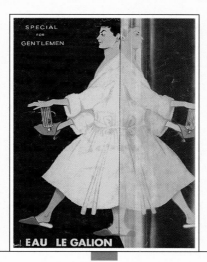

fumes to incite lust and indolence, characteristics which were detrimental to the energy of his troops. This marked the beginning of an odorously austere era which was to dominate men's perfumery until the end of the 1960s. Perfume habits were limited to a quick splash of toilet water after a shower or sport. And not just any toilet water. Only those with invigorating citrus top notes and woody base notes were considered fit for men. Flowers, musk and amber, all of which go into oriental fragrances, were definitely out. There was, of course, some resistance on the part of perfumers, for example Guerlain's Jicky, adopted by the aesthetes of *La Belle Époque* before women started wearing it. Caron's delightful vanilla-scented perfume Pour un Homme, Moustache by Rochas, with its mossy and citrus fragrances, and Vidal's Pino Silvestre, a classic of Italian perfumery, launched in 1945. In the United States, the warm notes of Old Spice by Shulton soon followed, while in Germany the musk notes of Tabac Original by Maurer & Wirtz was the big success of the 1950s. But it was not until Christian Dior produced Eau Sauvage that men finally had access to a toilet water which broke away from the heavy olfactory artillery of virility. Eau Sauvage was created in 1956 by Edmond Roudnitska, who not only dreamed of perfuming women with it, but even drew inspiration from the accords of another of his Dior creations, Diorissimo, a feminine perfume with a lily of the valley note. Eau Sauvage is a chypre blend which is treated with the same purifying rigor

Freshness is what men expect first and foremost from a toilet water, the indispensable accomplice for morning ablutions. This masculine ritual is depicted with humor in an advertisement for *L'Eau le Galion*, drawn by Maurel in the 1960s (above), and by René Gruau, who illustrated the sparkling sensuality of Christian Dior's Eau Sauvage in a cinematographic style (opposite).

as Diorissimo. It is both delicate and lasting and has daring floral notes which until then had been absent from men's toilet waters. As Roudnitska had hoped, as soon as Eau Sauvage appeared on the market it attracted as many female clients as male, thus starting the fashion for unisex toilet waters. In 1973, Paco Rabanne pour Homme became a new landmark, with its honeyed, animal notes, which added a sensuality hitherto absent from the masculine range. The magazine *Lui* participated in the campaign for its launch and for the last twenty years Paco Rabanne pour Homme has proudly led the men's fragrance market, despite the fact that rival products are far more numerous and varied now than when it started its career. In 1976, the American fashion designer Geoffrey Beene created a revolutionary cologne called Grey Flannel. A masculine perfume elegantly presented in a flannel-covered bottle, it has a strong violet smell, which some see as ambiguous and others as androgynous, but which is certainly resolutely individual. Its success encouraged other perfume creators, who finally began to explore new ground in the 1980s.

It is no longer possible to keep count of the articles and surveys devoted to the changes in men's "masculinity" over the past twenty-odd years. They all illustrate the extent to which men's attitudes towards perfume, and beauty products in general, have been transformed. More attention is paid to the body, virility is less codified and there is a visible sensuality, which is particularly reflected in advertising campaigns. There is the vital influence of men's fashions, which have become more colorful, varied and more seductive, all factors which explain the boom in men's perfumery which now represents

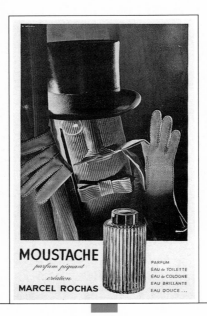

MOUSTACHE
parfum piquant
création
MARCEL ROCHAS

PARFUM
EAU de TOILETTE
EAU de COLOGNE
EAU BRILLANTE
EAU DOUCE...

From its publicity image, Caron's Pour un Homme would appear to be in the same category as Moustache, a woody fragrance launched by Marcel Rochas in 1949 (above), whereas in fact it leaves a far more intoxicating olfactory trail which associates lavender with sensual Bourbon vanilla, an accord which was considered the height of daring when the fragrance was first launched in 1934 (opposite).

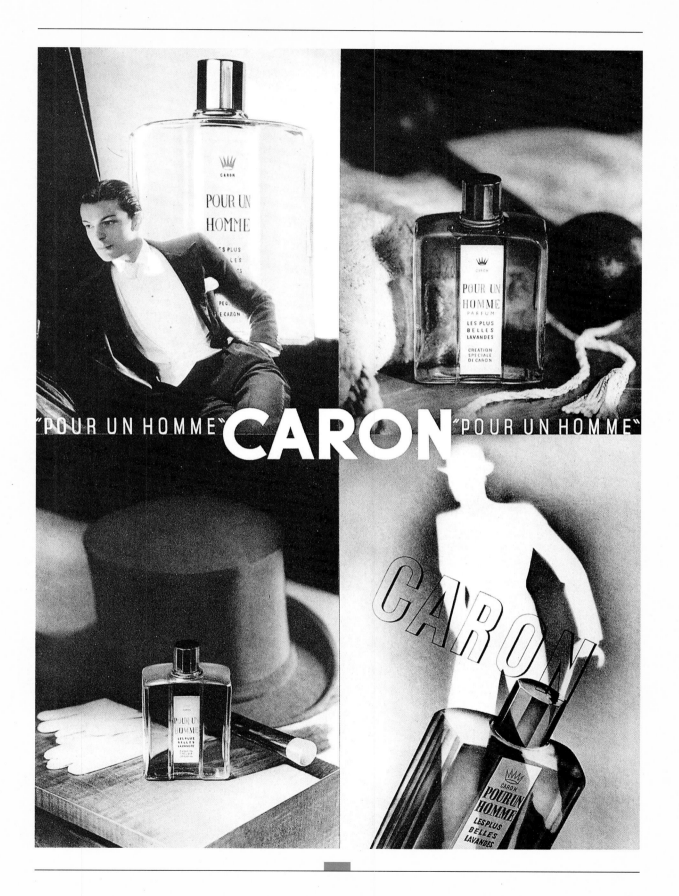

one third of the turnover of the various perfume companies and whose market share is constantly increasing. Perfumes for men have broadened their olfactory horizons: Davidoff's Cool Water with its fruity, flowery notes; the salty, refreshing notes of New West by Aramis and Kenzo pour Homme; a harmony of wood and amber in Obsession for Men by Calvin Klein and Paloma Picasso's Minotaure; or the resolutely vanilla note of Chanel's Egoïste. Nevertheless, the great classics are still favored by certain faithful clients.

PERFUMES FOR THE YOUNG

Whereas in many countries the birth of a child is an occasion for perfumed rituals (in Rumania the new-born baby is plunged into a bath perfumed with basil, mint, camomile and wild flowers, after which the bath water is emptied out at the foot of a rosebush, while in North Africa the midwife burns benzoin near the bed of the new mother to keep evil spirits away), the idea of perfuming babies is generally considered to be an aberration, even sacrilege. Babies are reputed to have a lovely smell, like a "pancake that's been soaked in milk," according to the wet nurse in Patrick Süskind's *Perfume*. Nevertheless, the idea slowly made headway and by 1950 Molinard had composed a perfume called Trois Bébés. But it was not until the 1980s that children's perfumery began to take off in certain children's boutiques, first provoking curiosity, then infatuation. The pioneering names—such as Le Petit Faune created by Monique Schlienger,

Eau de Bonpoint and Ptitsenbon, created by Catherine Painvin for Tartine et Chocolat in conjunction with the Givenchy perfume company—no longer have the monopoly on "junior perfumes." They now have to contend with other makes such as Shao-Ko ("little mouth" in Chinese), whose fragrances are cleverly presented in bottles representing Babar, Mickey Mouse, or Minnie Mouse which, when empty, find their way into the toy chest! According to Annick Goutal, children's perfumes possess all the characteristics of those for adults, with a few additional constraints. This self-made creator, an accomplished musician, first composed Eau de Bonpoint to accompany a range of children's clothes created by her sister, before putting her name to Eau de Camille and Eau de Charlotte. "A perfume for children," explains Annick Goutal, "must be as soft as a caress. It must respect the delicacy of young skin and pass a whole series of tests to guarantee its harmlessness. In order to avoid irritation, the alcohol content must be minimal, if not absent altogether. As to the fragrance, it should leave a perfumed veil which harmonizes with the child's natural odor. Eau de Bonpoint, with its accord of orange blossom and neroli top note, softened by rosewood and a trace of vanilla, was tested on all my friends' babies. Creating it was absolute bliss, because fragrances like these plunge you back into the innocence of childhood."

One country where women delight in children's perfumes is Japan. Japanese women shy away from heady western perfumes in favor of lighter, more modest fragrances. For this reason, exports to

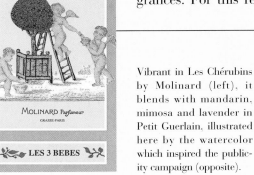

What could be more tender than a rose picked at dawn? This note is to be found in all children's fragrances, for its delicacy exalts the moving odor of a baby's skin in a natural and unobtrusive fashion.

Vibrant in Les Chérubins by Molinard (left), it blends with mandarin, mimosa and lavender in Petit Guerlain, illustrated here by the watercolor which inspired the publicity campaign (opposite).

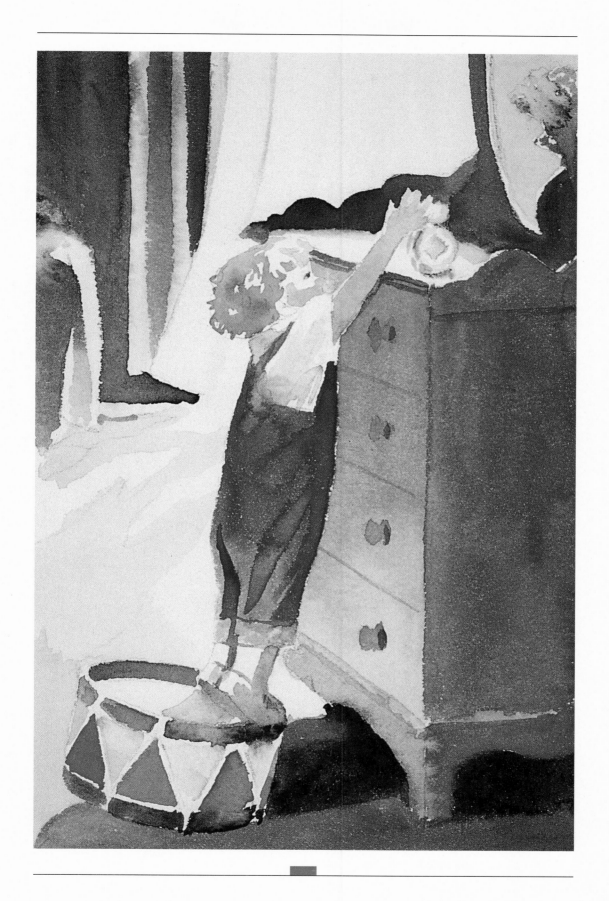

Japan account for almost half of Tartine et Chocolat's turnover!

As yet, children's perfumery only accounts for a small percentage of the profession's total activity. The fact, however, that magicians such as Jean-Paul Guerlain, the father of Petit Guerlain, Shalimar's deserving offspring, are setting their sights in the direction of the nursery, is a sure sign that this branch of perfumery can look forward to a rosy future.

DIFFERENT CHARACTERS, DIFFERENT PERFUMES

Why do we perfume ourselves, if not to express what neither clothes, nor words are able to do, in other words, that imperceptible element which belongs to the domain of the intellect? In Dominique Rolin's novel *La Voyageuse*, the author asks, "What is the deeper meaning of the simple yet magical expression 'to smell nice'? That intangible aura emanating from the skin embraces a hint of linen, a flashing image, a caress of silk and a musical rustle, in other words a direct and powerful link with the unsaid, the unperceived, the unimagined, the impossible and the intangible." Perfume is a garment which can envelop us, but which sometimes, without our knowing it, unmasks us. Psychologists have studied the links between characters and odors, and from their findings it appears that fresh, floral notes with immediate charm, such as Christian Dior's Diorissimo, appeal to extrovert, audacious personalities, whereas oriental, penetrating notes, like Estée Lauder's Cinnabar, suit less expansive women who prefer the mystery and intimacy of the tête-à-tête. The powdery notes which seem to shroud the body in a protective aura, like those of Jean-Charles Brosseau's Ombre Rose, are often chosen by emotional or narcissistic personalities, women who remain somewhat childish or those who are addicted to looking in the mirror. Floral-fruity notes, like those of Nina Ricci's Deçi-Delà, suit ambitious, optimistic personalities, while a powerful chypre trail, as found in Pour Monsieur by Chanel, attracts ambitious men fond of impos-

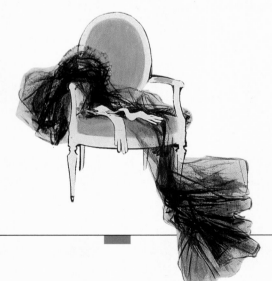

"She left a short while ago / and yet remains near me / with her perfume still / alive, still warm / from her body, so intoxicating . . ." As this fourteenth-century Chinese poem suggests, perfume is never as captivating as when it reminds us of the presence of a loved one, which is also the message transmitted by this publicity drawing, signed René Gruau, for Christian Dior's Diorama (above) and by this dreaming face portrayed by the fashion photographer Paolo Roversi for *Vogue* (opposite).

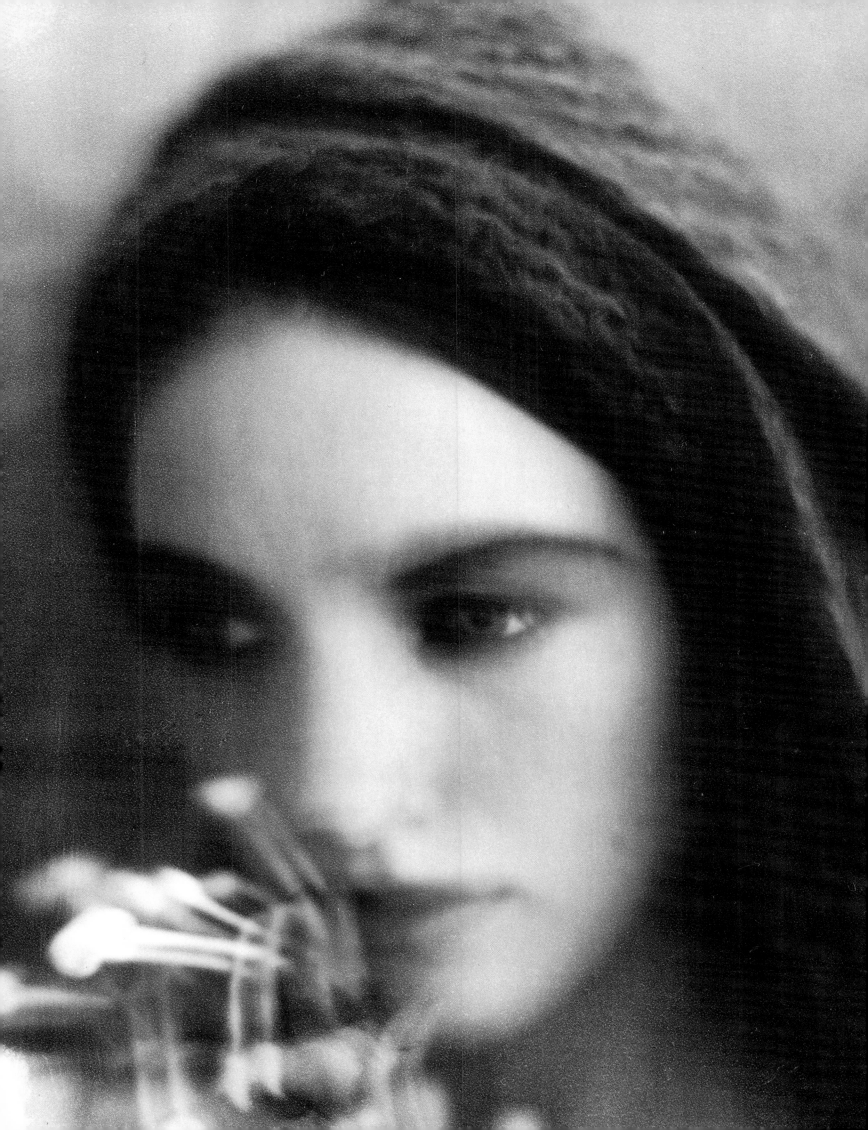

ing their point of view, and the balsam notes of Caron's Parfum Sacré find favor with more secretive personalities who like to venture off the beaten track. These comparisons and generalizations may appear cursory to some, but research in the psychology of odors is still very much in the embryonic stage.

Numerous other factors are liable to influence olfactory preferences, one of the most significant being diet. A study carried out by the perfumer Paul Johnson for the Robertet company showed that in Japan and Scandinavia, both great fish-eating nations, people generally find oriental notes, in which they detect an unpleasant smell of sweat, repellent. In America, by contrast, where meat consumption is at its highest, the same notes are extremely popular. Similarly, in Latin America, where the food is highly seasoned, people are attracted to spicy fragrances. Climatic factors are also influential; the higher the percentage of humidity in the air, for exam-

ple, the greater the receptivity to odors. The same perfume is not perceived in the same manner by a Chilean as by a German. Brazilian women, for example, are very keen on fougere perfumes, which in Europe are usually reserved for men's fragrances. Cultural influences are just as important. The Slavs are fond of the fragrance of the lily of the valley, which for them symbolizes the return of spring. In Muslim countries they have a preference for rose-water, used many centuries ago, by order of Saladin, to wash the walls of the Omar mosque, whereas they hate lavender because its camphor note reminds them of the burial rites practiced in their country. The idea a country or a culture has of a certain flower also influences perfume compositions. No French perfumer has yet dared to use the chrysanthemum, which can be seen in all French graveyards on All Saints' Day, whereas in Japan it is considered to be a symbol of power. For a long time, the intoxicating fragrance of the lily was excluded

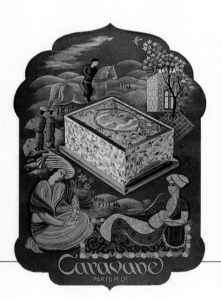

Like Milton, who in *Paradise Lost* evokes "Sabean odors from the spicy shore / Of Araby the blest," perfumers have constantly been inspired by the Orient, blending sandalwood, patchouli and musk to create opulent fragrances, members of the oriental blend family which includes Caravane, a fragrance by Bienaimé (above).

from perfume formulas, as it was considered that the flower's vocation was of a spiritual rather than a sensual order and that using it for hedonistic ends was an insult to the Virgin Mary, to whom the lily is dedicated.

CHOOSING A PERFUME

By stating that a woman who does not use perfume has no future, the poet Paul Valéry confirmed the stimulating and masterful virtues of perfume, which speaks for the timid, glorifies the temperamental and exalts the seductive. A perfume backed by a prestigious name can be reassuring, while a spirited one is stimulating: the choice of perfume is crucial. Before rushing out to buy a perfume, it is important to know that they are classified by families according to the essences they contain. The American Fragrance Foundation divides fragrances into nine basic groups (see The Connoisseur's Guide). The French classify them into seven families: *hespéridés* (citrus), *floraux* (floral), *fougères* (fougere), *chyprés* (chypre), *boisés* (woody), *ambrés* (amber/oriental) and *cuirs* (leather). Eau de Cologne is the most famous representative of the citrus family, composed of essential oils from lemon, bergamot and mandarin combined with orange tree components. The floral family is the largest group of all, comprising the single florals composed around one flower and the floral bouquets associating rose, jasmine,

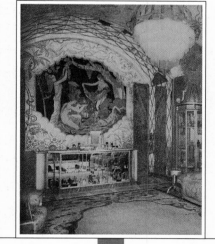

lily of the valley, tuberose, narcissus, etc. Also linked to this family are the blends known as floral-fruity, green floral, with its rustic accents, and the floral aldehydes such as Chanel N° 5. The fougere fragrances do not, in fact, evoke a fern odor, but contain accords of lavender, bergamot, coumarin and woody notes with an oakmoss base. Apart from Jicky by Guerlain, this family is mainly used in men's fragrances. Chypre, created in 1917 by the perfumer François Coty, gave rise to the chypre family, which are powerful perfumes based on accords of oakmoss. *Cistus labdanum*, bergamot and patchouli. Femme by Rochas and First by Van Cleef & Arpels come under this category. Men's fragrances are associated predominantly with the woody family, which combines opulent sandalwood and patchouli notes with the more sensitive cedarwood and vetiver, with a lavender-citrus top note. The amber family covers what are more commonly referred to as the "oriental" blends, which are suave, heady perfumes with predominant vanilla or animal notes such as musk. Yves Saint Laurent's Opium and Guerlain's Shalimar belong to this family. Finally, the leather family can easily be identified by its dry, somewhat smoky notes, similar to the smell of much-worn leather, which harmonize pleasantly with certain floral notes such as jasmine and rose. Tabac Blond by Caron and Bel Ami by Hermès both belong to this category.

A perfume should not be bought like a cake seen in a pastry shop window, even if it sometimes arouses similar

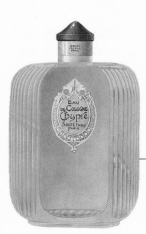

In the Richard Hudnut perfumery, opened in 1925 in Paris by this young American perfumer, the décor by Georges Barbier is like a precious wrapping for any women seeking the ideal perfume, one which as Colette put it, "surprises and makes strangers take note." A tender floral fragrance? Or the chypre trail of the Sauzé Frères' Eau de Cologne (opposite)?

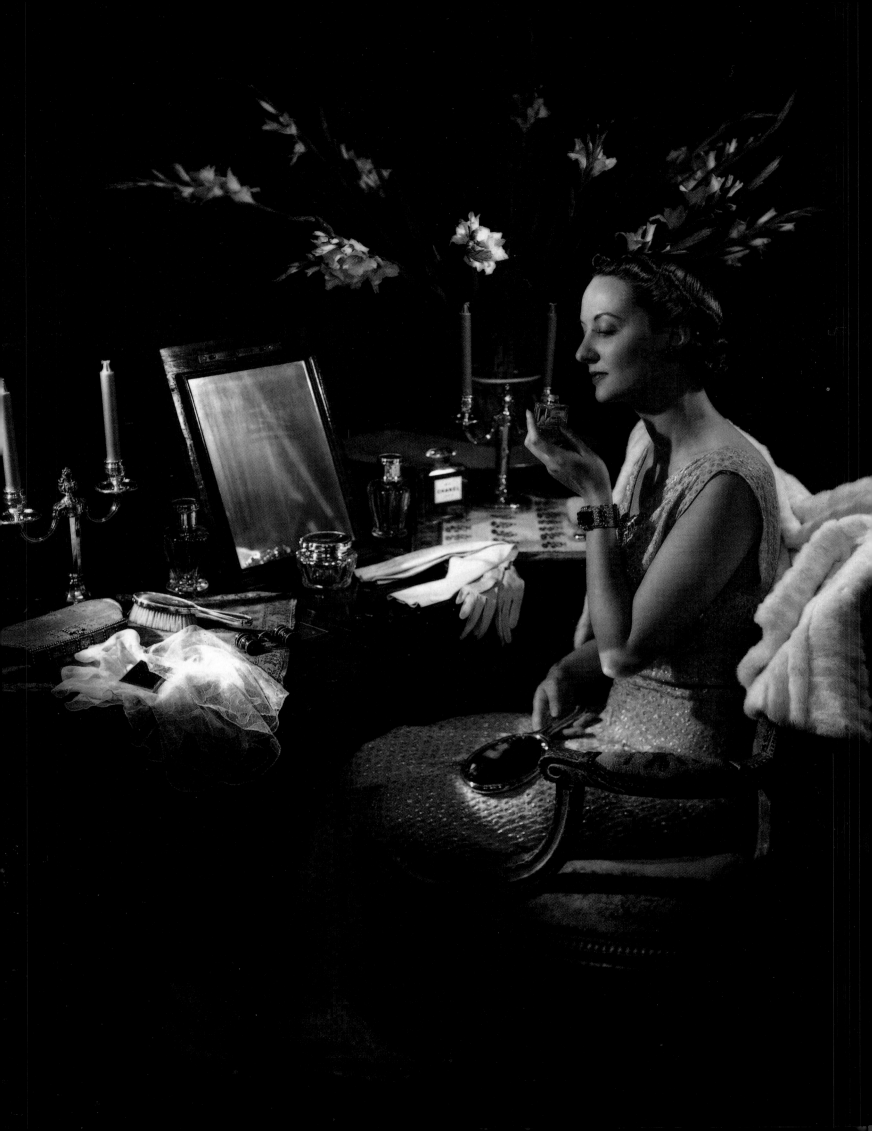

impulses. It should take time; perhaps dozens will be smelled before the buyer finds the one which suits their moods, desires and deepest impulses. A perfume chosen solely for its label procures a pleasure linked with the aura of a famous name which flatters its owner's ego. It makes her feel like a member of the elite, a woman of taste who is well-practiced in the art of attracting men. Moreover, it gives her assurance and is often the businesswoman's most discreet accomplice. The names of some perfumes are so attractive that one is tempted to buy them before even smelling them—a risk not worth taking. Dream-like names do not necessarily give an accurate idea of the perfume in question. In fact it is increasingly frequent practice for companies to choose the name before the perfumer has composed the fragrance. Buying the latest novelty is more a question of succumbing to the whims of fashion than catering to one's own emotions. The fascination may be intense, but is likely to be brief! Choosing the same perfume as your best friend can also lead to disaster. Although it is generally claimed that redheads exhale a milky odor, brunettes a musky fragrance and blonds that of almonds, each skin has its own particular smell and acidity, known as the pH, which is determined by sebaceous glands and eating habits. A person's odor can therefore vary during different periods of their life, particularly in the case of women because of the hormone cycle. A perfume will not smell the same on the

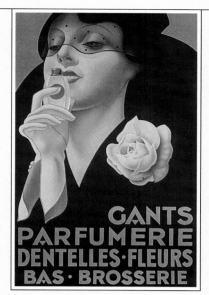

skin of a young girl as when it is worn by her mother.

Perfumes should be changed during the course of a person's life. The days are over when keeping to the same perfume was considered to be in good taste. The advice given by Stella Maris—a journalist of the 1930s who encouraged her readers to be faithful to one single fragrance with which they should perfume not only their body and clothes, but also all their personal effects such as writing paper, cushions, books and even their bed, so that "one single fragrance emanates from a person and everything they possess"—no longer stands. Modern women have understood that this type of olfactory tyranny might be excessive and the majority now use three or four different perfumes depending on the time of the day, the season, their mood, or the desire to surprise the one they love. "Perfumes are always new illusions," as the poet Rollinat wisely remarked.

Diversity does not, however, necessarily mean incoherence. A certain number of creators have created perfume collections based around central themes. The woody toilet waters by Serge Lutens for Shiseido, for example, contain the woody middle note of Féminité du Bois, which is then given either a fruity or floral trail. Meanwhile, the fashion designer Claude Montana has launched Suggestion, a presentation case of "three olfactory suggestions" all based around the same floral, musk heart.

The first waft of perfume from a newly opened bottle is so enticing! A moment of discovery to be savored eyes closed under a veiled hat, perhaps, as captured by this photograph of a Parisian model on the front cover of a 1934 catalogue of women's fashion accessories (above), or sat at one's table, already dressed and about to apply the perfume (opposite). But beware . . . according to the author Louise de Vilmorin, "Perfumes are cunning and, if treated with negligence, will throw your secrets to the winds."

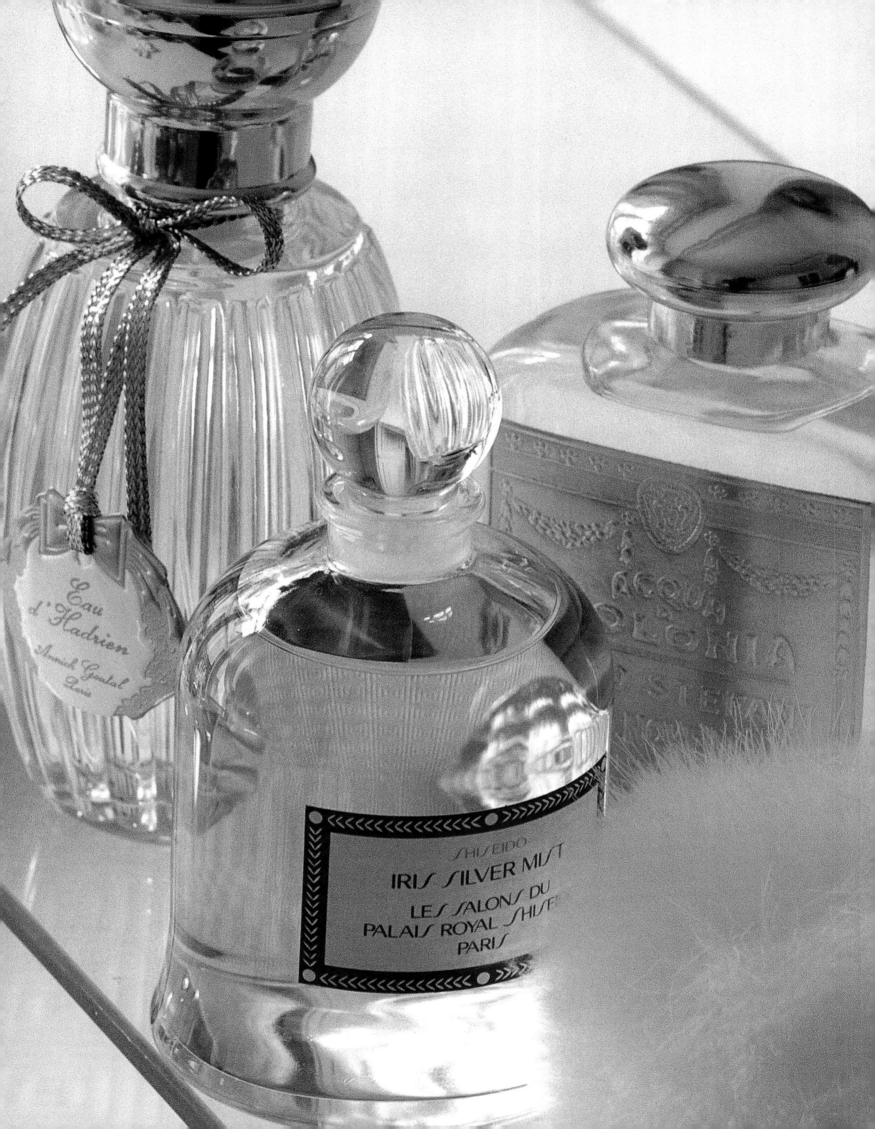

Each perfume envelops us in a particular aura. Going from one novelty to another and alternating very different types of perfume is like wearing various masks . . . tempting, but something which relies on knowing yourself well and respecting a few principles of harmony. Like creating a musical harmony from different notes, perfumes which are going to have to cohabit must get on well together. One way to ensure this is to choose perfumes which have notes or an accord in common. For example, one can alternate the suave vanilla note in Cacharel's Loulou with the more solar one in Laura Biagotti's Roma, and the candor of Weil's Bambou can also be found in the intoxicating Cabotine by Grès. Or else one can be flighty and yet faithful at the same time by trying various perfumes of the same make, like the Guerlain aficionados who go from Après l'Ondée, to L'Heure Bleue or Jardins de Bagatelle. Rose-lovers can try Yves Saint Laurent's Paris, Chanel N° 19, Caron's Bellodgia, Tea Rose by The Perfumer's Workshop, Evelyn by Crabtree & Evelyn, Rose Opulente by Jean-François Laporte, or Rose de Rosine created by Marie-Hélène Rogeon.

Like clothes, perfumes can be charming or unsettling depending on the circumstances, the season and the place. An oriental perfume, which is so intriguing in the evening, can inconvenience people if it is worn in the morning in a public place. In the United States, certain restaurants have notices up indicating that women wearing invasive perfumes will not be admitted. It is torture for the gourmet when a strong perfume kills the fragrant aroma of the dish he is about to taste. The author Colette had a strong dislike for these overpowering perfumes and more than once left her seat on account of them, either in a restau-rant, where they spoiled her appetite, or in the theater, where they distracted her from the play.

The seasons also have an influence on certain accords. The so-called gourmand perfumes, saturated with ripe fruit, are well suited to the richness of the fall, whereas in winter it is pleasant to protect oneself with the soft aura of powdery fragrances. The summer calls for cheerful floral perfumes and fresh toilet waters. It is possible to compose what is known as a "fragrance wardrobe." The secret of any successful partnership lies in mutual understanding

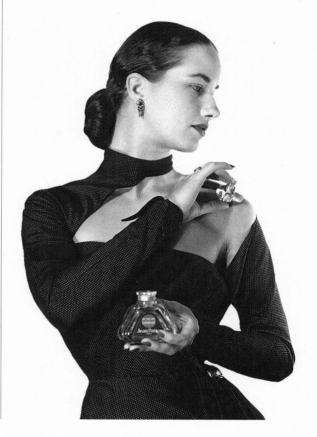

This model holding a bottle of Moment Suprême, created by Jean Patou in 1931, seems to suggest that perfume participates in the sensuous game of desire (above). One should not be misled by the innocent allure of perfume bottles, round like small children's cheeks. Under the innocent curves vibrate the sensual accords of Iris Silver Mist, created by Serge Lutens for Shiseido, Eau d'Hadrien by Annick Goutal and Santa Maria Novella's Acque di Colonia, with their notes of amber, heliotrope, sandalwood and ylang-ylang (opposite).

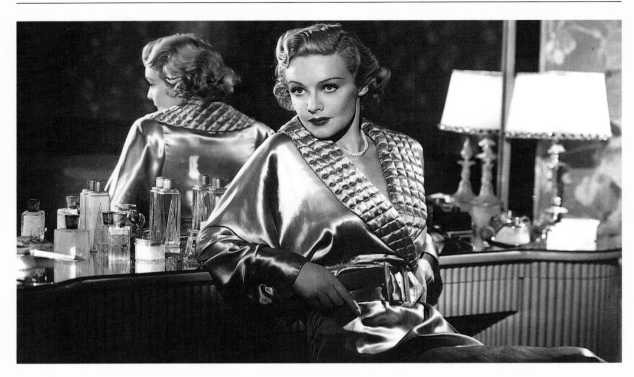

and respect. The same is true for perfumes. For example, a floral, a semi-oriental and a mild oriental fragrance form a perfect trio, which is also true for a fresh toilet water, a green fragrance and a floral fruity one.

FROM EXTRACTION TO EAUX DE PARFUM, BODY LOTIONS AND SOAPS

The extract, more commonly called perfume, is at the top of the fragrance hierarchy and is the inspiration and reference point for the whole line of perfume products. It is considered the noblest version of perfume because it contains top-qual-ity raw materials diluted in a solution of almost pure alcohol (96 percent), which provides the best acoustics for the heart and base notes. At the beginning of the century, the concentration of perfumed material in the extract rarely exceeded 15 percent, whereas nowadays it approaches 30. The extract, an object of desire, the ultimate symbol of luxury in its precious, traditionally sealed perfume bottle, the partner of exquisite moments and token of love, represents quality, tradition and the legend of a name. It is hardly surprising that the extract of Joy by Jean Patou, although too prohibitive for small budgets, represents 35 percent of the company's turnover, and that the perfume form of N° 5 leads Chanel perfume sales.

The extract is an object of desire, like the superb diamond perfume bottle for Trésor (right), launched by Lancôme in 1952. It is a part of the intimacy of a refined woman, personified here by the English actress Madeleine Carroll, the heroine of Alfred Hitchcock's movie *The Thirty-nine Steps* (above). Like a burning caress on the skin, the extract encourages our desire to attract. "I want to be courted," exclaimed Jeanette MacDonald, the heroine of Ernst Lubitsch's movie *The Merry Widow*, before taking Paris by storm (opposite).

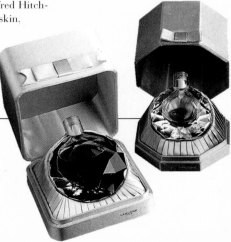

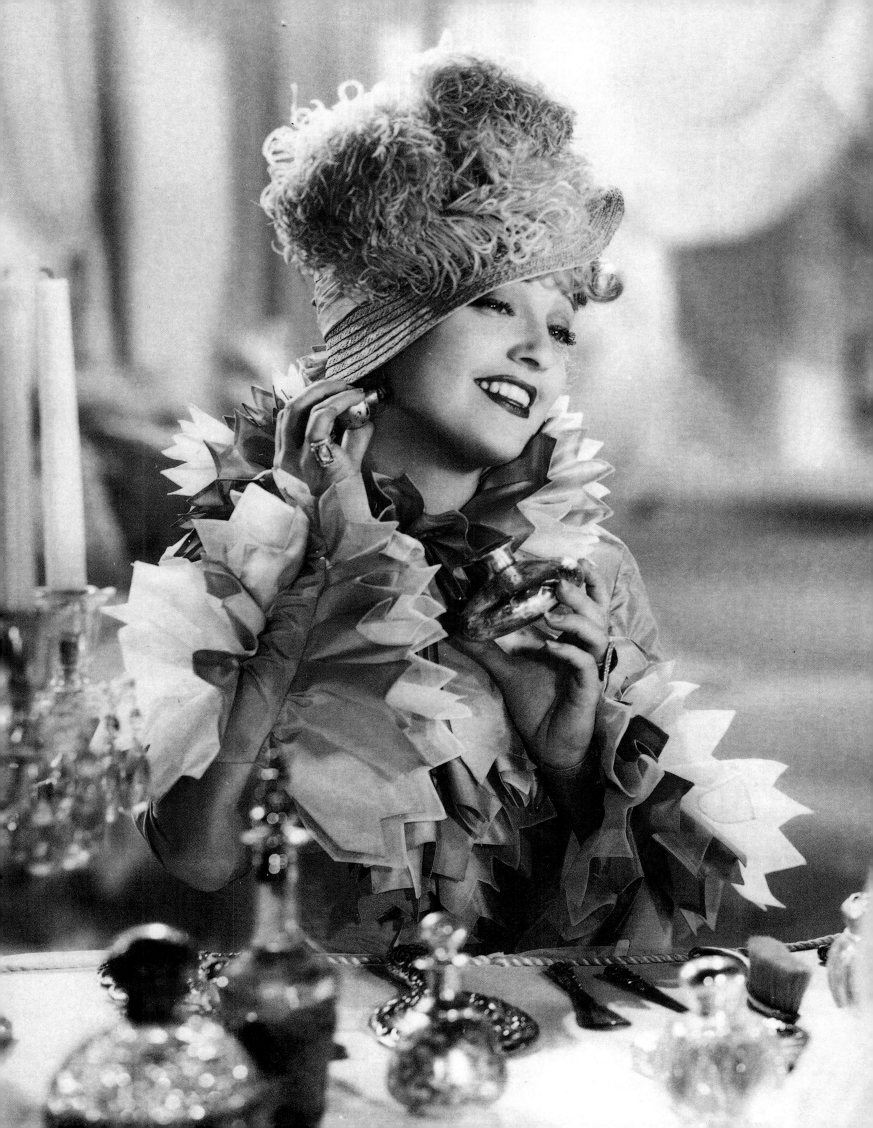

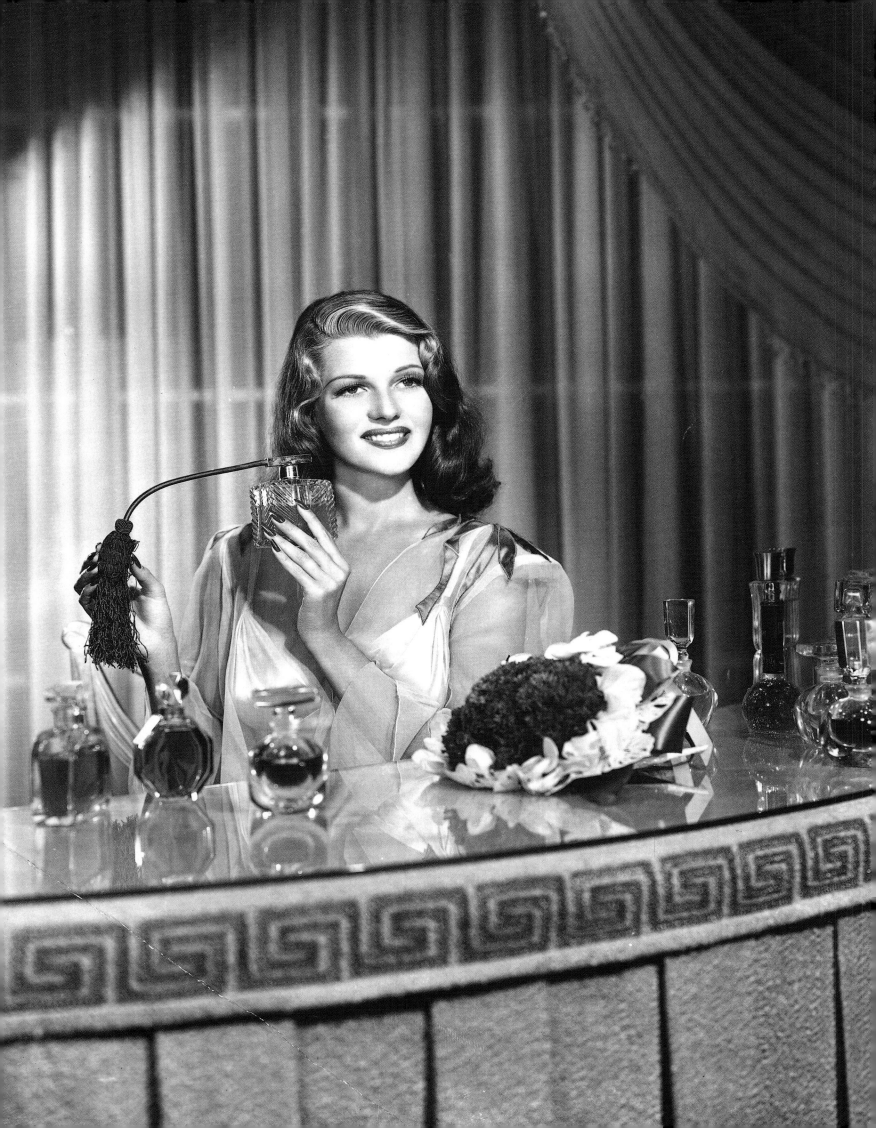

The extract, however, is no longer as universally popular with women as it was in the 1930s. Its price, its trail and fragility are ill-suited to a modern lifestyle. Hence the success of the less concentrated *eaux de parfum*, baptized *fleur de parfum*, *soie de parfum*, or *esprit de parfum*, depending on the make. Their arrival on the market in the 1970s coincided with the development of feminism. This was hardly a coincidence. Whereas the extract is the symbol of a certain femininity which conforms to traditional codes, governed by outward appearance and attraction, the eau de parfum, which can be worn in all places and on all occasions, is the constant companion of active, independent women. It is often sold in spray bottles, which enable one to apply Estée Lauder's "aerial" method: she recommends spraying the perfume a few inches in front of you and then stepping into the fragrance cloud, which has a far more subtle effect. Toilet water (eau de toilette) is less concentrated and, when worn, its harmonious notes are like a melody which leaves no trail. It is greatly appreciated by women who, as the fashion designer Pierre Balmain so charmingly put it, "Want to be different, but not noticed." Nowadays it is the refined partner of morning ablutions and provides a moment of pleasure after exercise.

Fragrant pleasures also exist in the form of creams, lotions and perfumed soaps. The professionals call them "body collections," but to attract women they use enchanting terms, such as "pearly spring," "subtle veil," or "fragrance caress." Sometimes they are launched at the same time as the perfume whose fragrance they share, or sometimes a few months later, like a delightful echo. These products offer a subtle, intimate form of perfume, which involve gestures reminiscent of ancestral rituals.

It would require more than one book to tell the complete history of the perfume rituals and customs of various populations and cultures through the ages. Some are better known than others. The Greeks rubbed different ointments on various parts of their bodies and wore floral crowns in order to avoid intoxication. In Rome, rejected lovers smeared marjoram balm on the front door of the house of their beloved. The young women of Constantinople chewed violets all day long in order that their skin should smell nice, whereas Louis XV's favorites rinsed their mouths with rose-water and perfumed their breath with iris powder. In India, women soften their skin with an ointment made from an aromatic root boiled in coconut oil. In the Sudan, they perfume their bodies by exposing them to the fumes of an aromatic wood, known as *talloh*, which is said to have a stimulating effect on the skin. There was never any question of the Japanese actually perfuming their skin, but they shroud themselves in the odorous aura which is given off from exotic wood shavings stitched into the hem of their kimonos. For many years, Europeans used to perfume themselves with powders,

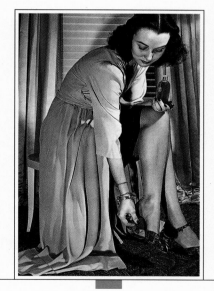

Like an intangible, bewitching cloak, a perfume shrouds the body and haunts the memory. It is the artful accomplice of seductive women, who are infinitely imaginative in this domain, like this young American woman in the 1940s who slips a perfumed sachet into her shoe (above). It seems that the curvaceous Rita Hayworth preferred the perfume spray and perhaps she also perfumed her gloves, in memory of the famous scene in *Gilda*, the movie which made her a star (opposite).

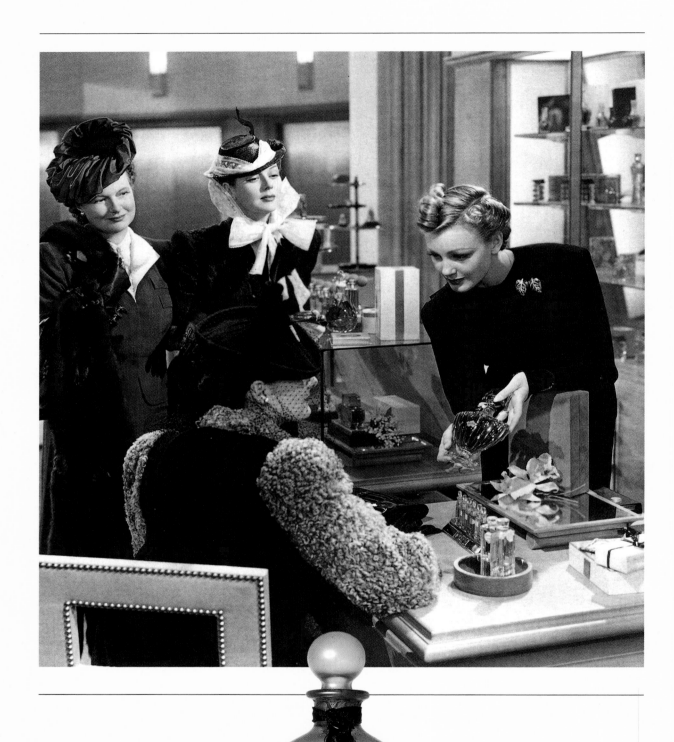

pomanders and gloves saturated with musk and amber, before turning to scented waters, then almost exclusively to perfumes. It was not until Estée Lauder launched her first perfumed bath oil that western women went back to that voluptuous, forgotten habit, and with such enthusiasm that nowadays it is out of the question to launch a great perfume without associating it with that charming quartet of talcum powder, cream, lotion and perfumed soap. Perfumed talc, so popular with the Anglo-Saxons, who use it in abundance at all ages, is no doubt the most delicate and thorough manner of perfuming oneself, for it envelops the body in a fragrant halo with a strong diffusive power, whereas perfume, in its alcohol version, concentrates its effect on precise zones of the body such as the neck, the nape of the neck and the wrists. And what could be more sensual than perfumed body creams? This perfume is a caress, a prelude to evenings of love, the accompaniment to intimate moments. Creams are almost as concentrated as eau de parfum and ensure a deep and lasting fragrance. Lotions have a low alcohol content and provide a rapid and discreet way of perfuming oneself, well adapted to the constraints of professional life and to active women who seek a certain understated refinement. Bath oils, on the other hand, are for relaxed weekends or those delicious moments of relaxation at the end of the day when you are free to dream of other worlds.

Discovering a perfume is an adventure, which, like great journeys, requires attention, emotion and patience. Choosing a perfume takes time. A perfume cannot be appreciated immediately on smelling it, for it takes a few minutes, sometimes more, for it to develop its entire olfactory symphony, which is certainly the case, for example, of a perfume with rich, complex notes. Perfume can only be tested on the skin if it is free from any fragrance, including the morning's perfumed soaps and cleansing milks. The best place is the pulse point on the wrist, where the veins give off a little heat which improves olfactory sensitivity. Apply a few drops and wait a while, above all without rubbing as this might change the odorous molecules. Good perfume stores have odorless paper strips known as blotter strips, which are used by creators for testing new perfumes. At Caron's, in avenue Montaigne, they sometimes spray perfume on clients' scarfs so that they can get used to the fragrance in the calm of their bedroom or living room, where the perfume harmonizes with their body, their mood and their secret dreams. Perfume must attract without the slightest reservation. A light peppery note, for example, hardly noticeable at first, might, in the long run, prove to be a source of inconvenience.

The morning is better suited to olfactory ceremonies. The body is rested and the senses more acute. Unless you have a highly developed sense of smell, it is not possible to test more than three perfumes at any one time. Any more than this and the odors become confused and one's sense of smell less receptive. It is best to smell two fragrances, choose one, compare it to a third and keep the favorite for another test on the following day. One has to have experienced the peaceful atmosphere of the perfumer's retreat and the silence of his laboratory to understand that fragrances develop best in serene surroundings. Crowded department stores or perfume stores on Saturday afternoons do not provide the necessary tranquillity for choosing a perfume. The right atmosphere is more likely to be found in

It takes a curious amount of self-control to resist the spell of the perfume bottle, the first thing one sees, the more so if the bottle is decorated in mother-of-pearl, like this fragrance created by Volnay, a perfumer long since forgotten (opposite, bottom). The perfume bottle, resting like a jewel in a case, is tempting even before one has smelled the fragrance. In this scene from the movie *The Women*, directed by George Cukor in 1939, a bottle of Guerlain's Shalimar is contemplated with interest by an elegant client accompanied by two friends (opposite, top).

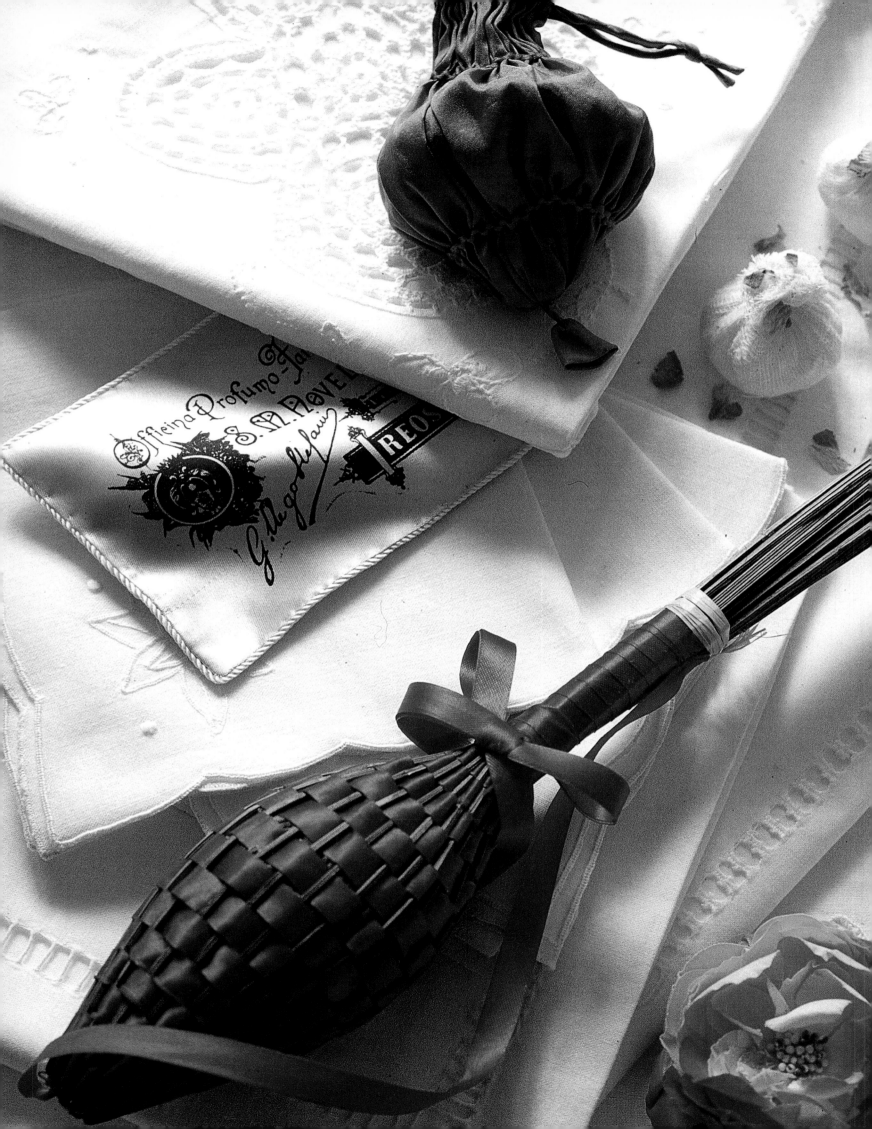

ENVIRONMENTAL FRAGRANCE

The ancients hoped to win the favor of the gods by burning resins and odorous woods. Priests burned vast quantities of incense on the top of the Tower of Babel, sending up fumes destined to reach and appease the easily offended gods. In antiquity, architecture employed the science of aromas and Chinese potentates had their sumptuous pagodas built in cedarwood, which they left unpainted in order to allow the creamy odors of the wood to diffuse into the air. European sovereigns yielded to the same frenzy and under the reign of the French king Francis I the walls of the Louvre were sprayed with floral waters by means of an indoor hose. Louis XIV, who ordered that a new fragrance be created every day for his exclusive use, employed a whole army of servants whose sole duty was to boil his shirts in a mixture of cloves, nutmeg, jasmine, orange blossom and musk. The height of refinement was reached at the court of Louis XV, where perfumed doves were released during official dinners and flew among the guests weaving a web of subtle intoxications.

It was around this time that the first fragrances for the home made their appearance in the houses of the aristocracy and the upper classes, in the form of potpourris in china or silver bowls. To begin with the petals and odorous wood shavings used in these mixtures were fresh and salt was sprinkled on them to preserve the colors and fragrances. Nowadays potpourris are made of dried flowers which are "reinforced" with essential oils. Pomanders (*pommes d'ambre*), whose spicy fragrances resemble potpourris, were worn from the Middle Ages on, either at the belt, or on chains round the neck. These hand-carved gold or silver balls contained ground amber, musk and odorous roots. The early examples have become collector's items, but their shape has inspired the perforated earthenware balls filled with amber (often synthetic) which are placed in cupboards or on side tables. As for the dried, clove-studded oranges, still made by French children at Christmas time, they are said to have been invented by a perfumer at the court of Henry III.

In England, home perfumes have been in vogue since the eighteenth century, but this is not the case in other European countries. Until the 1970s, in France perfuming one's living room was generally considered to be a refined, or even rather eccentric practice, exclusively reserved for aesthetes, or dismissed as a hippy craze when the fashion for incense sticks and cones brought back from the Orient came in. Home perfumes in France were therefore restricted to Berger lamps and Rigaud candles, the principle function of which was to dispel the odors of cooking and

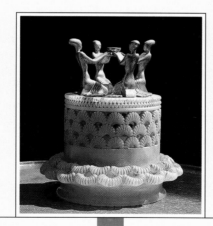

As suggested by this alabaster and gilded bronze perfume lamp, created by Armand Rateau in 1925, perfume is an offering (above). Perfuming bed linen brings an intimate touch of refinement to the home, illustrated here by a satin poutpourri sachet, muslin bags, a little cushion of Florentine iris powder, braided lavender tied with satin ribbons and an artificial rose made from aromatic materials (opposite, top to bottom).

tobacco. The mid-1980s brought the return of traditional values revolving around the home and the family, and with this came signs of change. The fashion for environmental fragrances was relaunched; people became armchair travelers, who, thanks to the rustic odor of a perfumed candle, could imagine themselves walking in a forest even when sitting in the heart of the city.

"Choosing an environmental fragrance," affirms the perfumer Jean-François Laporte, "is like creating an olfactory décor." This extremely demanding, imaginative perfumer brought environmental fragrances back into fashion in France in the 1970s by creating the first range of home fragrances. The idea came to him when staying with friends in Istanbul, in a palace on the Bosporus. Every evening, they lit a brazier in the living room into which were thrown pieces of perfumed wood, giving off a subtle odor which, rising up in wreaths, gently pervaded the room. On his return to France, he rushed to his laboratory, eager to try and compose home fragrances which would be as exciting as those he had experienced in Istanbul. And with what success! First there were the lovely apricot notes, as reassuring as rustic furniture, followed by the slightly dry, woody, or sometimes metallic notes, echoing the coldness of high-tech. Since then, the trend has been for fragrances which give the impression of being in the open air—sophisticated pastoral evocations which are so natural that if you close your eyes it seems as though the city has suddenly disappeared.

There are various ways of perfuming one's house in a more or less lasting fashion: scented candles, fragrant aerosols, potpourris of all sorts.

As to the fragrances, the choice can be overwhelming. Moderation is what Jean-François Laporte recommends first and foremost. "A home perfume must suggest an atmosphere without ever invading it. The setting must therefore guide the choice of the fragrance." For a cosy English living room, he advises a honeyed fragrance, whereas for a fresher, Provençal-style house, jasmine or lawn fragrances are well suited. A richer setting, in the Napoleon III style for example, calls for potpourri fragrances or a peony note. In rooms where cold materials such as glass and metal are predominant, a potpourri composed of spices, or a perfume spray with a Moroccan cedarwood base note, help to warm the atmosphere.

Other gadgets could be mentioned, such as the lavender bags embroidered by our grandmothers which they used to slip between the sheets, a practice which still has its followers, as do the pieces of cedarwood attached to clothes hangers, which not only perfume the cupboards but also keep away the moths! There are tender home fragrances in the form of perfumed porous stone hearts; the gourmand version, which consists of fragrant dried peach stones placed in bowls to perfume the atmosphere; and finally, the perfect housewife version in the form of fragrant powder sachets for vacuum cleaners, which transform carpets into fields of lily of the valley or lavender.

It is, however, to Greek monks that we owe the most poetic version of environmental fragrances, that of swathes of laurel and myrtle which are gathered at dawn and strewn over the stone floors of churches where, over the hours, they diffuse their heady fragrances like a religious chant.

The fragrance of happiness is without doubt that of a welcoming home where perfumed candles burn on low tables, while potpourris and clove-studded oranges enhance the secluded corners of bedrooms. A few examples of such products are leaves of lemon grass, small bundles of cinnamon tied with rafia, potpourris, a ball of cloves, and cinnamon-perfumed candles (opposite, right to left).

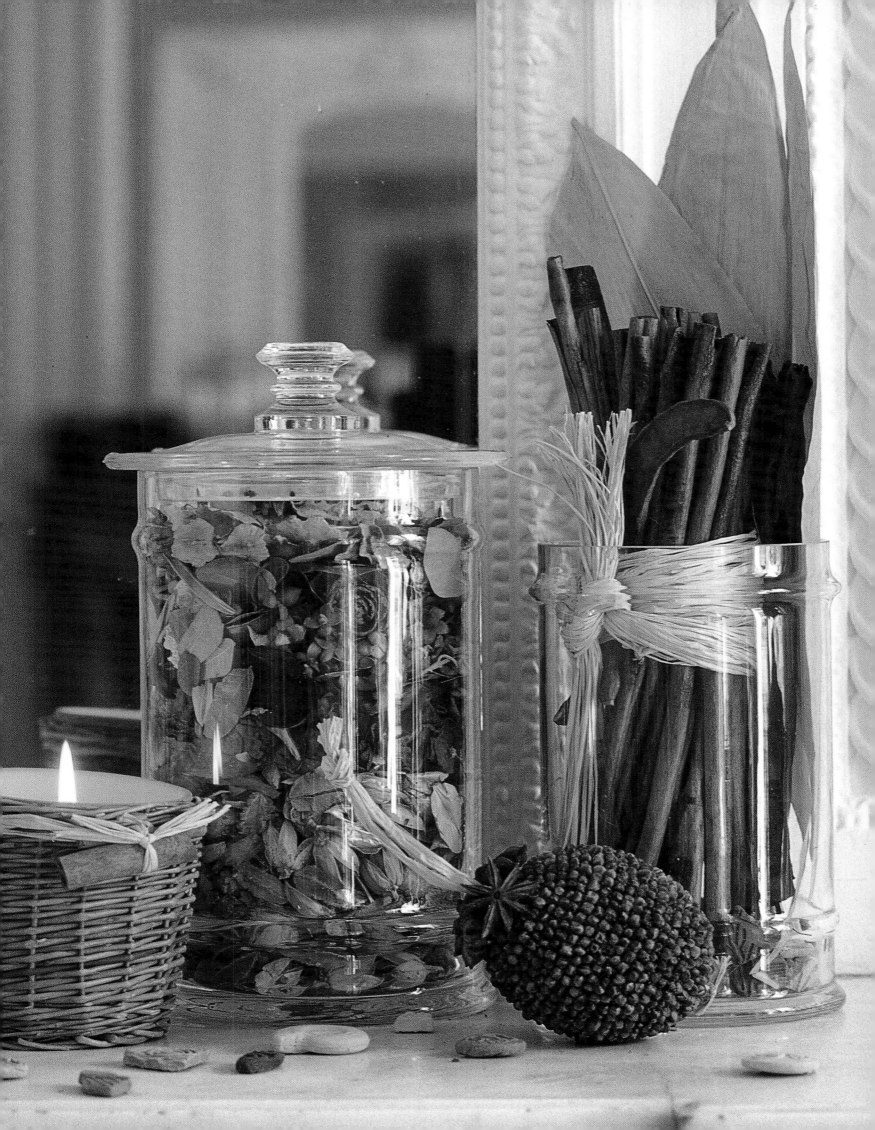

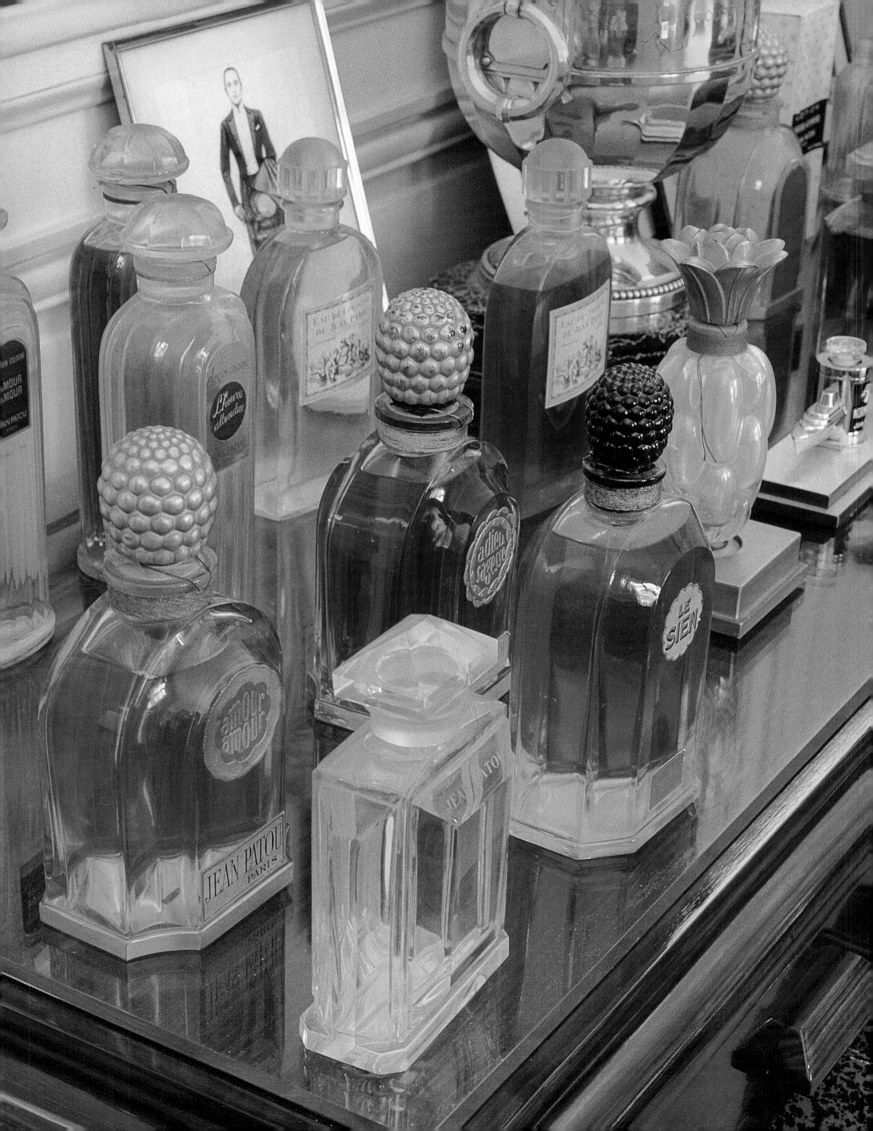

· 1,001 ·
PERFUME
BOTTLES

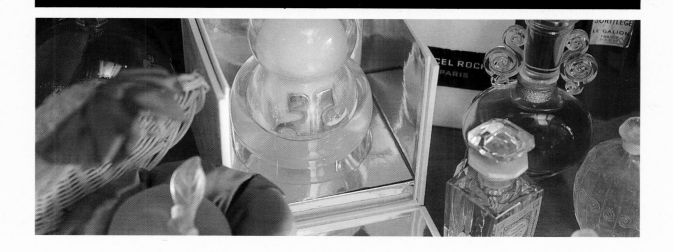

Creating new shapes and original silhouettes, exploiting the infinite subtleties of glass and its bright or intense colors, exalting the delicacy and brilliance of crystal and mastering every particularity, every possibility of the precious substance—such is the unique art of the perfume bottle designer. He alone has the gift for creating those fragile receptacles which sublimate and glorify the secret beauty of perfume.

In one dexterous movement the molten glass is removed from the heart of the blazing ovens and glows red in the darkness of the factory. By blowing exactly the right quantity of air into the pipe, the master glass blower transforms this heavy mass into a transparent, impalpable bulb. For the designer, taking part in the creation of something that has been constantly occupying his thoughts for several months is an emotional moment. At last, having imagined the perfume bottle in all its subtlety, measured its every detail, he is finally able to touch it, take it in his hands and appreciate its density, transparency and grain.

For the bottle designer, working with glass is a perpetual source of surprise and joy. A simple idea or sketch will suddenly transform the glass into a shell, a precious stone, opal or marble. Perhaps it was because of this gift of metamorphosis that the ancients attributed supernatural powers to glass and for this same reason that it has become perfume's privileged partner.

Glass and perfume, both of which are man-made products obtained through the synthesis of various elements, seemed destined to meet. In antiquity, fragrance containers were made out of various materials, including stone, alabaster, terra cotta and ceramic, later followed by precious metals such as gold and vermeil and then porcelain. The zenith of glassmaking (in Italy, in the fifteenth century) coincides with the first use of alcohol in perfume. No material, however, other than glass and crystal, has the ideal properties of stability and neutrality indispensable for containing a living substance in constant evolution such as perfume. And only glass and crystal have the flexibility and fantastic capacity of transformation which enable them to take on the most varied forms, colors and finishes and satisfy the most highly developed aesthetic requirements.

Years of intimacy have only served to strengthen this complicity and throughout their history perfume bottles have benefited from the development of increasingly sophisticated glass techniques. If, at the outset, they resembled objects in more common use, such as glasses, jugs and toilet utensils, they soon broke away, prompted by the value accorded to their precious contents. Although it is difficult to establish whether making perfume bottles was a separate art form, it is nevertheless clear that in every civilization and culture people have taken particular pride in mastering the techniques and knowledge needed to make these precious objects specifically intended for perfume. Although perfume bottles only represent a very small portion of the total use of glass, because of their perpetually innovative aesthetic requirements, they nevertheless contribute to the development of new glassmaking techniques.

The first known pieces of glasswork, in the

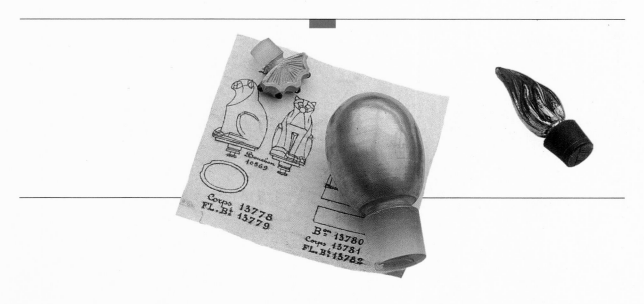

form of opaque-colored pearls used for jewelry, are Egyptian and date from about two thousand years B.C. Before the invention of the blowiron by the Phoenicians, at the beginning of the Christian era, the first perfume bottles were fashioned by winding molten glass around clay molds. Glass blowing not only meant a much finer substance could be obtained, but it also meant the bottle shape could be varied and refined. The Romans were the first to develop the production of perfume bottles on a large scale. Being great perfume lovers, they gave free reign to their imagination and produced intricately designed bottles with an appearance of patinated bronze and other metals or mother-of-pearl. The introduction of glass enameling by the Arabs was an important technical advance, but very soon the talent of the Venetians eclipsed all existing techniques.

As early as the thirteenth century, the Venetian glass blowers established themselves on the island of Murano, from where they proceeded to impress their art on the whole world. The lagoon, of course, provided exceptional raw materials, such as the extremely fine sand which gave the glass its particular transparency, but above all the Venetians had a glassmaking tradition which they were continually renewing and developing. In the fifteenth century, Venetian

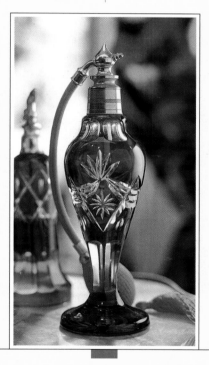

glassmaking was at its height and the possibilities seemed infinite. Glass was tinted with intense, deep colors, or decorated with delicate enamel motifs, made to look like frothy lace, precious stones or Chinese porcelain. It gradually became clearer and more refined until it acquired the appearance of *cristallo*, the crystalline glass for which Venice is renowned. The Venetians jealously tried to guard the secret of its production, but many craftsmen carried it away with them when they left the city and Venetian techniques soon spread all over the world, without, however, attaining that degree of perfection which only the purity of the materials found in its place of origin could ensure. This is how glassmaking came to be developed in Bohemia. There they produced a thick, extremely resistant glass, which was cut and engraved, giving birth to the famous Bohemian crystal. In the seventeenth century, it took on the ruby red tint discovered by alchemists, and was used to make decorative luxury objects, becoming a must among toilet articles.

Glass became an important commodity. In France, the arrival of powerful glass manufacturers contributed to the spread of a new savoir-faire which continued to develop centuries-old perfume bottle making techniques. When the large French glass manufacturers settled in Normandy, near the sandy expanses, rich in fire-

Today Jean Patou's perfumes (page 152) are sold exclusively in his boutique in their original perfume bottles, such as Amour-Amour (1925), Le Sien (1929), Vacances (1936) and L'Heure Attendue (1946). Collector's bottles can often be found in antique stores, like these bottles by Rochas, Volney, Ricci and Courrèges (page 153), or sprays (above), formerly used instead of flacons. As for the stoppers (opposite), these are also of interest to collectors.

wood, of the valley of the river Bresle, they not only renewed a tradition dating from the Middle Ages, but also developed the industries which today monopolize the worldwide production of perfume bottles. It was in Normandy that, in 1623, Pochet et du Courval, today one of the largest international glass manufacturers, decided to set up their premises, followed some years later, in 1665, by La Manufacture Royale des Glaces et des Miroirs (The Royal Glass and Mirror Manufactory), created on the initiative of Louis XIV's first secretary of state, Jean-Baptiste Colbert, which was subsequently to become Saint-Gobain-Desjonquères.

Soon, however, the discovery of lead crystal was to revolutionize the art of glassmaking and perfume bottles. In 1676, an Englishman named George Ravenscroft produced a mixture which enabled him to obtain an extremely pure glass. Crystal was a material so subtly malleable that henceforth nothing stood in the way of the designer's most elaborate requirements. Stimulated by this discovery, neighboring craftsmen worked tirelessly to reproduce this new substance, so incomparably transparent and refined. Les Cristalleries de Saint-Louis, created in 1586, which became Les Cristalleries Royales in 1767, and Les Cristalleries Baccarat, founded in 1764, created the most magnificent objects, with Baccarat establishing itself from the end of the last century as the greatest creator of perfume bottles.

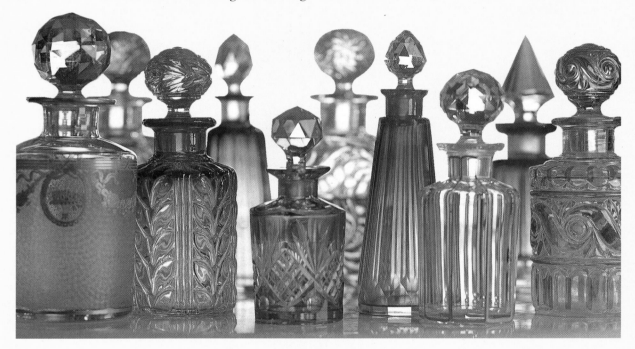

"Some scents can permeate all substances / even glass seems porous to their power," wrote Charles Baudelaire in "The Flask." Roses and jasmine, it is true, continue to haunt perfume bottles with their unforgettable presence (above). The magic of a long-forgotten era, when the art of toiletry was associated with the subtle fragrances of the iris and the violet, is illustrated in this painting by Georges Croegaert, entitled *In the Boudoir* (opposite).

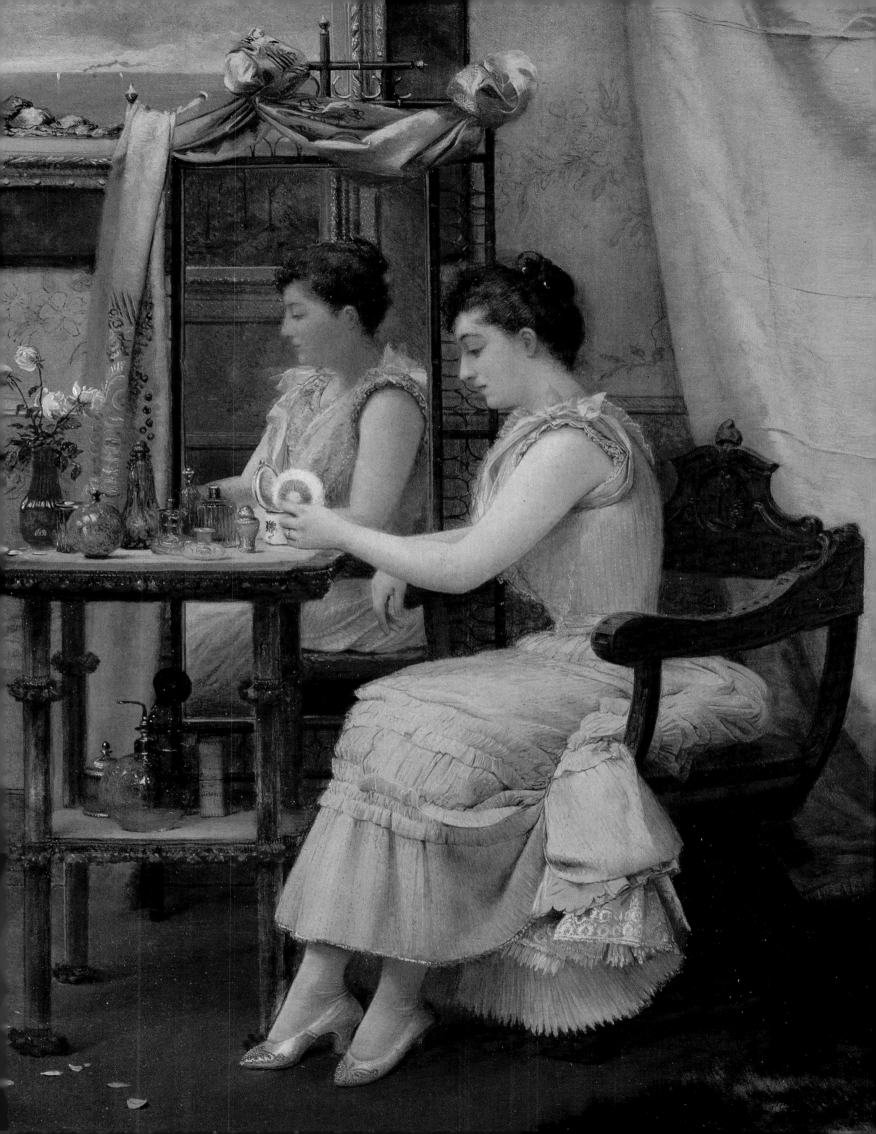

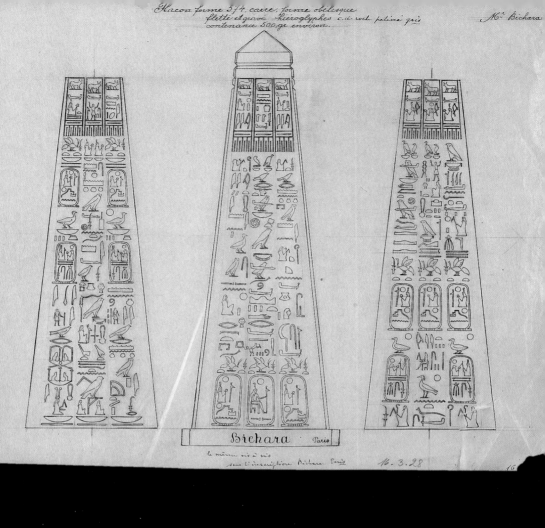

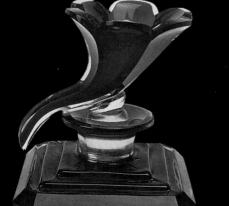

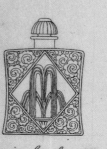

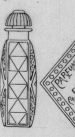

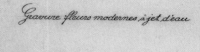

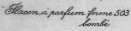

THE ART
OF THE PERFUME BOTTLE

Today when a creator designs a perfume bottle, its shape, color and style are inspired by the olfactory character of the perfume it is designed for. The relationship between a container and its contents, between the art of glassmaking and the perfumer, which seems obvious to us today, only came into being at the end of the nineteenth century. The powerful guilds which, until then, controlled each trade association, were governed by extremely strict rules and worked in a completely autonomous manner. The perfume produced by the French glove and perfume-makers guild was sold in dispensaries in plain glass bottles decorated with a colored label and wrapped in wax paper, and it was only in the fashionable woman's boudoir that it became united with the delicate perfume bottles, sold empty, which were created by the master glass blowers.

The abolition of the guilds during the French Revolution, allied with the development of industrialization and an increasing demand for quality products, facilitated the gradual rapprochement of the two trades. The proliferation of new perfume houses such as Lubin, Guerlain, Molinard and Houbigant stimulated innovative developments in the domain of perfume. Glassworkers began to create more refined perfume bottles and labels were decorated with motifs as elaborate as pictures, so as to set off the increasingly sophisticated fragrances to their advantage. The famous Guerlain flacon decorated with the royal bee motif was created by Pierre-François-Pascal Guerlain in 1853 for Empress Eugénie's Véritable Eau de Cologne Impériale, while a delicate bouquet of violets, hand-painted directly onto the glass, embellished the bottle for Roger & Gallet's Violette de Parme.

At the end of the last century, the development of Art Nouveau marked a radical break with the classical style and introduced an art inspired by nature. Émile Gallé triumphed with his milky, shadowy glass, weaving together somber arabesques, lazy spirals and mysterious flowers dotted with delicate insects. Objects which had previously remained somewhat formal in style were transformed into genuine works of art by talented artists, who revitalized and innovated glassmaking techniques and exploited new sources of inspiration for their motifs.

Among these artists were Antonin and Auguste Daum, Louis Comfort Tiffany, the American jeweler who developed iridescent glass, and the architect Paul Guimard, who created spiraling, sinuous perfume bottles for Millot's perfumes.

One of the revelations of the 1900 World Fair was the extraordinary talent of René Lalique. Lalique, who until then had been reputed for his work as a jeweler

"And half glimpsed images caress the surface of the glass!" This phrase of Maurice Maeterlinck's admirably evokes this magical substance which constantly unveils new mysteries, like these bottles of Eau de Cologne Surfine by Roger & Gallet (above). The most beautiful bottles are those made by the great glassworks: these are masterpieces from the Cristalleries de Saint-Louis (opposite).

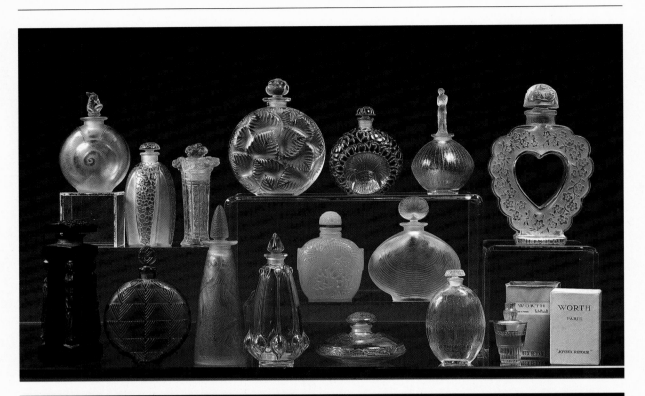

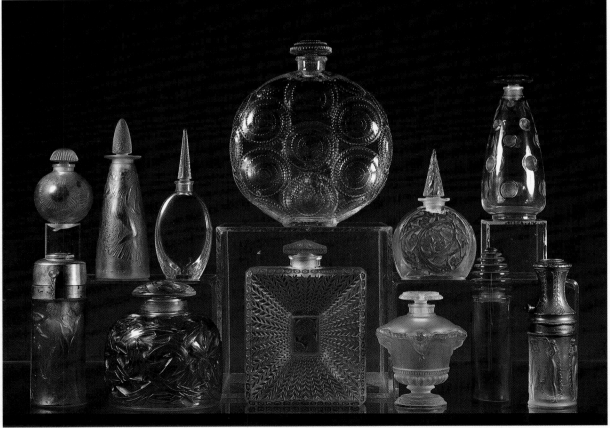

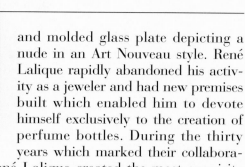

and silversmith, demonstrated a perfect mastery of this delicate art. The public was able to admire exquisite translucent dragonflies, milky roses, iridescent insects and delicate jewels made of glass and precious materials, which delighted women as discerning as the celebrated French actress Sarah Bernhardt.

What caught the attention of the talented perfumer François Coty, however, were a few exquisite perfume bottles made using the lost wax technique, one of which, created in 1893, was in the form of an iridescent amphora decorated with a fish motif. François Coty wanted the new fragrances he was creating to be presented in the most beautiful perfume bottles imaginable. His meeting with René Lalique proved to be decisive; he had finally found the man who would be able to express his audacious olfactory inventions in glass. L'Effleurt, produced in 1908, was their first joint creation. The Baccarat bottle, with its stopper in the form of an Egyptian scarab, was adorned with a pressed and molded glass plate depicting a nude in an Art Nouveau style. René Lalique rapidly abandoned his activity as a jeweler and had new premises built which enabled him to devote himself exclusively to the creation of perfume bottles. During the thirty years which marked their collaboration, René Lalique created the most exquisite perfume bottles for François Coty.

He drew inspiration from various sources, with nature proving to be an inexhaustible source for his exquisite flowers, his interlacing foliage and the insects—such as the stopper in the form of a bee for the bottle containing François Coty's Au Cœur des Calices—which were so popular at the time.

Thanks to François Coty's brilliant intuition, perfume bottles were no longer anonymous objects, but the expression of a particular mood, a state of mind. He was the first to conceive of the bottle and the perfume simultaneously, thereby paving the way for modern perfumery. François Coty set the example for many talented

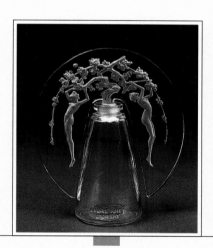

Two nymphs playing with branches decorate this perfume bottle created by René Lalique in 1913 for the Parfums d'Orsay (above). A fawn, as though in a dream, enhances L'Effleurt by Coty, the first perfume bottle he created in association with René Lalique, *circa* 1908 (top). Created for Houbigant, Guerlain, Worth, Molinard, Roger & Gallet and Nina Ricci, these Lalique bottles were recently sold in London at one of the annual sales organized by Bonham's (opposite).

people who were able to express their abilities both as designers and craftsmen. Under the influence of Art Deco, decoration came to be seen as the creation of a coherent, harmonious environment by a single artist developing the same theme in each of the objects within that environment.

The fashion designer Paul Poiret was the first to understand the importance of this movement. In 1911, he created two establishments in honor of his two daughters, Les Ateliers de Martine, which made decorative objects, and Les Parfums de Rosine. Paul Poiret was in fact interested in all forms of art, including fashion, textiles and textile design, painting, set design and decorative objects. The perfume bottles he created were inspired by this melting pot of influences. Associating materials as different as glass, crystal, fabrics, metal or paper in his compositions, he demonstrated that there were no longer any limits or restrictions to creation. Aladin, launched by Les Parfums de Rosine, was a perfect illustration of this philosophy, with its polished, repoussé metal bottle repre-

senting a combat between two monsters, its ivory stopper and fine chain, all in a presentation case covered with colored material bearing a Persian miniature motif.

From that moment on, the movement was launched and the most talented designers began to venture into unexplored territory. The first two decades of this century were marked by creations which rival one another in their poetic inspiration. Ernest Daltroff, the founder of the Caron perfume company, chose to pay perfume tributes to the happy moments of his life, and his bottles are distinctively poetic, delicate and innovative. Lace, sharkskin, silk flowers and woven straw are some of the materials which helped to make each of his perfume bottles quite unique. The most charming of them was no doubt La Fête des Roses in its black velvet presentation case lined with pink satin, which, when opened, unveiled a gilded, geometrically shaped crystal bottle lying in a sea of silk petals.

After an unproductive period during the First World War, the post-war years witnessed

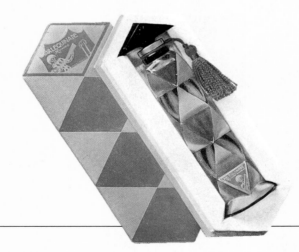

Arlequinade by Les Parfums de Rosine (1912) invites us into Paul Poiret's favorite games with words and bottles (above). En Avion, created by Caron (1930), leads us on the trail of Saint-Exupéry (opposite, top), whereas the hand-braided gold thread gracing L'Infini (1970) (opposite, middle) and Nuit de Noël (1922), with its sharkskin presentation case (opposite, bottom), reveal a world of luxury.

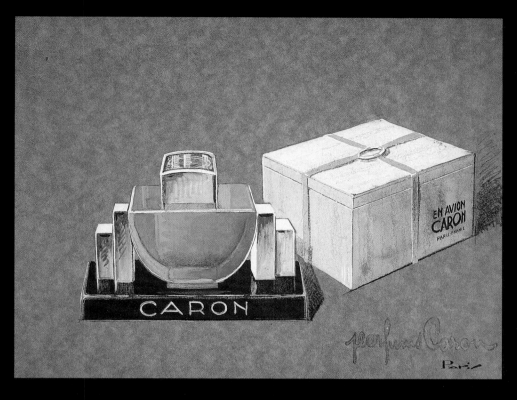

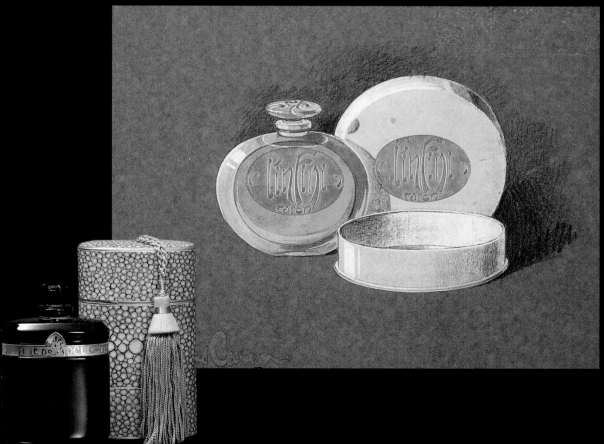

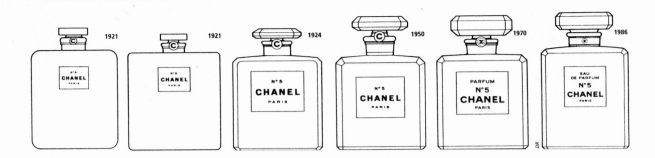

the arrival of perfume bottles which were so perfectly designed that they became archetypal landmarks in the history of bottle forms.

In 1921, Mademoiselle Chanel brought out a simple, flat, square perfume bottle with rounded corners and a chiseled stopper. At a time when exaggeratedly romantic bottles were still in fashion, N° 5 stood out as an exception. It was a model of perfect simplicity and pure elegance, reminiscent of the fashion designer's creations, which has never been equaled since. No concessions were made to romance whatsoever; the bottle is graced with a sober white label bearing the famous number and the name "Chanel" in black blocked lettering.

In 1925, the Exhibition of Decorative Arts set the scene for exceptional new perfume bottles. Among them was the magnificent Shalimar, designed by Raymond Guerlain, whose form, with its midnight blue stopper, evokes the fountains of the garden of Srinagar. Produced in a limited

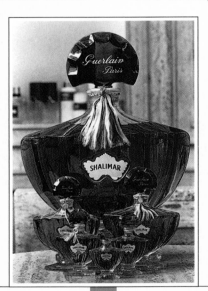

series in Baccarat crystal, this bottle is now one of the most famous of its kind.

In 1927, also in the Art Deco style, Armand Rateau designed the black sphere for Jeanne Lanvin's Arpège. The bottle, with its gilded, raspberry-shaped stopper, is decorated with a drawing of the fashion designer and her daughter Marie-Blanche, attributed to the artist Paul Iribe. Arpège, a fragile yet everlasting bubble suspended in space, symbolizes the whole magic of haute couture and perfume.

Two doves, symbols of peace and love, interlaced on a generously contoured perfume bottle was how Robert Ricci imagined L'Air du Temps. It was designed by Marc Lalique in 1947. Known all over the world, the bottle represents eternal femininity and the return of a certain romanticism. Due to the constraints imposed by mass production, for a time the two doves had to be replaced by a single one, but recently they have been reunited.

The Chanel N° 5 perfume bottle has been modified five times since its creation in 1921, so as to reflect the times (top), whereas the bottle for Shalimar by Guerlain (above), inspired by the exoticism of the Orient, has, on the contrary, remained unchanged since its creation in 1925. "Miracle of elegance, living perfume," wrote Louise de Vilmorin about Lanvin's timeless Arpège. Its famous sphere, decorated with a design by Paul Iribe representing the fashion designer and her daughter Marie-Blanche, was designed by Armand Rateau (opposite).

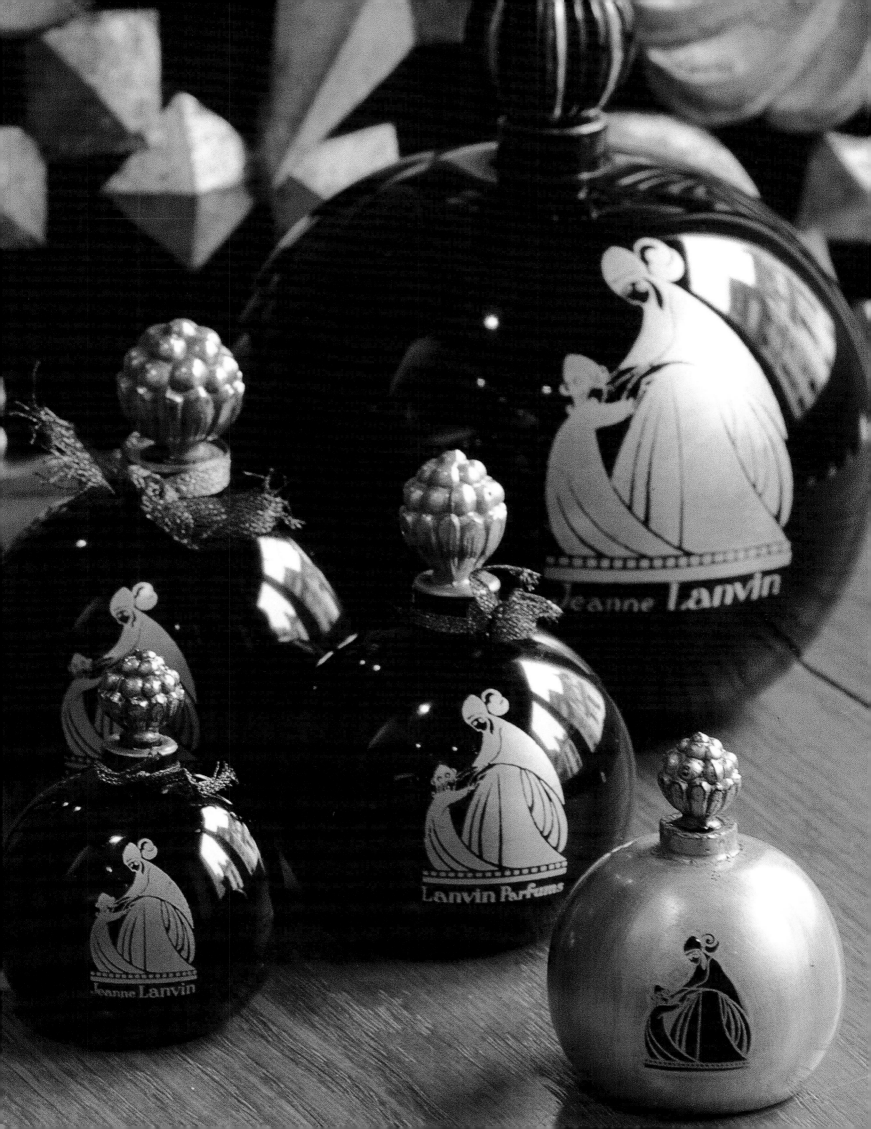

THE PERFUME
BOTTLE: IMAGE OF A MAKE

From the 1950s, the designer's approach was radically modified by changes in the perfume industry. Perfume lost its exclusive and elitist associations and gradually became an important commodity. Whereas in the past it had been the attribute of ladies of doubtful reputation, it became more intimate and more easily available, aimed at attracting people with very different personalities from all walks of life. Perfumers became more and more interested in the desires and needs of both men and women. Creating a perfume became a more subtle, structured process, carefully thought through at every stage. This was the beginning of the marketing era. Henceforth all perfume companies wishing to create a new product had to ask themselves who their clients were and how they should be approached.

The perfume bottle was invested with new value. Whether in department store windows or in magazines, it had to be eye-catching and enticing. The whole spirit of the brand was condensed into a few cubic inches of glass or crystal. The bottle had well and truly become a product of communication and general consumption, combining genuine aesthetic qualities with economic requirements. Perfume had to be charming, attractive and, of course, reasonably priced.

The question was how to reconcile the aesthetic with economic considerations, how to bridge the gap between the purely artistic domain and that of industrial production. This delicate task was put in the hands of specialists, designers whose training revolves around these two factors, the mastery of both the aesthetic and the technical aspects involved in the mass production of art objects.

The technical constraints confronting artists at the turn of the century were nothing compared to those now imposed on contemporary creators. The industrialization of production methods and profitability are at the center of all modern creations, and in order to continue producing perfume bottles of which they can be proud, designers are constantly obliged to find new methods to circumvent the limits imposed on them.

François Coty had sensed the importance of the role of these creators when, in 1934, he entrusted the creation of perfume bottles to Pierre Camin, who had been trained at the École Boulle, Paris's prestigious decorative arts college. The same is true of Armand Petitjean, the founder of Lancôme, when he chose Georges Delhomme, who had also worked with François Coty, as artistic manager and bottle designer, a responsibility which he held for many years. Apart from Chanel, who still employs an "eye", Jacques Helleu, who spends his time creating, supervising and improving the company's public image, and Guerlain, who, in 1974, entrusted Robert Granai with the creation of the perfume bottles and the packaging of other beauty products, nowadays most bottle designers are independent and work for a variety of companies. They are the privileged interlocutors and translators of the fashion designer's or perfumer's ideas. Unlike the artist, who imposes his personality and his style on his work, the bottle designer remains

Extremely precise drawings are necessary for the creation of a perfume bottle. These dimensions enable the glassworker to create the mold for elegant perfume bottles, such as Valentino pour Homme, created by the designer Pierre Dinand (opposite).

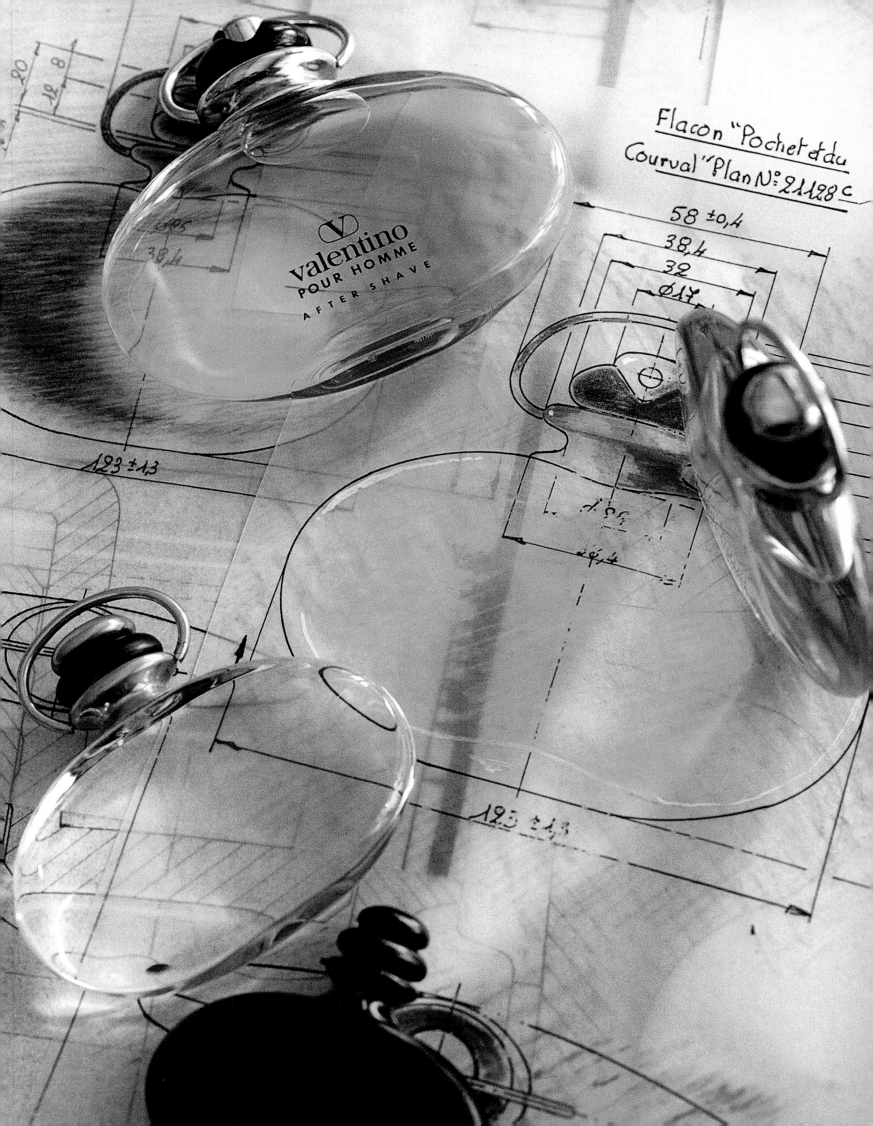

backstage. As one designer, Joël Desgrippes, remarks, "A bottle designer puts his talent at the service of a creator or a make, in order to be able to create an object which suits their style and their image."

Today, a handful of designers, for the most part French, are responsible for bottle production the world over. For thirty-five years now, Pierre Dinand has been designing exceptional perfume bottles for the most famous fashion houses, including Yves Saint Laurent, Givenchy, Valentino, Armani and many others, seeking to translate their unique style, personality and spirit. Of his three hundred and more perfume bottles, he is particularly attached to Opium, the result of a fascinating collaboration with the fashion designer Yves Saint Laurent, for whom he designed the bottle in the form of an *inro*, a small Japanese tobacco box, which he lacquered in rich colors. He is also fond of two perfume bottles he designed for Calvin Klein, the American fashion designer: the polished sensual form of Obsession, and the contrasting geometrical purity of Eternity.

The sculptor Serge Mansau is another celebrated bottle designer. He is fascinated by forms found in nature—his sculptures are haunted by the forms of minerals and plants—and his perfume bottles evoke objects accidentally fashioned by the wind and the sea, like the forms he imagined for Kenzo: stones and flowers for Kenzo pour Femme, a wad of leaves for Parfum d'Eté and bamboo tinted by the reflection of water for Kenzo pour Homme.

As for Joël Desgrippes, his fascination for the identity and history of the various makes of perfume led him quite naturally to the creation of perfume bottles. He studied graphic art and likes to create symbolic objects, magical perfume bottles which communicate a company's style and unique personality and character. From a single detail or a particular technique, he is able to build up a powerful image. In this way he created jewel bottles for the jeweler Boucheron, one of which was a ring, the symbol of eternal alliance, hollowed out to contain the perfume and set with a sapphire blue stone. He also created the bracelet for Jaïpur, which is made of no less than thirteen pieces, combining rock crystal and gilt, in the heart of which lies the invisible perfume, like a well-guarded secret.

Be they in Paris, New York, Milan or Tokyo, perfume houses as different and as prestigious as Tiffany, Oscar de la Renta, Sonia Rykiel, Bulgari and Salvatore Ferragamo, as well as stars like Elizabeth Taylor, all place their trust in these designers.

The designer is first given a precise outline of the perfume's intended market, as it is important for him to know what aesthetic and social bracket his product is aimed at, and for what type of woman or man the new perfume is intended. His research begins by trying to enter as fully as possible into the spirit of the make which entrusted him with the conception of its new perfume, and to explore all the subtleties of the designer's or stylist's personality. The techniques relating to other activities with which these perfume companies may be involved can also be a source of inspiration. Everything has the potential to provoke an idea: the famous Hermès scarf, for example, which inspired 24

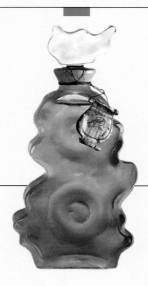

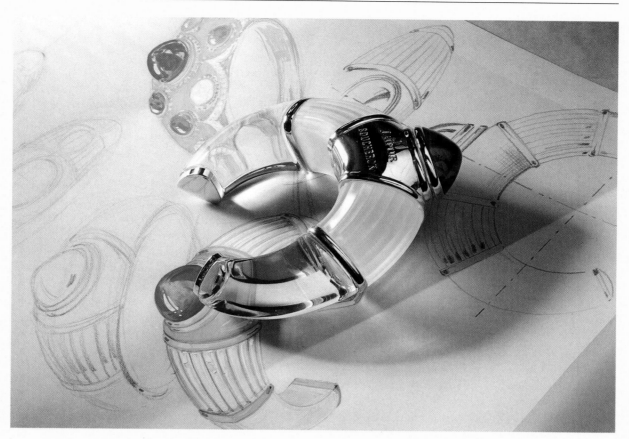

Faubourg, the association of colors and cheerful, baroque materials employed by Christian Lacroix which come together for C'est la Vie, his own perfume; or there again certain jewelers' unique manner of setting precious stones or of using gold and silver. The designer travels all over the world and is constantly looking for new ideas. He is influenced by all trends, by fashions inspired by everyday life and by the tendencies he senses in the air. The designer has to be in touch with the times, because a perfume bottle is always the reflection of current trends. And then there are those objects picked up here and there, like a piece of pottery on the beach, a glass bead in a souk, a piece of wood rubbed smooth by flowing water, or a piece of metal found on the ground . . . the most insignificant object can sometimes be the starting point for a creation.

Gradually the designer's ideas take shape and sketches follow one after the other. Thousands are drawn, some of which are discarded mercilessly, others carefully kept.

This magical form, a symbolic bracelet concealing the fragrance Jaïpur by Boucheron, is the result of the brilliant encounter between the world of jewelry and that of design, between Alain Boucheron and the designer Joël Desgrippes (above), while the bottle for Cantilène by Revillon, designed by the artist Fernand Léger, flaunts a resolutely baroque form (opposite).

Hundreds of sketches of perfume bottles are pinned up on the studio walls—a whole series of silhouettes, colors and materials. Gradually certain forms emerge as being stronger, more powerful and more significant than the others. The designer, assisted by volume specialists, retouches them with almost invisible strokes, modifying a curve, the fineness of the bottle neck, or a fold of the glass: each detail is carefully thought out and measured down to the last fraction of an inch. Prototypes of the designs are produced in foam or plexiglass, which are then proposed to the perfume houses. One model, or maybe more, is singled out: a sphere-shaped bottle, for example, seems to attract particular attention, so it will have to be improved, proportions and certain details decided on, in order to ensure its success. The work and reflection continue for days on end, even nights. The material is sculpted with knives and final dimensions are noted for the glassworkers by means of a caliper rule. After several weeks, maybe months of work, a choice is finally made. This is the one! This is the bottle! It is almost as though the perfume is already shimmering behind its deep, seductive glass walls!

THE BIRTH
OF A PERFUME BOTTLE

Nowadays the majority of perfume bottles are produced by glass manufacturers such as Pochet et du Courval, Saint-Gobain-Desjonquères, BSN or Bormioli and the whole process is completely automated. The demand for perfume bottles has become so great that, in order to adapt to the market, the glass manufacturers have acquired machinery which is capable of producing hundreds of bottles an hour.

The birth of a perfume bottle is always an exceptional moment. Glass blowing by compressed air, a method introduced in the 1930s, followed by the installation of automatic assembly lines in the 1970s, adopted by most of the large glass manufacturers, have revolutionized a trade which, until then, had been entirely manual. Today there is a striking contrast between the huge factories, the technology used, the immense ovens, the deafening din of the machines, the violent, inhuman beauty of the various automated systems and the crystalline fragility of the perfume bottles, which emerge still languid from the heat of the steel molds in which they have been

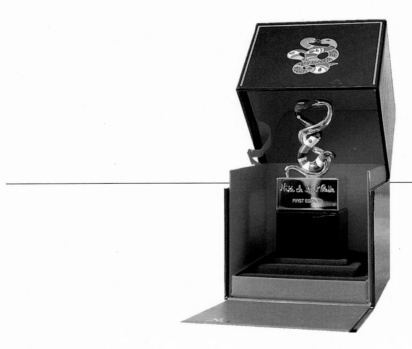

fashioned. The Pochet et du Courval factory is like an alchemist's cavern. A mixture of sand, soda, lime and cullet are melted in the blast furnaces, forming molten gobs which then drop into the molds which mechanically and uninterruptedly release colonies of perfume bottles. These are conveyed through a special tunnel designed to lower the temperature of the glass progressively to prevent it from cracking. Conveyor belts transport them to the various workshops, where each bottle will receive the undivided attention of skilled workers who, with their expert vision and manual dexterity, are responsible for the finishing touches, decorating the bottle with beautifully colored enameling, for example, or adorning it with a gilt motif.

The most highly reputed crystal manufacturers, such as Baccarat, Lalique or Saint-Louis, are always the favorite choice when it comes to deluxe editions, such as the bottles used for extracts, or those issued in limited numbers.

Whereas in Venice the mists and the slow pace of life prepare one for the ancestral skills of the master glassworkers of Murano, it is with some surprise that one discovers the Lalique crystal factory in the discreet little village of Winger-sur-Moden, in Alsace. It is hard to imagine that in these vast, light buildings men and women are in constant contact with molten glass. Earthenware ovens, linked together in a honeycomb pattern, blaze in the ardent gloom and the master glassworkers, with the age-old gestures of traditional craftsmanship, extract, by means of a long hollow rod, the requisite quantity of molten crystal for the perfume bottle. With one breath they blow the exact amount of air required into the molten gob and with a flexible gesture of the wrist they make the bulb expand, gradually thinning the material out until the crystal goes clear. The perfume bottles, as yet untreated, are slowly cooled using water and then conveyed on wagons to the cutting workshops. Some need to be trimmed, some will be polished, while others will be sanded. The workers handle bottles, sometimes weighing more than two pounds, with unfaltering precision and all the while the crystal dust shrouds men and machines in a white veil. A few yards away, in clean, light workshops, women in white overalls trace refined motifs onto the perfume bottles; a paintbrush delicately deposits a drop of blue enamel onto a motif, stoppers are gilded and the undersides of the perfume bottles are numbered and engraved with the Lalique name.

During the entire duration of the various processes, all eyes and hands scrutinize the crystal, watching out for the almost invisible hairline crack which would bring a premature end to the bottle's existence and force it to join the piles of broken crystal near the exist which glisten like mounds of snow.

Alongside the delicate processes used to create these exceptional bottles, glassworkers are constantly improving techniques in order to obtain new colors and forms. Each creation is a challenge. Producing glass of an intense, deep red is not as simple as one might imagine. It is the most difficult color to obtain, especially if one wants it to be warm and generous like the red of the bottle for Venise by Yves Rocher or Guerlain's Samsara. Gradations of color are also extremely difficult to

Paradise and original sin are universal themes which haunt perfumes, like these two intertwined serpents by the artist Niki de Saint-Phalle, symbolizing the bond between beauty and passion (opposite).

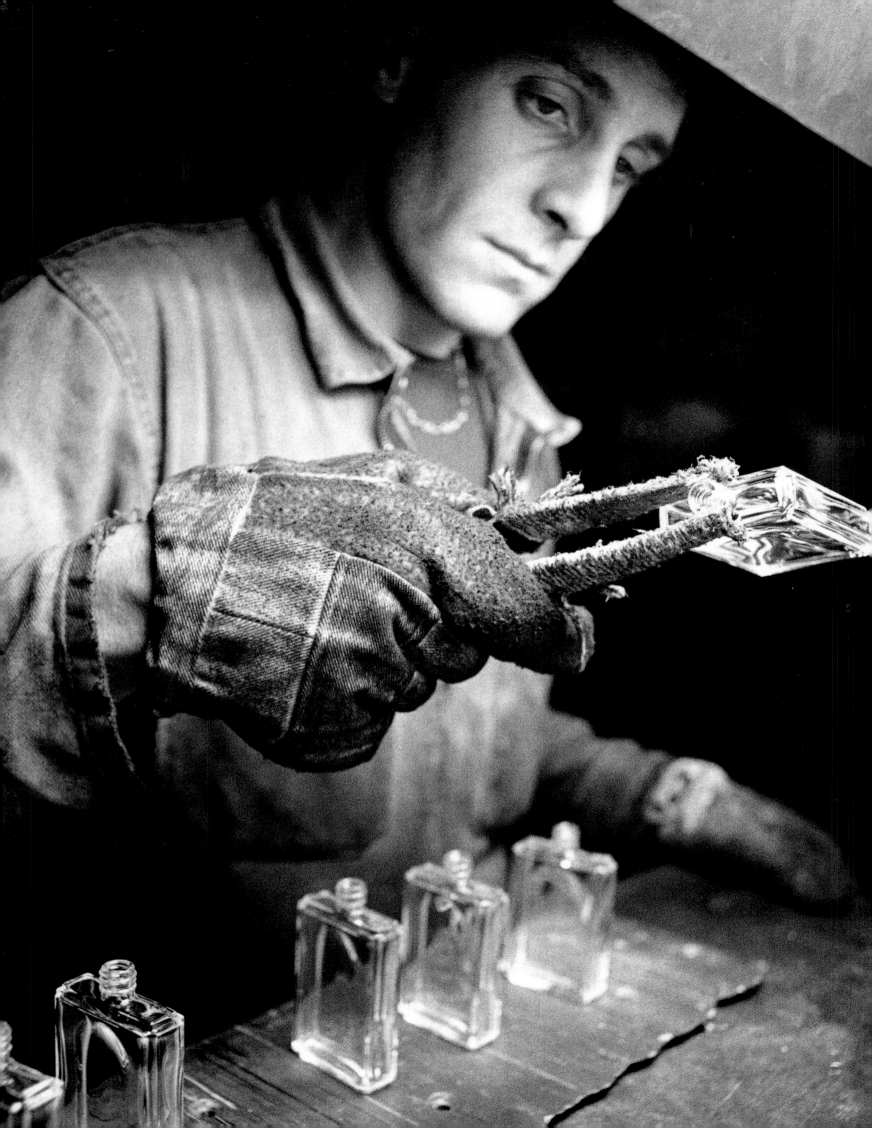

obtain since the pigments have to be distributed in exactly the right quantities through the glass. For this purpose a spraying technique is used which, by covering the bottles with a thin film of transparent or opaque enamel or paint, enables the desired color and effect to be achieved. This was the method employed for Dune by Christian Dior. Glass can also be frosted, as is the case of the bottle for Private Collection by Estée Lauder, or partially frosted, as with Nina, by Nina Ricci. Some perfume bottles, although mass-produced, are nevertheless decorated by hand, like the royal-bees bottle which Pochet et du Courval have gilded by hand for Guerlain since 1853.

Although glass is the only substance which is not denatured or spoiled on contact with the perfume, these bottles make abundant use of skillfully treated plastic or metal ornaments which give them extra beauty. The extraordinary progress made in these domains, notably that of plastics, has led to the development of substances of high quality and great flexibility, the appearance of which is often very similar to that of glass. Metals can also be used in various ways, such as the geometric metal casing on Calandre by Paco Rabanne, the metal flasks containing Cacharel pour Homme or Globe by Rochas, and the metal corset which encircles the bust-shaped bottle by Jean-Paul Gaultier. Sometimes other materials are used, such as the rubber tubing covering Joël Desgrippes' glass perfume bottle for French Line by Revillon.

A few final details still need to be attended to. For the deluxe models, some perfumers, such as Guerlain, Lalique, Nina Ricci and Chanel, still resort to the traditional labeling and sealing techniques, as does Jean Patou, who continues to apply these finishing touches to the bottles for Joy and 1000 in their extract form. In the company's premises in Levallois, just outside Paris, the bottles are cleaned using alcohol and air before being filled with perfume. Each stopper is then adjusted individually, by hand, by the emery technique, i.e. adjusting the ground glass stopper to the bottle neck by friction, in order to obtain a perfect fit. The neck of the bottle is then covered by a fine, damp, membrane made from animal intestine called a *baudruche*, which ensures that it is perfectly airtight. A gold thread is wound around the membrane and tightly knotted. The perfume bottles are then adorned with bows, ribbons, pendants or tassels which are tied round the bottle necks like scarfs, giving them a charmingly attractive appearance. Finally, they are placed in presentation boxes, which in turn are protected by cellophane.

The presentation box, whether for a prestige model or for general consumption, plays a decisive role. It must be eye-catching so as to stand out from the hundreds of closely packed boxes on the store shelves. A whole universe of color, materials and graphic style is compressed into a few square inches. The important thing is that the packaging is seductive, as for Guerlain's L'Heure Bleue, which is romantically set in imitation woven straw, for Safari by Ralph Lauren, in its impression of crocodile skin, the evanescent flowers of Cacharel's Anaïs Anaïs and the oriental minaret of Nuits Indiennes by Jean-Louis Scherrer. Sometimes the box is so beautiful or so much part of the perfume bottle itself (like

Nothing is too beautiful to contain perfume. In the creation of a perfume bottle each gesture counts, and great accuracy of vision and sleight of hand are necessary to attain such perfection. This glassworker (opposite) controls each perfume bottle as it emerges from the furnace.

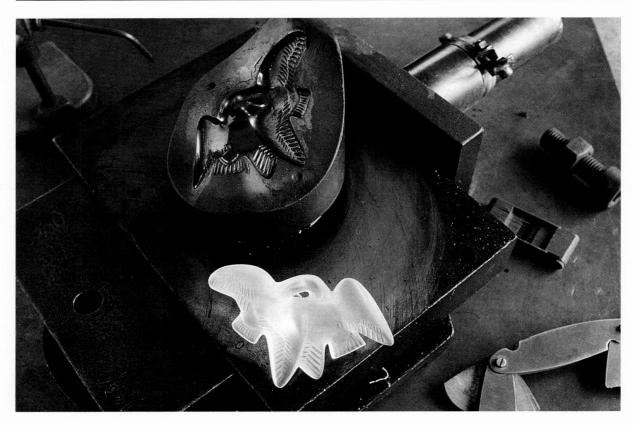

Jean-Paul Gaultier's "food can" and the plexi-glass cube for Montana's Parfum de Peau), that one is loathe to throw it away. Sometimes soft, rustling tissue paper is placed between the box and the bottle, like the calyx around Kenzo, or the paper around Amazone by Hermès, folded using origami techniques to look like a scarf.

Perfume bottles have always reflected the fashions and fantasies of the day. The 1970s, for example, witnessed the triumph of geometric forms and the use of new materials; the 1980s introduced asymmetry, deconstructed forms and new, artificial materials and colors; the 1990s, galvanized by the approach of a new millenium, are dominated by a baroque spirit of fantasy and fun.

Nowadays, if there are universal codes which dictate a bottle's style each country is nevertheless governed by its own particular aesthetic tastes. In the Middle East opulent forms and rich materials are in favor, whereas in Japan they prefer simple, natural forms. As for the Russians, they remain faithful to traditional scenes, with characters and landscapes inspired by their country's cultural heritage.

When crystal meets steel, when a refined substance encounters the industrial universe, the result can be an object as fragile and precious as these intertwined doves, who tenderly protect L'Air du Temps by Nina Ricci (above).

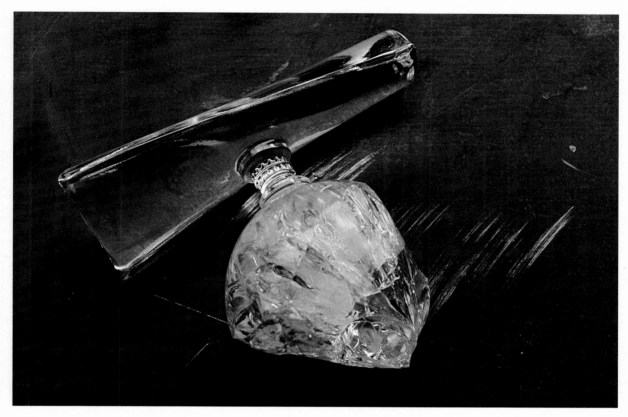

The universe of the trademark, its history, its particular style and its evolution are represented by signs and symbols easily identifiable by the consumer. The bottle for Givenchy's Fleur d'Interdit, with its delicate motifs, puts the accent on transparency and softness. Like a ruby red moon, the bottle for Guerlain's Samsara evokes a conscious, asserted femininity. Romantic, love-struck women will be attracted to Kashâya by Kenzo, with its iridescent bottle in the form of folded leaves, the stems at the top attached by a narrow strap forming the stopper, evocative of hidden secrets. Men with a pronounced classical style will tend towards the traditional, masculine bottle of Paco Rabanne pour Homme. Femininity and high fashion are represented by cascades of draped material, as in the case of the magnificent Diva by Ungaro. The very young will eagerly outstretch their hands for Petit Guerlain or Babar by Shao-Ko. The most refined will look towards the jewel bottles by Van Cleef and Arpels, Cartier, Bulgari, Tiffany and Boucheron, which illustrate their own particular style, a mixture of precious materials, rigor and purity of forms.

Perfume bottle stoppers are miniature works of art which are modeled with extreme care. This stopper has just emerged from the furnace; the rough base will be sectioned, shaped and polished so as to fit perfectly into the bottle neck (above).

A PASSION FOR COLLECTING

It is not without a certain satisfaction that the designer observes the increasing number of perfume bottle collectors. Nowadays most perfume lovers systematically keep the bottles of the perfumes they purchase, while others become collectors. Formerly a perfume was the affair of a lifetime. Standing imposingly on the dressing table, the bottle became the image of a person, it epitomized their personality. A person 'became' Femme by Rochas, Arpège by Lanvin or Pour un Homme by Caron.

Over the last ten years or so the number of perfumes we use has multiplied. Hence, no doubt, the desire to hoard them up in order to demonstrate the various subtleties and facets of our personalities. In this way, a woman can state she is classic like N° 5, changeable like Tocade by Rochas, with its yellow, green and red stoppers, or a femme fatale with Estée Lauder's Youth Dew. Keeping bottles is also a way of recalling events from the past, as each one carries within its crystal walls memories of distant landscapes, tears or laughter.

Collecting perfume bottles is a game which is easy to get caught up in. Someone who owns a bottle of Lancôme's Trésor, for example, might little by little try to acquire all the models, from the miniature to the extract. Or they might receive Jean Patou's Colony, created in 1938, as a gift, and suddenly find themselves wanting to possess all the perfumes which reflect that bygone age—which can still be found in the Jean Patou boutique in Paris. As soon as a new perfume is launched, perfume lovers are on the lookout for it. One woman actually admitted to us that she collected all the new extracts as they come out.

Some amateurs collect the Boucheron ring and bracelet bottles, which they carefully keep in their presentation cases. Others make secret gardens out of the stones, leaves and bamboo of Kenzo's bottles, while still others compose fantasy landscapes with the interlaced snakes in brightly colored enamel by Niki de Saint-Phalle. The Jean-Paul Gaultier addicts try to collect all the corsets in their various shapes and colors. Others amuse themselves by composing perfume meals with Azzaro's Oh La La! champagne glasses, or the raspberry, mandarin and cherry-colored bottles of Nina Ricci's Deçi-Delà. The stars on Thierry Mugler's bottle for Angel dazzle and reflect in the collectors' eyes, enticing them to create whole constellations of them.

There is a great attraction for perfumes which were at the center of a scandal, like the bottles for Champagne by Yves Saint Laurent, on which the forbidden name was concealed by a stroke of red lipstick. Limited and numbered editions, created to mark exceptional events, are immediately snapped up. Caron celebrated the centenary of the Statue of Liberty with a Baccarat crystal perfume bottle representing the famous statue enclosed in a gilded cage representing the scaffolding which surrounded it during its restoration. One thousand copies of Jean Patou's Normandie, created in 1935, have recently been produced, while Ungaro's Diva celebrated its tenth birthday by gracing its bottle with a stopper in ruby-colored crystal. Every Christmas, Paloma Picasso's perfume dons a new outfit, once taking the form of an amphora mounted on a gilt stand; Eau d'Hermès was brought out in a

Régine de Robien's boutique is popular with collectors of flacons, in particular those created by Lalique, for example Cyclamen by Coty, Narkiss by Roger & Gallet, Au cœur des Calices by Coty, and Le Corail rouge by Forvil (opposite).

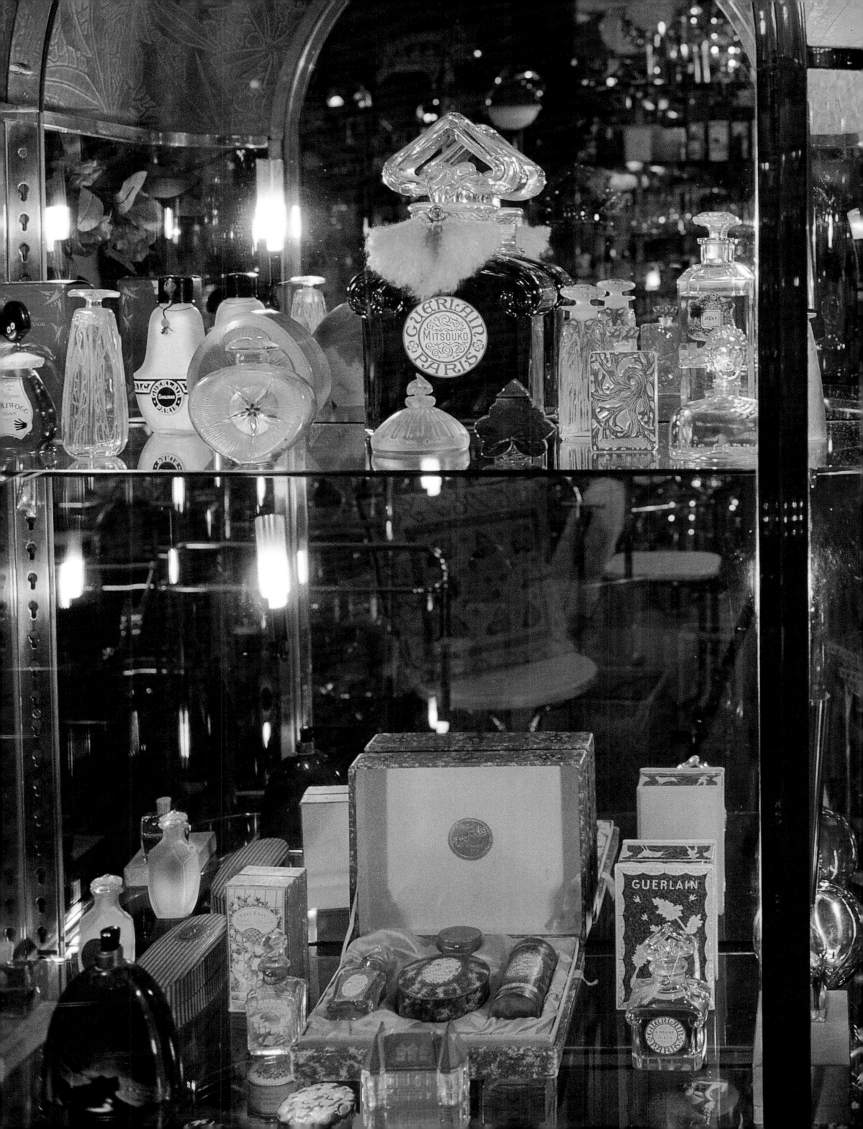

Baccarat bottle engraved with a horseman; the doves on Nina Ricci's L'Air du Temps took on a new color, and Diorissimo returned to the wonderful Baccarat crystal bottle surmounted by a bouquet of flowers in gilded bronze which had been created for it in 1956. Then, of course, there are the sheer follies for the very wealthy collectors, such as the Boucheron ring, which the jeweler produced in a luxury version—a dizzying combination of gold and rock crystal with a blue-lacquered stopper, set with diamonds and four pear-shaped sapphires.

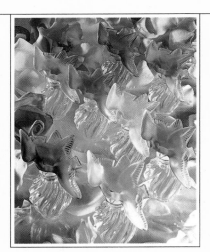

The fascination for contemporary perfume bottles is linked to the discovery of their predecessors and it is to Régine de Robien, an interior decorator and bottle collector, that we owe this recent craze. About fifteen years ago, in the vicinity of the Saint-Sulpice church in Paris, she opened her boutique, Beauté Divine, offering a whole universe of toilet articles. It was an immediate success. For the first time perfume bottles that everyone remembered, but that no-one had thought of keeping, were on show in a store window. Some collectors discovered with delight the dream-like bottles of Paul Poiret, Caron and Schiaparelli, testimony to a little-known, forgotten art. In 1986, the first perfume bottle auction took place at the Hôtel Drouot and Régine de Robien was appointed expert. Prices rose and collectors got carried away. Perfume manufacturers who, by ignorance or negligence, had squandered their heritage, tried to buy it back. Real treasures were discovered,

such as Roger & Gallet's Partir, a perfume bottle in the form of a compass card in a presentation case representing a galleon, and J'appartiens à Miss Dior by Christian Dior, a bottle representing a dog sitting on a yellow cushion in its superb case in the form of a kennel. Other examples were the beautiful Lancôme bottles in their presentation cases conceived in the style of stage sets, like Marrakech, created by Georges Delhomme, a bottle encircled with gold thread standing out against a palm tree décor, Kypre, in its case reminiscent of oriental cloisonné enamel, and Spoutnik, a delicate opalescent bottle in the shape of a moon.

Who could resist the charm of Elsa Schiaparelli's Roy Soleil, a perfume bottle designed by Salvador Dali representing a sun decorated with little gold flames enclosed in a golden conch shell, or the humor of Snuff, a pipe-shaped bottle nestling in its box on a bed of wood shavings, or of Zut!, two pretty legs allegedly belonging to Mistinguett revealed by a dress which had slipped to the ground, or of Sleeping, a Baccarat bottle in the form of a candleholder with a candle and a red flame serving as a stopper, or there again of Shocking, a glass bust with a tape measure knotted around it?

Perfume bottles also appeal to our love of the exotic and the mysterious, like Chu-Chin-Chow, a round-faced Chinese man sitting cross-legged, created by the perfumer Bryenne, or the Chevalier de la Nuit by the perfumer Ciro, representing a torso in opaque

A designer's audacity is reflected in the perfume bottles he creates: to collect them is to preserve the expression of this incredibly refined, daring, and often witty form of creativity for future generations. Nina Ricci, for example, celebrated the success of L'Air du Temps—which continues to make hearts beat ever since its creation in 1948—by giving the bottle's famous doves new colors (above).

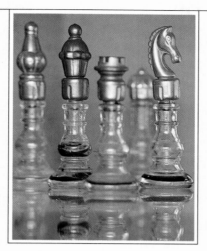

black glass topped by a plume. The Orient transmits its poetry and exoticism to Kobako by Bourjois, a bottle decorated with chrysanthemums in a Bakelite case with a black base, to Subtilité by Houbigant, a Baccarat buddha complete with gold ring and to Isabey's Bleu de Chine, a lantern-bottle decorated with an enamel floral design in a case guarded by a mandarin surrounded by dragons.

Well-informed collectors have good reason to be jubilant. Chanel N° 5's bottle has been modified five times since its creation in 1921, admittedly almost imperceptibly, but nevertheless sufficiently to prevent it ever going out of fashion. Miss Dior brought back a bottle dating from 1945, the year of its creation, and both the perfumes and bottles of Balmain's Vent Vert and Soir de Paris by Bourjois have been radically transformed, although still keeping a certain spirit of the past.

Many collectors have become involved in something which started out as a mere hobby. Perfume bottles have become Madame Jolanda Gallarotti's unique passion. She lives in Switzerland and has a collection which numbers several thousand. She is particularly interested in the crown-shaped bottles created by Prince Matchabelli, a perfumer of Slav origin who was very successful in the United States, and she has assembled several hundred of his bottles in all different sizes and colors.

"The further you progress in a collection," explains Francis Touyarou-Grabe, a designer for Nina Ricci and also a fervent collector of perfume bottles, "the more demanding you become and if at the outset you tend to buy somewhat indiscriminately, you soon realize your mistakes." Ideally, of course, all collectors want to find the sealed bottle in its presentation case, but it can happen that they come across something exceptional and in that case there is no hesitation. Francis Touyarou-Grabe's fetish perfume bottle is the sphere-shaped form of Arpège by Lanvin in turquoise-colored Sèvres porcelain, of which only one hundred were produced.

Sometimes collection mania takes a hold of perfume bottle designers, as is the case of Joël Desgrippes, who began by bringing together a few picturesque bottles from the 1960s, including the amusing Avon perfume bottles representing themes from life, like the wedding couple. He finally took to frequenting antique dealers and salesrooms, favoring poetic bottles reminiscent of forgotten emotions.

As Régine de Robien points out, although perfume bottles have recently entered the sacrosanct domain of antiques, collecting them remains first and foremost a question of the heart. Rediscovering bottles of bygone days has brought the value and quality of contemporary creations to the attention of the general public. It has also had the effect of underlining the aesthetic value that perfume represents today. Perfume has everything needed to captivate and seduce us for many centuries to come!

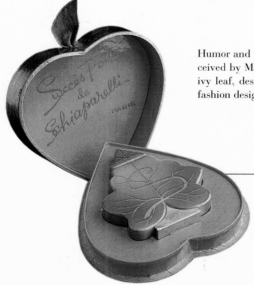

Humor and poetry are no strangers to perfumery, as illustrated by this chess game conceived by Mary Chess in which the pieces are perfume bottles (above), or this ceramic ivy leaf, designed in 1952 by the artist Peynet for Elsa Schiaparelli, the great Italian fashion designer and friend of the Surrealists (opposite).

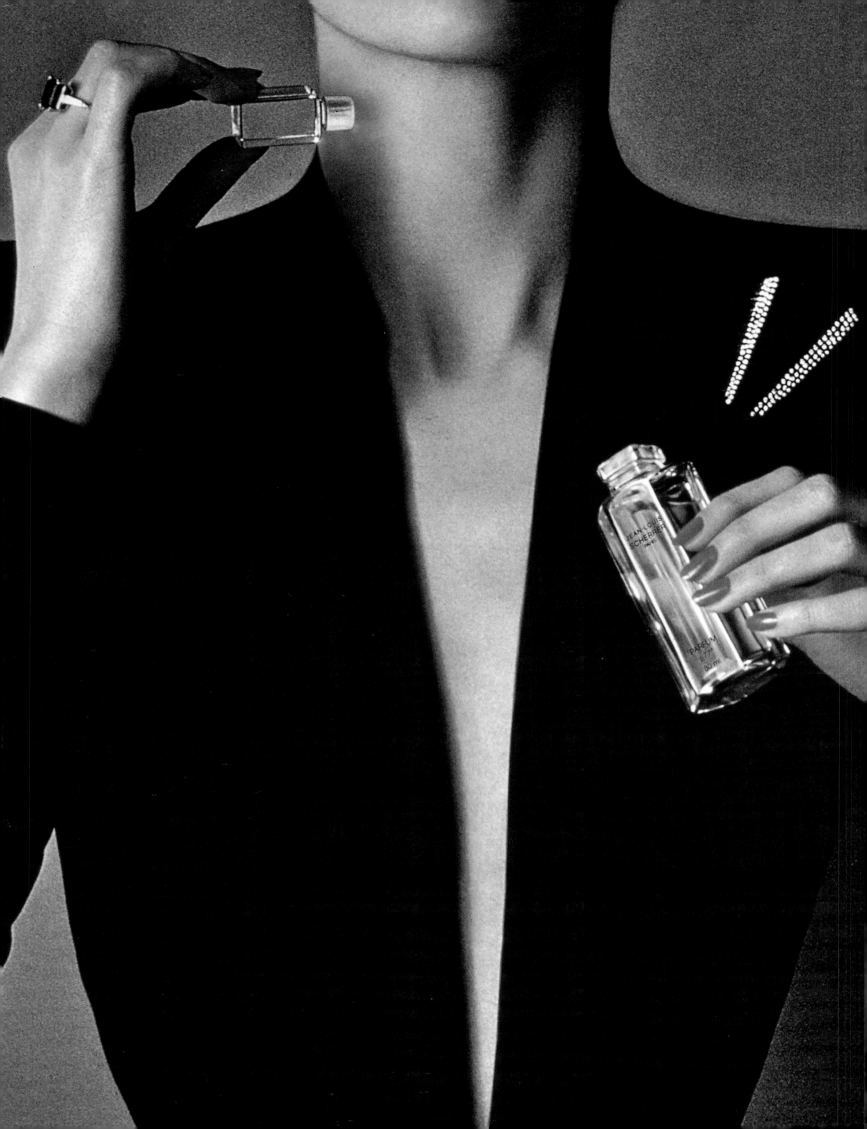

· THE ·
IMAGE
OF
PERFUME

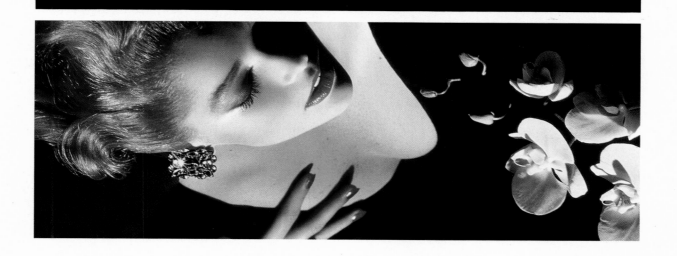

What words are capable of capturing the inexpressible subtlety of perfume? What images can portray its irresistible, elusive charm? The challenge seems impossible and yet it must be met. Perfume is not merely an odor, it is a universe which concerns the imagination as much as the senses, the wish to dream as much as the wish to be noticed. The language of perfume is made up of a series of codes, signs, words and images—created by advertising, magazines, photographs and films—which open onto the world of dreams, romance and fantasies.

Once again Mademoiselle Chanel bent over the blotter strips she held in a fan between her fingers, then, indicating the one her perfumer, Ernest Beaux, had dipped in the fifth phial, she exclaimed, "That's the one, I shall call it N° 5!" Why that particular number? Was it, as some people suggested, to do with a childhood memory, that of the strange mosaic design patterned with numbers which decorated the floor of the boarding school where Coco Chanel had spent her adolescence? Certainly, Coco never denied being superstitious. In any case, the number five seemed to augur well; the perfume was launched on May 5, the fifth day of the fifth month of the year. One thing is certain, within the space of a few seconds, "the exterminating angel of the twentieth century" as the writer Paul Morand called her, had propelled perfume into modernity.

NAMING A PERFUME

Until the arrival of N° 5, perfume names had centered around the languorous semantics of two main themes: flowers and love. The floral inspiration seems all the more obvious since flowers, the raw material of perfumery, evoke a whole symbolic system around the themes of virginity, virtue, innocence and chivalry, reproduced in the language of flowers which, though lost in part now, was familiar to women in the past. To receive Les Paquerettes by Roger & Gallet, was to hear "I dare not love you," and to offer Victor Vassier's Violetta Tatiana suggested innocent love. Around 1910 everyone was crazy about three of François Coty's perfumes, namely Rose Jacqueminot, Muguet des Bois (lily of the valley) and Jasmin Corse. One of Godet's perfumes is called Envois de Fleurs (sending flowers) and one of Guerlain's first perfumes, Jardin de Mon Curé (my vicar's garden). Houbigant owes his first big success to Quelques Fleurs and Caron to Narcisse Noir (black narcissus) and to

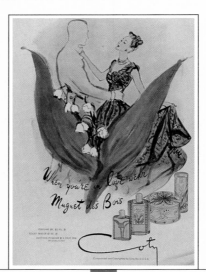

Fleurs de Rocaille (rock garden flowers). This particular trend might seem somewhat outdated and yet it still inspires perfumers, from Nina Ricci's Fleur de Fleurs and Guerlain's Les Jardins de Bagatelle, to the latest perfume by the American fashion designer Carolina Herrera, christened quite simply Flore.

No other domain cherishes the theme of love more than that of perfume. Perfume is the partner to the senses, the favorite attribute of romantic

François Coty, who opened a boutique in New York as early as 1913, exported all his perfumes to the United States. This publicity drawing for an American magazine praises the powers of the fragrance Muguet des Bois, created in 1936, and suggests, "When you're in love wear Muguet des Bois!" (above). Whether one chooses to exalt the fragrance, as in this advertisement for Jean-Louis Scherrer's first feminine perfume (page 180), or this photograph revealing the sensuality of Yves Saint Laurent's Opium in 1984 (page 181), the objective is the same: to create an image that has force.

women and seductresses and the first gift that lovers exchange. It is the indelible symbol of past love affairs and follows the cultural trends of seduction. The first decade of this century celebrated the raptures of innocent love, for example, Premier Oui (first yes) by Arys, Guerlain's Pour Troubler (to arouse), Baiser Suprême (supreme kiss) by Monna Vanna and Vertige (dizziness) by Coty. The perfumes of the twenties exalted the inconstancy of love with Amour-Amour and Adieu Sagesse (farewell wisdom) by Jean Patou, Flirt by Pinaud and Roger & Gallet's Miss Flirt, whereas the double meaning of Lubin's Ouvrez-moi (open me) and the invitation of Eteignons Tout (put out all the lights), skillfully skirt round the dictates of prudishness. In the 1920s, the Fionet establishment dared to launch a perfume called Jouir (meaning both "to enjoy" and "to climax"), to which the prestigious American magazine *Harper's Bazaar* gave ample coverage and which subsequently inspired the title of a novel by Paul Marguerite. In 1991, Estée Lauder's Spellbound brought the apparently obsolete tenderness back into vogue, and inspired a proliferation of romantically named perfumes which, as in the case of Eternity by Calvin Klein or True Love by Elizabeth Arden, seemed determined to exorcise the sensual excesses of the preceding decade.

Poison by Christian Dior and Obsession by Calvin Klein, the two great successes of the 1980s, were not the first, however, to fish in the troubled waters of seduction. In France, the fashion designer Paul Poiret (yes, Poiret again!) was the first to venture into this domain with Fruit Défendu (forbidden fruit). In America, until the 1940s perfume was daring and wicked, and it was with a taste for scandal that Adrian, fashion designer to the Hollywood stars, launched Sinner, inspired by Jeanne Lanvin's My Sin. That was followed by Fabergé's Aphrodisia, Scandale by Lanvin, Tabu by Dana and Givenchy's L'Interdit (forbidden). The perfume by Guy Laroche, J'ai Osé (I dared), is a contemporary of the French women's liberation movement and the protests of May 1968. By daring to use the name of a forbidden substance, known to provoke a state of ecstasy, Yves Saint Laurent's Opium went one step further, restoring a sultry and provocative aura to perfume which it had, to a certain extent, lost.

The name of a perfume is not only there to identify or reflect a fragrance and provide a taste of what is to come, but it must also fan the consumer's desire, liberate their fantasies and carry them away, like a concert, a film or a novel, so as to let them experience the ecstasies of a Baudelaire, who stated, "As other souls to sea on music go, / Mine, o my love! upon your scent sails on." From the outset, perfume has never ceased to explore the themes of exoticism and escapism. What could be more appealing or evocative than imaginary lands and untrodden plains? Many perfume names draw their inspiration from this repertoire, such

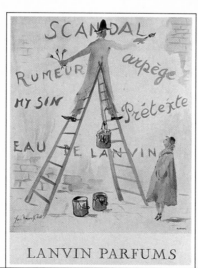

In 1949, Lanvin published a publicity booklet about perfumes entitled *L'Opéra de l'odorat* (opera of the sense of smell). Colette wrote a sensual preface devoted to the fragrances of her childhood and Louise de Vilmorin contributed a series of delightfully impertinent poems, illustrated with much humor by Guillaume Guillet (above).

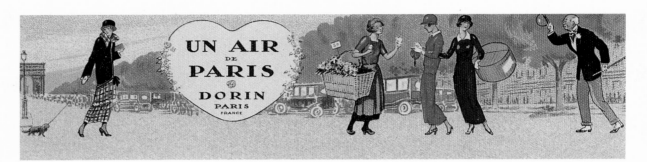

as Caron's Yatagan (a Turkish saber), Farenheit by Christian Dior, Paco Rabanne's Ténéré (a desert in Algeria) and Safari by Ralph Lauren. From the nineteenth century, with the influence of Orientalism which inspired so many painters, the magic of the Orient literally made perfumers' fortunes. Fashionable women flocked to the opening night of *Madame Butterfly*, their furs scented with Roger & Gallet's Jade or with Kobako by Bourjois. Shades of the Orient appear all through Guerlain's history. The perfume called Liu reminds one of Princess Turandot's unfortunate slave from Puccini's opera. Mitsouko was inspired by a popular novel, published in 1919, which tells the story of a love affair between a Japanese girl and a British naval attaché during the 1905 Russo-Japanese war. The name Samsara is taken from Sanskrit and means 'the way of wisdom'. And what does it matter if Babani's Daimo does not figure on any map! The most beautiful paradises are imaginary. Nowadays, 'away' is not so far away and holidays in Asia have become almost commonplace. Perfume, however, upholds the exotic, glorifies far-off lands, encapsulates myths. Estée Lauder's Cinnabar, Byzance by Rochas, Jaïpur by Boucheron and Kenzo's Kashâya still make us dream!

The alluring image of the French capital, which has long been hailed the center of elegance and pleasure, appealed not only to Yves Saint Laurent—he dedicated a magnificent rose bouquet named Paris to the city—but also to several of his predecessors. In 1919, the perfumer François Coty created a fragrance called Paris which was intended for the English market, followed later by Guerlain's Paris Nouveau and Lancaster's Mademoiselle de Paris, presented in a glass Eiffel Tower. There were other tourist routes, such as Avenue Matignon by Rochas, Rue de la Paix by Guerlain and Rue Royale by Molyneux, all names which reveal the perfumers' international ambitions. In this respect, the success story of Soir de Paris by Bourjois deserves a mention. Nothing predisposed the Bourjois establishment to producing perfumes, since it was known for its makeup and more especially for its compact face powder. They set up an office in New York and from there contemplated how they might conquer the American market. The solution was not going to be simple, since competition in the makeup sector was fierce. So why not with perfume? The American perfume industry was still nonexistent and the "Made in France" label the height of prestige. They decided to launch a perfume

Whereas Un Air de Paris, created in 1921 by the Dorin perfume house (above), is forgotten today, Soir de Paris, launched just eight years later, is still the signature perfume of the Bourjois company (opposite). This magnificent spray of Bulgarian rose, tuberose and powder-scented carnation made its entry in astonishing cobalt blue livery with harmonious curves. The bottle for the extract was rapidly joined by a range of fragrances in bottles of various sizes as well as a line of makeup products (opposite).

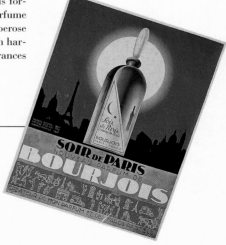

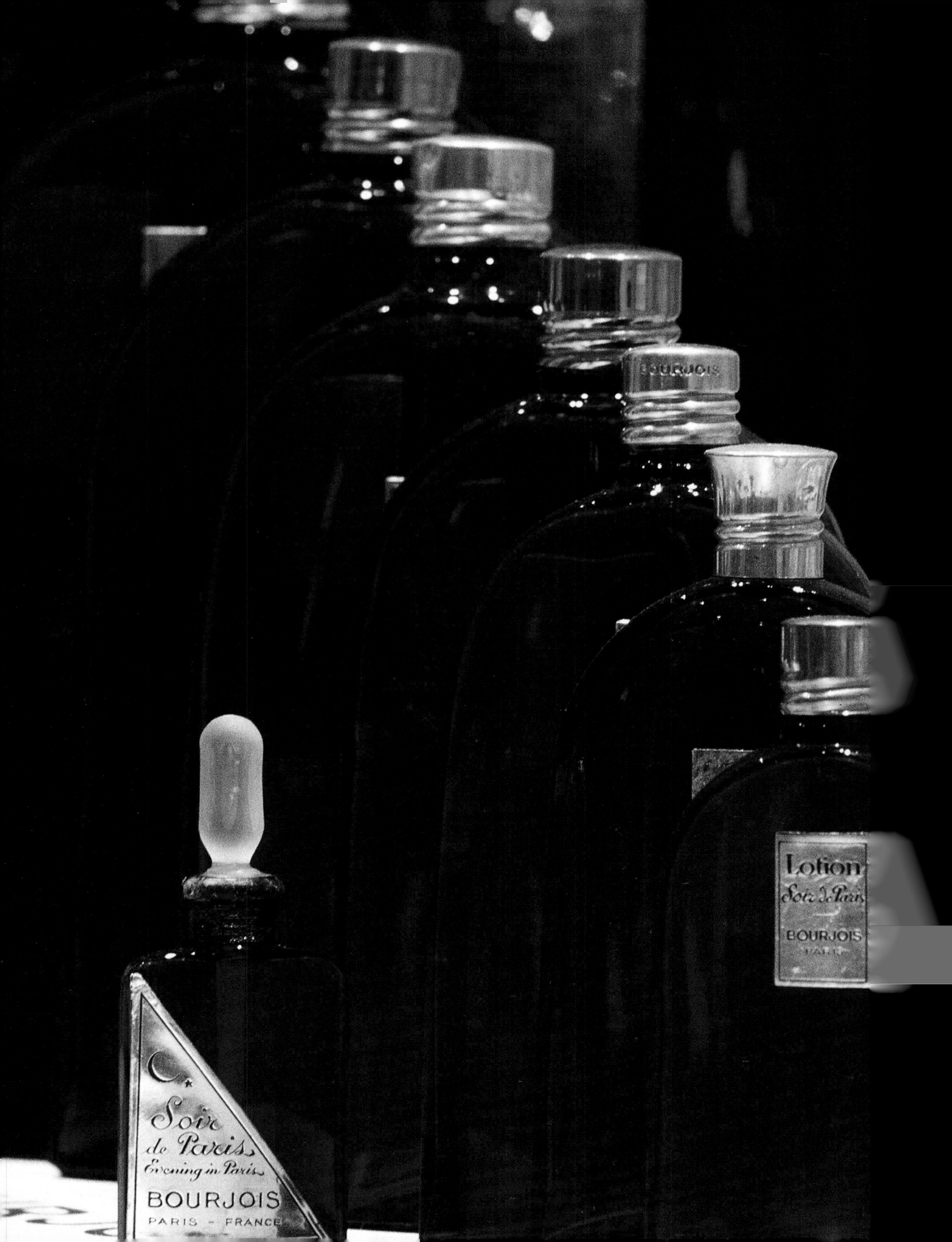

which was sufficiently Parisian to attract the Americans, for whom the French capital evoked visions of luxury and refinement, and yet sufficiently American for them to be able to feel familiar with it. The result was Evening in Paris (only when it was launched in Paris did it become Soir de Paris). The means employed to ensure its success were considerable, especially for the time. There were posters portraying a mythical Paris and perfect Parisian women, special offers, a limited series of presentation cases in which the perfume was accompanied by miniature replicas of Parisian monuments, not to mention Marcel Carné's film *Quai des Brumes*, which consecrated the perfume in 1938 by showing the hero Jean Gabin giving it as a gift to Michèle Morgan, his leading lady.

"Perfume," says the fashion designer Pierre Cardin, "is a memory which never fails." It does indeed mark the memorable events in life, for a fragrance is always there to remind one of first meetings, romances or weddings. It is hardly surprising, therefore, that certain perfumers had the idea of launching "commemorative perfumes." Financially, this was a clever move since it saved on the cost of promotion which was provided by coverage of the event the perfume was celebrating. With his perfume Normandie, Jean Patou celebrated the inaugural crossing of that magnificent transatlantic liner on May 29, 1935. For the occasion, the bottle, in the shape of a steamship, was offered to all first-class passengers. Today, the same bottle is a

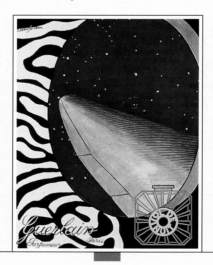

rarity much sought after by collectors. Patou did not stop there; Vacances reflected the elation following the granting of the first paid vacations for workers in 1936. One should also mention Vol de Nuit (night flight) by Guerlain, which was conceived in 1933 as a tribute to Antoine de Saint-Exupéry and the Air France company created the same year. The much awaited liberation of Paris was fittingly celebrated in 1945 with L'Heure Attendue (the awaited hour) by Jean Patou and Nina Ricci's A Cœur-Joie in the following year. In 1956, while the young jet set were swinging their hips in the cellars of Saint-Germain, the perfume company Scarlet, now forgotten, brought out Cha Cha Cha, and the Marquay company, which has also sunk into oblivion, changed the name of one of its perfumes from Coup de Feu to Rock-'n'-Roll.

The fact remains that creations such as these, perfectly in harmony with their day and age, run the risk of becoming outdated in a relatively short space of time, whereas all perfumes in fact aspire to handing their name down to posterity. As a result, some perfume names are not connected with any particular period or atmosphere, but exert their charm merely by their sonority, such as Balahé by Léonard, Habanita by Molinard and Vivara by Pucci. Others, like Escape by Calvin Klein and Wings by Giorgio Beverly Hills, evoke the intangible quality of perfume. There are also those which trace the pattern of the sun, moon and stars across one's memory. The daylight shines in Lumière (light)

The smoked glass perfume bottle for Guerlain's Vol de Nuit, with its cut-off corners and propeller motif, is an intrepid invitation to travel (above). Caron's perfume En Avion is magnificently represented in this 1945 poster, inspired by the exploits of the aviator Jean Mermoz (opposite, left). Originally the perfume was to be called Carlingue; however, the name was considered incompatible with Caron's international ambitions, as underlined by this poster of the *Normandie* liner (opposite, right). Worth perfumes also dominated the 1930s. For Dans la Nuit, René Lalique created an astonishing star-spangled, midnight blue perfume bottle, which was later used for Je Reviens (opposite, bottom).

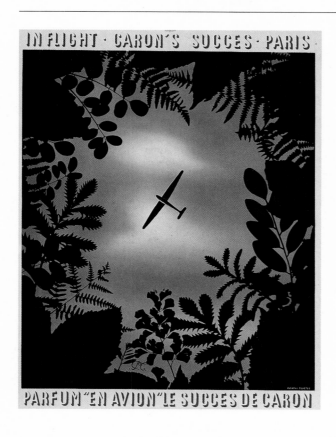

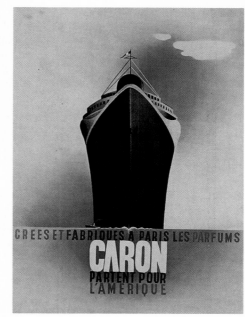

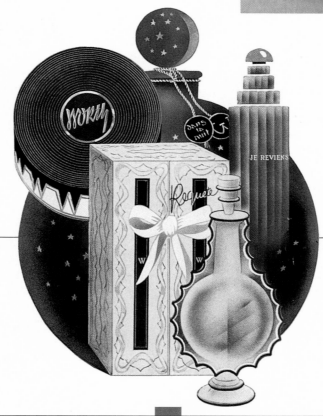

by Rochas, Jour (day) by Féraud and Clair de Jour (daylight) by Lanvin, counterparts to those vibrant perfumes which pay tribute to the magic spells of the night, that theater of attractions and transgressions which exhales the fragrances of nature and bodies and inspires perfumes which evoke rare moments stolen from ecstasy, such as Nuit de Noël (Christmas night) and also Nocturnes by Caron, Lancôme's Magie Noire (black magic), Nombre Noir (black number) by Shiseido, Dans la Nuit (in the night) by Worth, Ungaro's Ombre de la Nuit (shadow of the night) and Karl Lagerfeld's Sun Moon Stars.

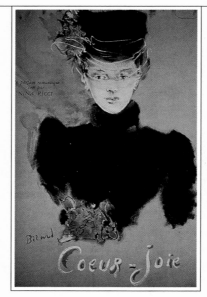

Poles apart from these mysteries, there are those names which float lightly like soap bubbles, like high-spirited retorts, such as Ciao! by Houbigant, Elsa Schiaparelli's three perfumes Zut!, Snuff and Shocking!, Christian Lacroix's C'est la Vie!, Loris Azzaro's Oh La La! and Nina Ricci's Deçi-Delà, a mischievous reference to the famous melody from André Messager's opera, *Véronique*. These are playful names that ring out like an exclamation, easy to remember and to pronounce in other languages and, above all, charmingly enticing.

Finding a name for a perfume nowadays can be something of a problem. Gone are the carefree years when Caron could name one of its creations Royal Bain de Champagne, without bringing down the wrath of the corporation of that celebrated beverage, as the Yves Saint Lau-

rent perfume company discovered. Today, names, from the most attractive to the most commonplace, are the subject of complicated regulations and protective measures. Companies now exist which register names, terms and expressions with the unique aim of selling them later at exorbitant prices. The registration of copyright, which was initiated to combat the abusive use of well-known trademarks, has become a source of profit for shrewd people who are quick to register a name which they think the prestigious brands are likely to buy. If registering a name is a relatively costly process, the purchase of a name can cost up to $200,000! By means of a data bank, it is possible to verify whether the name has already been registered. If that is the case, the interested party is obliged to direct their research along other channels, a

Nina Ricci's first perfume, A Cœur-Joie, was launched in 1945. The artist Christian Bérard, who designed the first poster, seems to have been particularly inspired by the exquisite femininity of this fragrance (above), whereas the drawing evoking Royal Bain de Champagne, a perfume created by Caron for a Californian millionaire, simply shows the perfume bottle, which is an exact replica of this festive beverage (right).

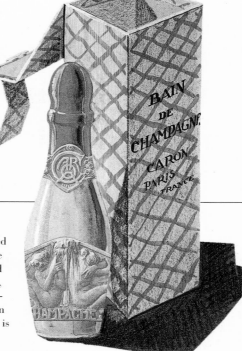

process which can take months. All things considered, using one's patronymic, or even a simple initial, like Y by Saint Laurent or KL by Karl Lagerfeld, provides an attractive solution, frequently adopted by famous fashion designers and creators, which helps to make their name known to a wide public and allows them to export it without the problems of translation. In this day and age, successful perfumes can be found all over the world. They require a name which is easy to pronounce and remember, and above all one which does not suggest any ambiguity, as is the case of Guerlain's Samsara, which in some Middle Eastern countries means an easy woman. It is easy to understand why certain perfume manufacturers resort to the computer, which from one single word, enables one to obtain about one hundred others with the same syllables and sonority—which was how, from the French word *mariage*, Givenchy found the name Amarige.

Perfume slogans first appeared at the turn of the century and were at the root of the success of certain perfumes such as "Joy. The costliest perfume in the world . . ." The slogan, a distinctive phrase or motto, acts on the subconscious and is conceived to stimulate desire and encourage people to make purchases. The creator of slogans, the key man in publicity agencies, is a virtuoso of sonorities and innuendos who endeavors to establish a bond between the product and the consumer, to stir up desire by

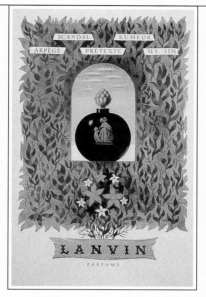

creating an atmosphere of intimacy. For example, "Opium. Sensuality to the extreme"; "Miss Dior. Definitely very Dior"; "Wings. Set your spirit free." Humor and play on words are very welcome, such as, "When he's lost his heart and then his head, the French say he's . . . Insensé," and "Angel. Beware of angels . . ." The fashion designer Yves Saint Laurent, who was prevented from christening his perfume by the name of Champagne, mischievously called it his "Tribute to the woman who sparkles!" Some put the emphasis on rhythmic names, while others place the accent on mystery, such as "Incognito. The fragrance of intrigue." There is no such thing, however, as a miracle solution. The slogans one remembers are often the simplest, for example, "Pour Monsieur. Elegance is timeless" and "Eden. The forbidden fragrance."

FROM THE POSTER TO FASHION DESIGN

When God created Adam, he first created his eyes, the mirrors of the soul and the windows onto the world. Of our five senses, sight seems to us to be the most precious, the most immediate, the most important, yet in the end it is the most misleading, for under the pretence of appealing solely to our reason, it surreptitiously sets our imagination in motion.

"Arpège, a musical perfume, offering a bouquet of fresh and warm notes. A prodigious success, it evokes both flowers, fruit, fur and leaves," wrote Louise de Vilmorin, a great admirer of this particular fragrance. A picturesque image which no doubt inspired this poster for Arpège, printed in 1946 (above).

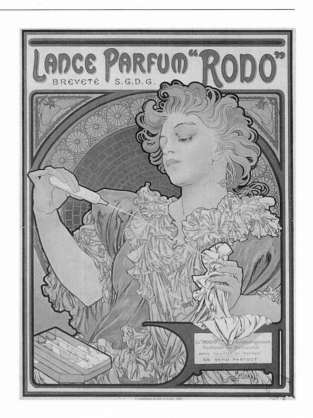

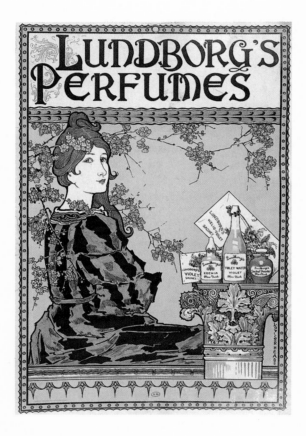

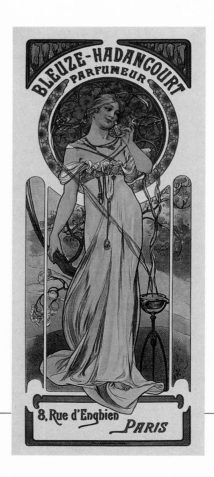

Very early on, perfumers realized all the advantages that images could offer them. Associating perfume with a particular image is to give it personality, make it more attractive, even before its fragrance has been inhaled. The commercial poster made its appearance around 1830 in the form of a small, black-and-white lithograph, intended, at the outset, for new literary publications. The first perfume labels, conceived at the same period, represented flowers and portraits of romantic women. They were only a few inches high and the printing was sometimes of inferior quality.

It was Jules Cheret, born in 1836, who was destined to become the future father of the modern poster, which was to give perfume a much wider public. He was a lithography virtuoso and developed new presses which could produce large format prints, in color, at reasonable prices. His workshop printed about a thousand posters which adorned the building site hoardings for Haussmann's vast Parisian renovation program. The *Belle Époque* is considered to be the golden age of posters and the Czech artist, Alphonse Mucha, as one of its most talented representatives. He was publicity designer for the actress Sarah Bernhardt and the first poster he created for her was drawn in a characteristically exuberant design of pastels and curves. In 1898, the perfumer Rodo asked him to design a poster extolling the merits of his "perfume launcher," a sort of syringe for rapidly perfum-

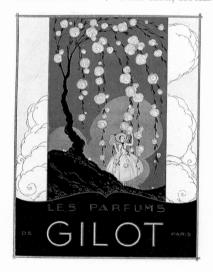

ing linen. In 1900, the perfumer Houbigant entrusted Mucha with the decoration of his stand for the World Fair. It caused a sensation and it was not long before all the celebrated perfumes of the period took to using posters. Sometimes the popular woman/flower theme inspired allegorical scenes, sometimes more familiar settings portraying a woman sitting at her dressing table putting on perfume. In 1905, or thereabouts, Leonetto Capiello, the Italian caricaturist, created his first posters for the Daver perfumes. His sense of humor and distinctive style of drawing brought new life to poster art which was to dominate the profession for nearly twenty years.

The 1920s witnessed the decline of poster designers in favor of fashion artists. Top-quality perfumes were in vogue and advertisements began to appear in women's magazines, in the form of charming little scenes composed by the favorite artists of the fashion designers, such as Sem and, notably, Paul Iribe, who sketched Paul Poiret's, Jeanne Lanvin's and Coco Chanel's most beautiful models for *La Gazette du Bon Ton*. Later on Salvador Dali and the painter Christian Bérard took an interest in the medium and they created some memorable advertisements for the Italian fashion designer, Elsa Schiaparelli. Schiaparelli worked mainly with Marcel Vertès, a painter of Hungarian origin who illustrated Colette's novels and whose unrestrained style, marked by his humor and candor, brought a new freshness

Perfume posters reflect the main pictorial trends of the time. This poster for the Gilot perfume house, which was creating perfumes in the 1920s, shows the stylistic influence of Art Deco (above). This is a far cry, however, from the opulent allegories of *La Belle Époque*, the undisputed leader of which was the artist Alphonse Mucha, who designed this advertisement for the Rodo "perfume launcher." Based on women who are half vestal virgin, half enchantress, his posters elevated perfume to the status of a sacred object (opposite).

to a discipline which had become somewhat conventional.

The real change, however, was brought about by the artist René Gruau. Born in Venice in 1910, his light-hearted vision and his signature flanked by a little star graced the world of fashion and perfume for over forty years. In 1932 he settled in Paris, still going by his original name Renato de Zavagli. He immediately turned towards fashion drawing, signing with the pseudonym of René Gruau. In the 1940s, the fashion designers Pierre Balmain and Jacques Griffe entrusted him with his first perfume posters, but it was with Christian Dior, a childhood friend, that the osmosis proved to be the most complete and lasting. Their collaboration began in 1948 with the birth of Miss Dior. The name had just been found and Dior, wildly enthusiastic, immediately asked Gruau to create the poster for this first perfume, giving him carte blanche to design it as he wished. The result was an image of a swan with a pearl necklace and a black velvet bow tied round its neck. The poster traveled internationally for many years. This was followed by the jubilant

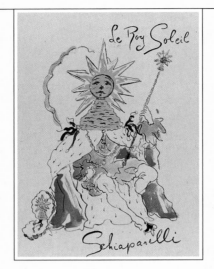

women Gruau created for Diorella and the irresistible man in a white bathrobe for Eau Sauvage. Gruau's talent for sketching dynamic poses, his daring compositions, humor and glamor, seemed immune to the vagaries of fashion. Yet all this was forgetting the increasingly invasive presence of photography. The two most recent Dior perfumes, Poison, followed by Dune, bypassed the honor of having their image created for them by this last ambassador of the charm of illustration.

THE ART OF PHOTOGRAPHY

Nowadays perfume means photographs. Their reign is absolute and undisputed. To charm is to be photogenic. Lanvin, in 1932, was one of the first perfume houses to understand this. Robert Bresson, then a young photographer, took the first photographs of the round, black bottle. The formal beauty of their composition transformed them into genuine works of art. Perfume was elevated to the rank of a sacred object, as is clearly illustrated in another photograph in

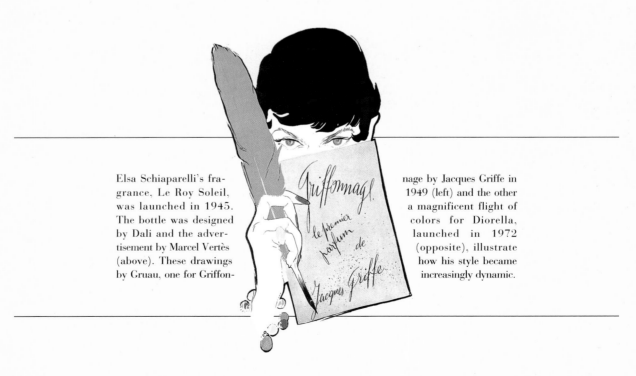

Elsa Schiaparelli's fragrance, Le Roy Soleil, was launched in 1945. The bottle was designed by Dali and the advertisement by Marcel Vertès (above). These drawings by Gruau, one for Griffon- nage by Jacques Griffe in 1949 (left) and the other a magnificent flight of colors for Diorella, launched in 1972 (opposite), illustrate how his style became increasingly dynamic.

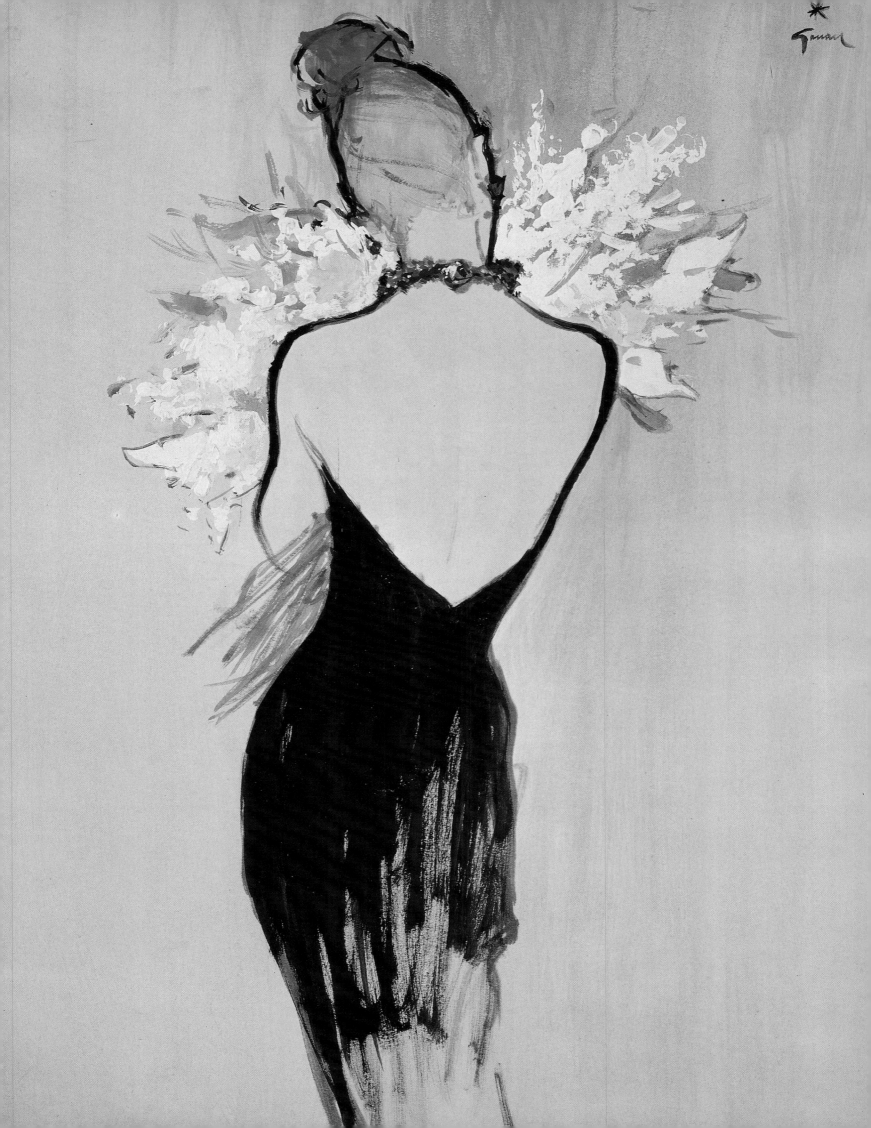

which the bottle is held by the hands of a woman whose face is invisible, a mysterious vestal virgin draped in a garment reminiscent of antiquity.

All the great names in photography have trained their cameras on perfume, including Erwin Blumenfeld, Henry Clarke, Irving Penn, Richard Avedon, David Bailey, Jean-Loup Sieff and Peter Knapp, to mention just a few. Certain associations proved lasting; Yves Saint Laurent's Opium, for example, has been linked with Helmut Newton's glossy eroticism for nearly twenty years. As for Sara Moon and Cacharel, Anaïs Anaïs owes its whole identity to the English photographer's tender yet dynamic vision. Photographs imprint their personality on a perfume. The romanticism of David Hamilton, who, in the 1970s, created the setting for L'Air du Temps, has nothing in common with the more austere vision of the Mexican, Enrique Badulesco, who, in 1993, created the artwork for the publicity campaign for Nina Ricci's legendary perfume, accompanied by a revealing slogan, "Why not move with the times?"

One way of ensuring that a perfume's image keeps up with the changing times is to back new talent. Dominique Issermann is the inspired representative of a group of young photographers who introduced a completely new vision of fashion at the end of the 1980s. She started off by modernizing the romanticism of Nina Ricci before moving on to Christian Dior. Her mission was to update the image of Eau Sauvage, which had, from the outset, been closely associated with the images drawn by René Gruau. The end result was the superb black-and-white photograph of a bare-chested man with a provocative and sensual presence.

The most exemplary case is, nevertheless, that of N° 5 which, thanks to a carefully studied visual strategy, has not aged at all. Jacques Helleu, Chanel's art director since the 1960s, was inspired by the famous retort given by Marilyn Monroe when asked by an indiscreet journalist what she wore in bed. She replied: "Chanel N° 5." What greater seal of approval could a perfume wish for than the heartfelt utterance of a world-famous film star? From then on, Chanel decided to make N° 5 the modern attribute of the ideal woman by associating it with role models who were famous either for their beauty or for the roles they played in movies. The idea was to choose a new woman for every era, international stars who incarnated the dreams of seduction of women from all over the world. In 1965 they chose the actress Ali MacGraw, who became famous with the film Love Story. In 1968, it was the turn of the cover girl Lauren Hutton, in 1970 Jean Shrimpton, the oracle of the pop years, followed by the French film star Catherine Deneuve from 1967 to 1977. Since 1986, they have turned to another French actress, Carole Bouquet, and the top model Claudia Schiffer. The image of Chanel N° 5—the silhouette of a star in the hands of master photographers such as Henry Clarke, Irving Penn, Richard Avedon and Helmut Newton—has succeeded, just as its creator had always wanted, in providing a consistent reflection of modernity.

Until the 1960s, publicity photographs portrayed perfume in all its splendor in the rigorous perfection of a still life, or the impeccable glamor of women in studied poses. They offered no social code except one of luxury, represented by a mink stole or a dress by a famous designer.

In contrast to Anaïs Anaïs, Loulou appeals to the more audacious and strong-minded woman. Launched by Cacharel in 1987, Loulou—a gentle litany of musk, heliotrope and vanilla—diffuses an assertive yet pure sensuality. The English photographer Sara Moon associated it with this face which seems to tremble as if awaiting a kiss (opposite).

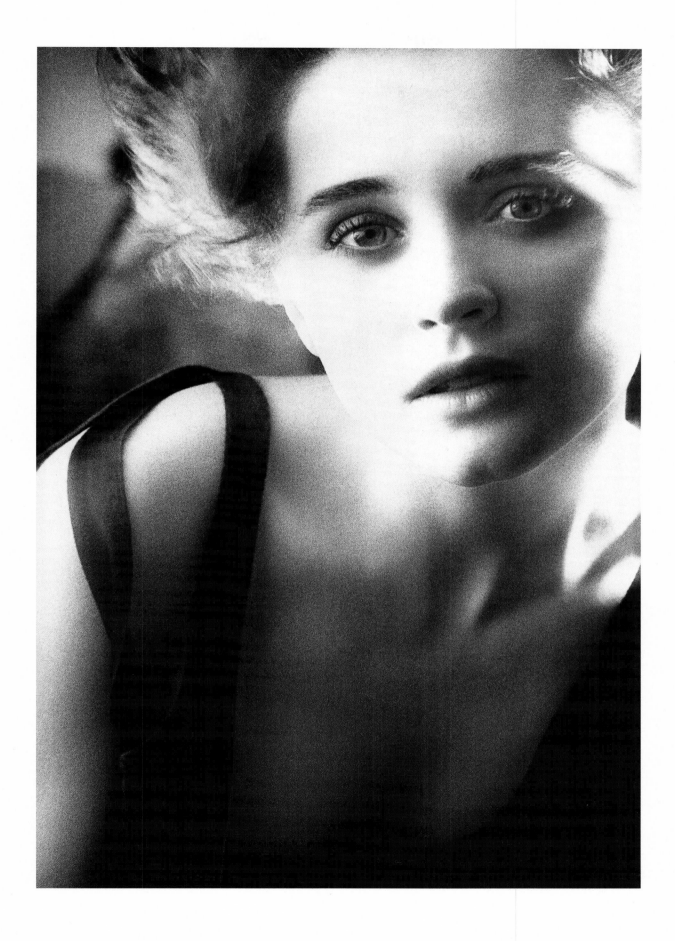

Everything changed in 1971 with Yves Saint Laurent's publicity campaign for the launching of his perfume Rive Gauche. The photographs portray the sort of young, lively and cheerful women one sees in the street—independent, liberated women who, according to the slogan, are "unpredictable." Perfume became a reflection of its age, of the collective aspirations of an era. It was no longer a mere accessory to seduction, but a testimony of its time. It was an attitude, a choice of lifestyle. In the 1970s and 1980s, a style of advertising, based on the concept of representing a "slice of life," became generally accepted. It presented a variety of images of men and women based on a few stereotypes, such as the sporty type, the insolent woman, the romantic, the adventurer, the seducer, etc. With Fidji by Guy Laroche and the image of a naked woman on an island, a sort of modern Eve clasping the perfume bottle as a mother would clasp her child, perfume went beyond outward appearance to delve deep into the female subconscious, portraying a somewhat idealistic vision of femininity which reconciles mistress and mother and tender and passionate love.

"Without perfume, skin is speechless" proclaimed a publicity campaign run by the Comité Français du Parfum, illustrated by the photograph of a naked man and woman in a passionate embrace. The body is good for sales: the body of a star, the perfect body, muscles as hard as a rock, radiant curves enthroning a perfume, the sanctuary of the bosom where the love elixir rests. An image of ritualized, excessive virility is also popular, as in the first publicity campaign for Drakkar Noir by Guy Laroche, which shows a perfume bottle clenched in a man's fist on which a woman's hand lavishes a suggestive caress. Calvin Klein had already shocked America with his publicity campaigns for his fashion designs, one of which showed a woman in jeans on top of a lion, which provoked an angry reaction from the Women Against Pornography association. He caused offence again with his first perfume, Obsession, launched in America in 1985, which used a photograph showing a naked couple on a swing. Sometime later a photograph for another campaign dared to show the revels of a woman with two men.

Can eroticism maintain its provocative force in a society which renders nudity and the sexual act commonplace? Once the force of desire has worn itself out with so much banality, what language is left to be used? One solution is to resort to derision and humor, using the clichés most commonly associated with virility, seduction and luxury. To promote the perfumes Coco, Egoïste and Egoïste Platinum, Chanel gave carte blanche to Jean-Paul Goude, the provocative and controversial organizer of the bicentenary celebrations of the French Revolution in 1989. The choice was a courageous one since there was a risk that Jean-Paul Goude might tarnish the company image by violating the unwritten codes which ensured its prestige. Yet he brought great enthusiasm and talent to the project. For the perfume Coco, he dressed the young actress Vanessa Paradis as a bird swinging on a perch in a cage, while for Egoïste Platinum, he poked fun at men by portraying a man boxing against his own shadow, and for Egoïste he showed an arrogant lady's man hounded by his past conquests. The gamble paid off: the derisive messages did not go unnoticed and had a most salutary effect on sales.

"A perfume is nothing without skin, it is the encounter between the two which is magical," states Giorgio Armani, the Italian fashion designer. The publicity campaign for Acqua di Giò was illustrated by this image taken by the well-known fashion photographer Patrick Demarchelier. Its chaste sensuality, reminiscent of drawings by Ingres, is nevertheless very much in keeping with modern times (opposite).

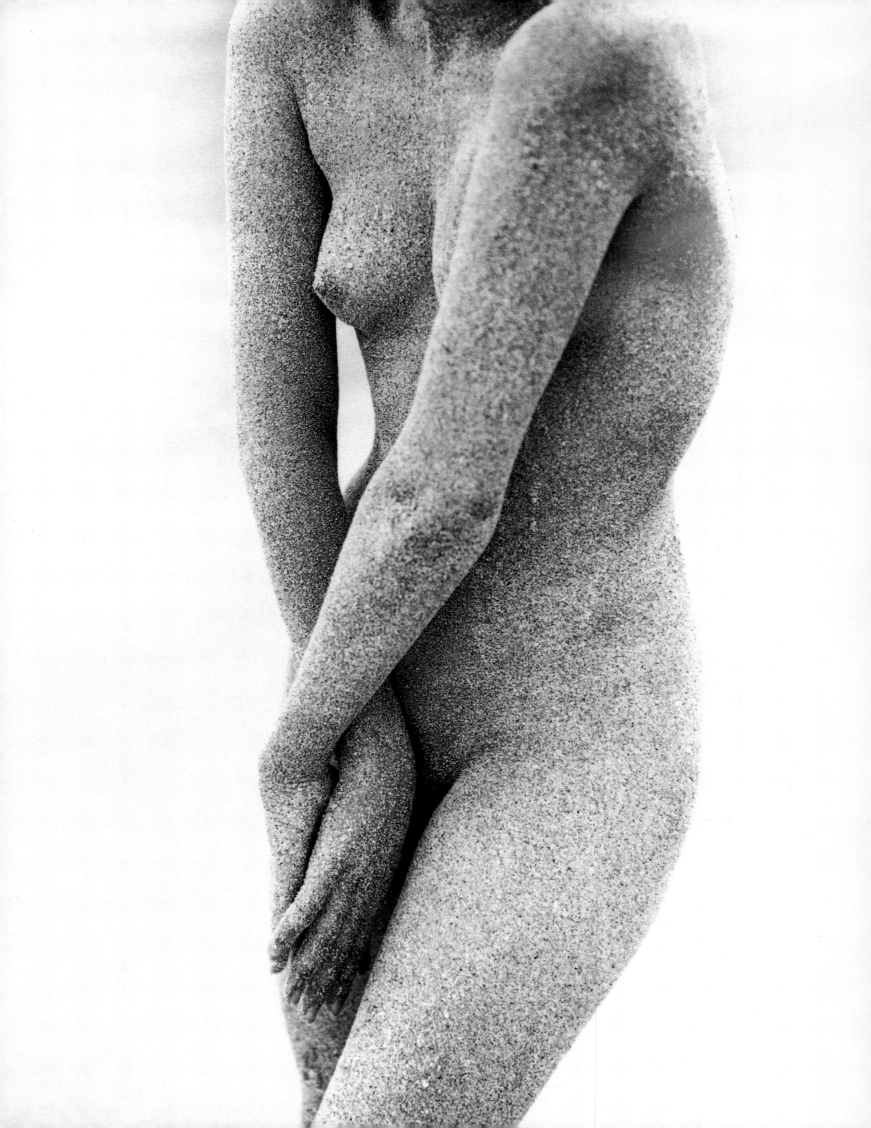

What is the best way of building up an international reputation for a new perfume? If it is by making it known to a maximum number of consumers in a minimum amount of time, then the answer is by making a film. The television advertisement has proved an efficient follow-up to existing forms of publicity. Producing a short film requires an enormous capital which, in the case of a well-known make of perfume, might represent up to 15 percent of its estimated turnover! The aim is to present a lasting image of a new perfume in thirty seconds (the average length of an advertisement). Perfume company art directors will go to any expense—employing shock images, trick effects, extraordinary locations and famous actors—to ensure the success of their latest creation. Fabulous contracts, tailor-made scenarios and colossal budgets are involved as in the case of full-length feature films. The most famous film directors have taken to their movie cameras, including Roman Polanski for Chanel's Antaeus, David Lynch for Yves Saint Laurent's Opium and Giorgio Armani's Giò, Andrei Konchalovski for Byzance by Rochas and Martin Scorcese for Armani pour Homme.

Due to the constraints imposed by the client, some directors disguise their individual professional style, while others have been inspired by their encounter with perfume. There were the special effects and the robots in the film that Ridley Scott, creator of *Alien*, directed for Chanel N° 5. For the designer Jean-Paul Gaultier's first perfume, the photographer Jean-Baptiste Mondino, known for his record sleeves and pop videos, created a fantasy film, with a deafening soundtrack, featuring chattering young beauties and a mystical sixty-year-old woman . . . a disturbing, resolutely new vision which greatly contributed to the success of the perfume.

Publicity films for well-known perfumes are, like the product, aimed at worldwide audiences, something which creates considerable difficulties. Attempts to reconcile opposing tastes and cultures and their various taboos can lead to a rather banal result, unless the accent is placed on emotion, one of the most widespread human values, or on the universality of certain legends, such as the film for Eden by Cacharel, which, to a soundtrack of twittering birds and burbling streams, evokes the sensual meeting between Adam and Eve.

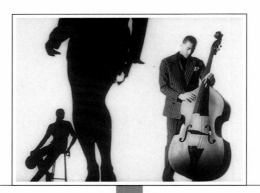

How can the cinema help a new perfume capture the attention of its public? It can draw the viewer into a powerful sequence of complementary images and music, such as the film created by Yves Saint Laurent for the launch of his perfume for men, Jazz.

Although a strategic element of a campaign, the short film is only one of a series of investments. Promoting a perfume involves millions of dollars and budgets are increasing every year. The $17.5 million budget for launching Guerlain's Samsara in 1989 was considered colossal at the time, but is a figure which has long since been exceeded.

Promoting a new perfume involves all forms of media—television, radio, cinema and billboards. The cost of publicity space is becoming more and more expensive due to the increasing number of new perfumes. This has resulted in the widespread use of scent strips in magazines, those narrow bands of paper sprinkled with microscopic perfumed capsules. All one has to do to sample the perfume is to tear the strip out of the magazine and rub it against one's skin. The make Giorgio Beverly Hills initiated this technique for their first heady perfume. The perfume companies' infatuation for this practice has become somewhat excessive in the United States and in some magazines there is a scent strip on every fourth page!

The story of perfume has no end. New fragrances are constantly being brought out, names which will perhaps be the classics of the future. Meanwhile, the prestigious perfume houses continue to work with passion and patience, upholding a delicate balance between tradition and modernity. From one decade to the next, the history of the classic, now legendary perfumes, gains in intensity and mystique. Generation after generation, they attract men and women, giving them a taste of eternity.

There are more words, more images that could be shown, but let us leave the essence of perfume where it is—elsewhere. It is in every home, in every room, in every life, for perfume is, above all, an intimate experience, only revealing its true self when in close contact with the skin, when married with feelings for which it becomes the vehicle and the mirror. Will we be faithful to it? What secrets will we confide in it? What love affairs will it accompany? No-one can predict the full story of a new perfume, but it will certainly involve the soul and the body, the heart and its emotions, the love of life, sadness, the radiance of happy days, reflections of the past, memories, secrets and those elusive feelings which only the subtlest of our senses can unveil.

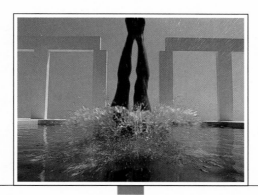

The moving image has become essential for the launch of a new perfume. This film directed by Herb Ritts for Guy Laroche (above) was made for the launch of Horizon. The iris is a key ingredient in great perfumes such as Chanel N° 19 and L'Heure Bleue by Guerlain (page 200). This label was created around 1913 for the eau de Cologne Inoubliable, launched in Moscow in 1864 (page 201).

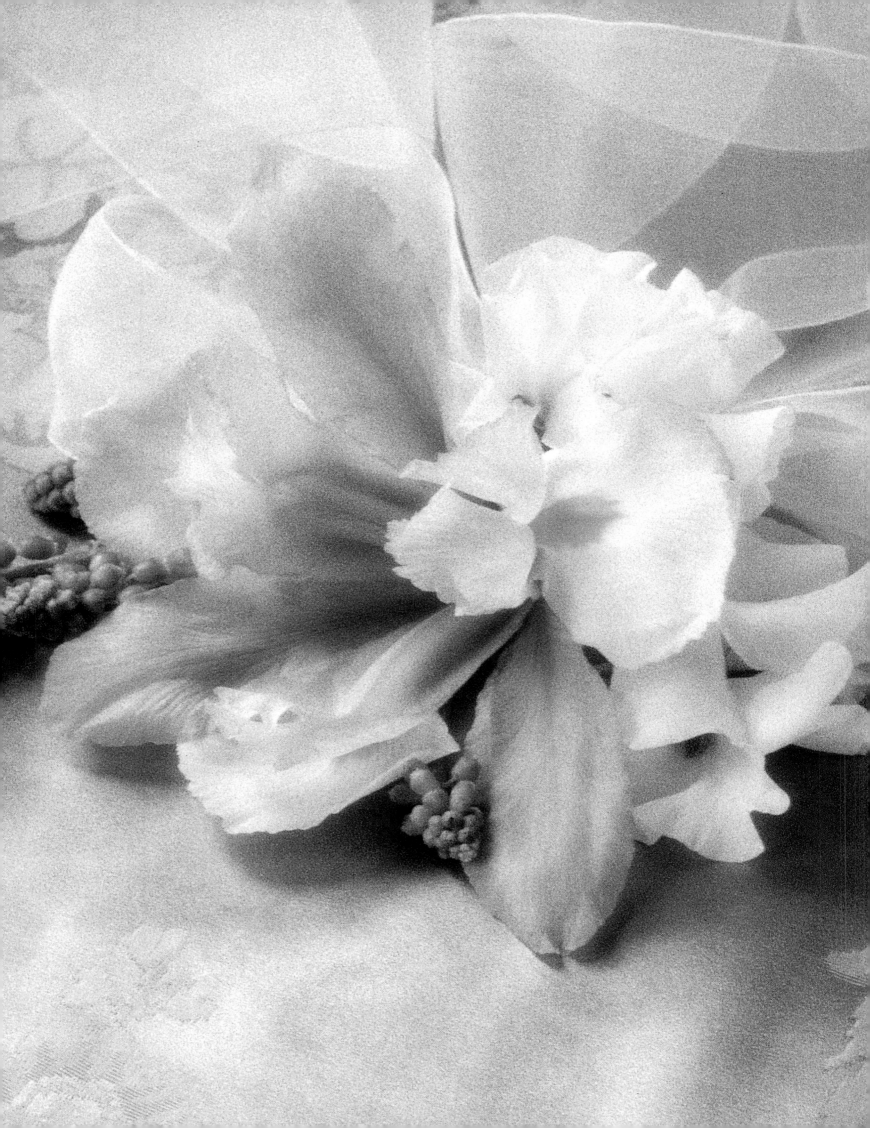

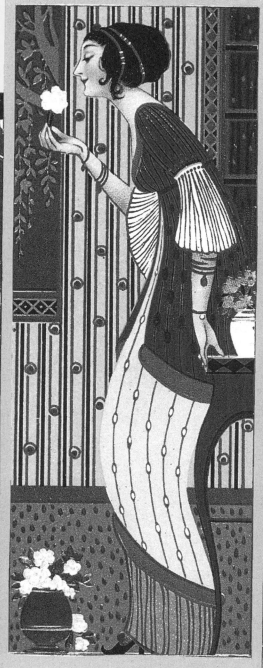

THE CONNOISSEUR'S
GUIDE

SELECTED ADDRESSES

This guide, although not exhaustive, offers practical information on the various aspects of perfumery. The addresses listed have been chosen for their prestige, originality, or simply for their charm and beauty. Our aim is to give perfume-lovers a starting point from which to explore the fascinating world of perfume for themselves.

The reader will find the addresses (in Paris, the French provinces, England, Italy and the United States) of specialized perfume stores, many of which are mentioned in this book, which sell original fragrances with blends different from those usually found in the better-known perfumes on the market. The guide also offers information on where to buy antique and contemporary perfume bottles, and gives the addresses of museums and schools where you can learn about the history and techniques of perfumery, or be introduced to the fine art of the perfumer. In addition to this handy directory, The Connoisseur's Guide contains a list of the main fragrances classified by family, a glossary of terms, a bibliography and, finally, a few tips on how to perfume oneself, that sensual art which endows the body with a little more soul. . . .

PERFUME STORES

The simplest and most obvious places to buy perfumes are department stores and specialist boutiques. Department stores stock most of the well-known brands and each make has a separate stand for its fragrances, staffed by one or more sales assistants specially trained by the manufacturer to advise clients and help them to find the product which suits them best. Customers should take their time and wander from one stand to another, asking to sample the perfumes on blotter strips. If necessary, they should go outside to smell the fragrances in a more neutral atmosphere.

In addition to the department stores, there are a variety of smaller, more specialist boutiques where one can choose a fragrance in a more relaxing environment. Many of these boutiques, especially in Europe, have been around for generations, if not centuries. These smaller premises, often beautifully decorated, make choosing a perfume a real pleasure and allow one to make a selection at leisure in a delightful atmosphere of "pleasure, peace, and opulence."

Paris

ANNICK GOUTAL
14, rue de Castiglione,
75001 Paris. Tel: (1) 42 60 52 82
The various boutiques of this perfumer are like enchanted islands in the heart of Paris. They can be recognized at a glance by the ivory-colored walls festooned with golden ivy and the femininity of the traditional velvet or gold drawstring purses from which emerge the butterfly stoppers

of the 1924 flacon which Annick Goutal has chosen for all her perfumes. Her fragrances contain subtle, lasting blends and are produced using the best-quality raw materials. Sables, for example, is inspired by the flowers which grow wild on sand dunes. Passion, a composition of tuberose, vanilla and jasmine with a strong animal note, is a personal favorite of Annick Goutal's. Her greatest success is Eau d'Hadrien, a symphony of Sicilian lemon, mandarin and cypress.

L'ARTISAN PARFUMEUR
24, boulevard Raspail,
75007 Paris. Tel: (1) 42 22 23 32
The Artisan Parfumeur boutiques, with their opulent emerald and black décor, are reminiscent of a nineteenth-century perfumer's laboratory. These boutiques propose a range of men's and women's toilet waters and spray or heat-diffused room fragrances. The ever-changing range of perfume objects is quite unique, one example being the Boule d'Ambre sculpted by a potter. The toilet waters and home fragrances, such as Mimosa pour Moi, Vanilia, L'Eau de L'Artisan Parfumeur and Parfum de Feuilles, are inspired by scents from nature and various olfactory landscapes. The most popular home fragrance, Mûre et Musc, an avant-garde gourmand perfume, is a subtle combination of sparkling freshness and enveloping warmth. The most promising fragrance, Premier Figuier, created in 1994, also contains audacious accords inspired by the various facets of the fig tree (woody, green, fruity and milky) and is as delicious as cool shade on a hot day.

BOUCHERON
134, avenue Victor Hugo,
75016 Paris. Tel: (1) 47 55 81 87
It was in 1988 that the celebrated jeweler of the Place Vendôme launched its own perfume, a superb floral bouquet enhanced by a sandalwood note, in a magnificent bottle in the form of a ring. Its success led to the creation of a men's fragrance, Boucheron pour Homme, and a second perfume for women, Jaïpur, concealed in the heart of a bottle in the form of a sapphire blue and gold bracelet. These three exceptional fragrances are displayed in a luxurious boutique with crystal showcases and blue lacquered pillars.

JEAN-CHARLES BROSSEAU
26, rue de l'Université,
75007 Paris. Tel: (1) 40 15 98 72
In 1981, this discreet milliner, highly regarded by fashion designers, launched a new fragrance with nostalgic flights of rose and vanilla. Called Ombre Rose, it was an immediate success. Two other perfumes followed, Ombre Bleue, a more summery fragrance, and Ombre d'Or, with a woody undertone. The fragrances only have a limited distribution, so it is best to go straight to the boutique in the rue de l'Université, where they can be found among the hats, berets and other delights created by Jean-Charles Brosseau.

CARON
34, avenue Montaigne,
75008 Paris. Tel: (1) 47 23 40 82
This boutique, one imagines, is how a lady's boudoir at the turn of the century might have been and is one of the most beautiful perfume houses in Paris. Soft lighting enhances the charm of the various toiletries on sale: swan's down powder puffs, lacquered compacts, crystal and opal flacons, sable makeup brushes, dressing table tidies in Sèvres porcelain, to name but a few. The service is friendly and advice readily offered on the perfumes sold exclusively in this boutique, these being Narcisse Noir, Nuit de Noël, Fleur de Rocaille and Parfum Sacré, as well as on the twelve old fragrances presented in antique-style urns in Baccarat crystal and in Art Deco bottles. Some fragrances, such as N'Aimez que Moi, a rose note tinged with iris and violet, created in 1916, and Tabac Blond, composed in 1919, the ancestor of our modern leather note, date from when the establishment was founded. The mimosa note of Farnesiana, created in 1947, and the white flower notes of French cancan, composed in 1936, are extremely popular. At Caron's, choosing a perfume is taken very seriously, which is why they offer to perfume client's scarves or handkerchiefs, so that they can appreciate the fragrance in the comfort of their own home before coming to a decision.

CHANEL
29, rue Cambon,
75002 Paris. Tel: (1) 42 86 28 00
Mademoiselle Chanel founded her fashion house in this outwardly rather austere building in 1910. The upper floors still house some of the workrooms and fitting rooms, as well as her private apartment, which has been left just as it was when she lived there. The ground floor consists of a vast boutique where black lacquer and mirrors form a backdrop to the display of ready-to-wear fashions, beauty products and the various Chanel fragrances. Four fragrances created in the 1920s by the perfumer Ernest Beau, are available exclusively at this address: N° 22, an accord of Provence rose, tuberose and Grasse jasmine created in 1922; Cuir de Russie, a perfume with warm animal notes launched in 1924; Gardenia, a white flower bouquet with a delicate green top note created in 1925; and Bois des Iles, a whisper of sandalwood, tonka bean and vetiver somewhere between bitter almonds and gingerbread, which dates from 1926.

CRABTREE & EVELYN
177, boulevard Saint Germain,
75006 Paris. Tel: (1) 45 44 68 76
This boutique, with its parquet floor and hand-painted floral wallpaper, is fresh and charming. Here one can buy the floral talcs, body lotions and soaps and corresponding toilet waters, all in pretty Liberty-print boxes, for which this English perfume house, founded in 1976, has become renowned. The same floral inspiration is to be found in Crabtree & Evelyn's two fragrances, Gardenia, a heady accord of white flowers, and

the newest creation, Evelyn, which reproduces the fragrance of the Evelyn rose, created specially by the famous English botanist David Austin.

CREED
38, avenue Pierre-Ier-de-Serbie,
75008 Paris. Tel: (1) 47 20 58 02
The Creed family has been composing fragrances since 1760, when an English tailor, James Henry Creed, founded the establishment in London. He was soon supplying Queen Victoria and a multitude of European Royals with his products. In 1853, the Empress Eugénie encouraged him to open a shop in Paris and Creed opened a boutique not far from the Champs-Elysées. Here, in a glass and white marble décor, between two eighteenth-century statues, are displayed Creed's traditional fragrances together with those that he composes from natural essences in his laboratory in Fontainebleau. The formulas are weighed, mixed and macerated in vats and filtered by hand. His most popular fragrances are Green Irish Tweed, created in 1986, which evokes the verdant Irish countryside, and Fantasia de Fleurs, which was created for Elisabeth of Austria. Creed also creates perfumes to order, a process which takes about six months and for which the minimum order is ten liters of perfume.

CHRISTIAN DIOR
30, avenue Montaigne,
75008 Paris. Tel: (1) 40 73 54 44
The grey décor of this elegant boutique is an ideal setting for the celebrated Christian Dior perfumes. Diorama and Diorling can be purchased only at this address, where collectors can also acquire the Baccarat or Saint-Louis crystal perfume bottles, including the very beautiful model for Diorissimo.

DYPTIQUE
34, boulevard Saint Germain,
75005 Paris. Tel: (1) 43 26 45 27
It was in 1961 that the English painter Desmond Knox-Leet, now deceased, opened a boutique in Paris proposing the first "Made in England" potpourris and pomanders, as well as a delicate toilet water called Ombre Dans L'Eau. He also created a range of perfumed candles, of which there are now thirty-four kinds, the most popular being Cannelle. Bois Ciré, the most recent model, gives off the comforting smell of mellow, polished wood.

GRAIN DE BEAUTÉ
9, rue du Cherche-Midi,
75006 Paris. Tel: (1) 45 48 07 55
Since 1977, Odile Ménardier has been selling English perfumes in a boutique filled with Victorian chests of drawers, embroidered cushions and "Made in England" porcelain and silver curios. Available here are fragrances by Floris, Geo F. Trumper and a wide range from Penhaligon's, which she considers to be the ultimate English perfumer. For men she recommends Blenheim Bouquet, originally created for Sir Winston Churchill, and for women, the same company's delightful Victorian Posy. Penhaligon's room fragrances, presented in spray or essence form, are well worth trying: Morning Glory for the spring, Summer's Cup for summer, Forest's Robe for the fall, and Winter Garden for the winter.

GUERLAIN
68, avenue des Champs-Elysées,
75008 Paris. Tel: (1) 47 89 71 84
The fans of this renowned perfume house frequent the Champs-Elysées boutique, which was opened at the turn of the century on the ground floor of a town house specially built for the Guerlain family, who lived on the first floor. The boutique, with its Carrara marble floor and Bohemian crystal chandelier, is unchanged. The legendary flacons are displayed in discreetly lit recesses, where one can admire the great classics Shalimar and L'Heure Bleue, as well as the lesser-known Après l'Ondée, created in 1906, Liu, in its 1929 black and gold Art Deco flacon, and Mouchoir de Monsieur, which in 1905 had already become a great success. Today's fashionable men come here to order the replica of the one-and-a-half-liter extract bottle, which can be filled with toilet water, eau de parfum, or, the ultimate luxury, with perfume, an absolute folly at a mere five thousand dollars! The famous one-liter flacon with the white or gold bee motif is more reasonably priced and one can have it filled with one's favorite toilet water and engraved with one's initials. Eau de Verveine, no longer in the catalogue, is available to order. Also worth visiting is the beauty salon on the first floor, which was decorated in 1939 by Christian Bérard, Jean-Michel Frank and Diego Giacometti.

HERMES
24, rue du Faubourg-Saint-Honoré,
75008 Paris. Tel: (1) 40 17 47 17
Opened in July 1994, the "fragrance area" in the center of the Faubourg-Saint-Honoré boutique is decorated in the style of a drawing room, with a sea-green sofa and light wood paneling setting off the celebrated Early American silk scarf, whose design also figures on a collection of perfume sprays. The complete range of this prestigious establishment's perfumes is displayed in recesses suffused with light. It includes Calèche, which still heads sales, Amazone, Parfum d'Hermès and the most recent arrival, 24 Faubourg, of which the king-sized bottle of toilet water is practically impossible to find elsewhere. Atomizers in grained leather or metal engraved with a scarf design, designed for the women's fragrances, are sold exclusively at this address. Men have not been forgotten either, with Equipage, Bel Ami, and Eau d'Hermès, a unisex toilet water created by the great perfumer Edmond Roudnitska. Hermès also offers Eau de Saint-Louis, a citrus fragrance which is presented each year in a new flacon designed for the Saint-Louis crystal manufacturers. Collectors take note!

LANCOME
29, rue du Faubourg-Saint-Honoré
75008 Paris. Tel: (1) 40 17 47 17
The Lancôme premises have recently been completely renovated and the six classic Lancôme fragrances can now be admired in a magnificent new décor. For men Lancôme offers Sagamore, a woody fragrance with a subtle vanilla note, and Balafre, decidedly more spicy; for women, O Intense, Magie, Sikkim and the superb Climat, a whirl of rose, narcissus and summery notes which is sold in a replica of the bottle designed for it in 1934 by the artist Georges Delhomme.

JEAN-FRANÇOIS LAPORTE,
MAITRE PARFUMEUR ET GANTIER
84 bis, rue de Grenelle,
75007 Paris. Tel: (1) 45 44 61 57
Jean-François Laporte's wonderful fragrances are displayed in a setting which seems to come straight out of Casanova's memoirs, with its Tiepolo-style painted ceiling, Cordoba leather walls and raspberry-tinted windows. Inspired by the olfactory tradition of the seventeenth century, when perfumers were also glovers, he has created subtle, intimate perfumes, such as Secrète Datura, which are radically different from other fragrances on the market today, favoring the opulent accords and vibrant harmonies so highly prized by Proust and Baudelaire. The best-selling perfume is Rose Muskissime, an audacious combination of rose and exotic fruit with an ardent musk trail. Men tend to opt for the delicately woody note of Iris Gris.

OCTÉE
53, rue Bonaparte,
75006 Paris. Tel: (1) 46 33 18 77
Josiane Daudon, who opened this spacious boutique with its light parquet and shelving, considers that every woman is unique and that her perfumes should therefore be unique as well. She therefore invented an original concept: twelve numbered fragrances divided into three main groups, the voluptuous, the light and airy and the floral-gustative (which includes the astonishing Note 4, a chocolate fragrance with a violet undertone), and a series of nine concentrated essences. These latter can be used neat, as extracts, but can also be used to individualize the fragrance that the client has chosen. Customers thus have a choice of 108 fragrances.

OFFICINA PROFUMO-FARMACEUTICA DI SANTA
MARIA NOVELLA DI FIRENZE
Chez Amin Kader
2, rue Guisarde,
75006 Paris. Tel: (1) 43 26 27 37
The fashion designer Amin Kader is now the sole distributor in France of the perfumes and beauty products of the Santa Maria Novella pharmaceutical perfumery. This exquisite boutique means that Parisiennes can at last buy the eau de Colognes, toilet waters and perfumes produced

---

THE TEN MOST
PRESTIGIOUS FRAGRANCES

Numerous new fragrances are launched every year and choosing among them can sometimes be overwhelming. The ten most popular and famous perfumes in the world, however, remain classics which never go out of fashion. They are listed below in chronological order:

L'Heure Bleu, by Guerlain
N° 5, by Chanel
Shalimar, by Guerlain
Arpège, by Lanvin
Joy, by Patou
Femme, by Rochas
Miss Dior, by Christian Dior
L'Air du Temps, by Nina Ricci
Opium, by Yves Saint Laurent
Trésor, by Lancôme

in Florence. For the home this boutique proposes the long-forgotten Armenia paper and an irresistible potpourri, neither too sweet, nor too bland, nor too floral, which is also available in sachets for perfuming linen.
(See "Perfume Stores, Italy")

PARFUMS DE ROSINE
Jardin du Palais Royal,
43, rue Montpensier,
75001 Paris Tel: (1) 42 60 47 58
Colette, who lived nearby, would have appreciated this trim little store with Tyrian pink walls and pretty console tables decorated with roses. Its owner Marie-Hélène Togeon, a descendant of Panafieu, perfumer to Napoleon III, wanted to capture the spirit of the Années Folles. Three perfumes are available here: La Rose de Rosine; La Coupe d'Or de Rosine, which is a charming accord of vanilla and red fruits; and the sensual Mea Culpa de Rosine, her latest creation.

JEAN PATOU
7, rue Saint-Florentin,
75008 Paris. Tel: (1) 44 77 33 00
It was in the rue Saint-Florentin that Jean Patou opened his first boutique in 1925 and the perfumer's new premises in the same street feature furniture designed by Louis Sue and André Mare, who were Patou's interior decorators in the 1920s. The fragrances are displayed in a revolving bar and include Joy, 1,000, Patou pour Homme and the twelve original Patou perfumes which have recently been revived. Collectors will appreciate the limited edition of numbered replicas of the original Colony crystal bottle, which is in the form of a pineapple and one thousand of which have been made.

PATRICIA DE NICOLAI
69, avenue Raymond Poincaré,
75016 Paris. Tel: (1) 47 55 90 44
In less than ten years this young woman, a descendant of Pierre Guerlain, has become a highly regarded perfumer. The blue and white striped boutiques display her popular perfumes, such as Sacrebleu, Number One, and Petit Ange, a toilet water for babies, the bottle of which can be engraved with the baby's name. For men there is the popular New York, with its spicy-peppery note. Exclusive perfumes can be created, but orders take at least six months to prepare.

LES SALONS DU PALAIS ROYAL SHISEIDO
5, rue de Valois,
75001 Paris. Tel: (1) 49 27 09 09
The décor of this boutique, located under the arcades of the Palais Royal, with its moons and a fantastic bestiary created by Serge Lutens, the artistic director of Shiseido, was hand-painted by specialists from the Historic Monuments Foundation. The scores of fragrances Lutens has composed are based on four central themes, Les Eaux Boisées, Les Somptueux, Eaux Anciennes and Bois Sépia. The fragrances are sold in traditional-style perfume bottles which can be engraved. The boutique also has a magnificent collection of antique perfume bottles.

YVES SAINT LAURENT
Institut de Beauté,
32 rue du Faubourg Saint-Honoré,
75008 Paris. Tel: (1) 49 24 99 66

DEPARTMENT STORES:
GALERIES LAFAYETTE
40, boulevard Haussmann, 75009
Paris. Tel: (1) 42 82 34 56
LE BON MARCHÉ
24, rue de Sèvres, 75007 Paris.
Tel: (1) 44 39 80 00
PRINTEMPS
64, boulevard Haussmann, 75009 Paris.
Tel: (1) 42 82 50 00

French provinces

PARFUMERIE FRAGONARD
20, boulevard Fragonard,
06130 Grasse. Tel: (16) 93 36 44 65
The Fragonard perfume house, named after the painter Jean-Honoré Fragonard, who came from a family of perfumers, opened in Grasse in 1926. It perpetuates a certain traditional style of perfumery, exemplified by the charming, simple notes of the toilet waters, classified in eleven women's ranges and two men's ranges. The Fresh Flowers category comprises three fragrances, namely honeysuckle, mimosa and vervain. The violet, rose and carnation fragrances figure in the Heady group, while the Bewitching range is composed of magnolia, jasmine and lily of the valley. The Naturals represent a very sound investment, with a selection of lemon, lavender and vanilla fragrance waters, as well as an eau de Cologne dating from 1926, when the establishment was founded. Some of these fragrances are produced on the premises and the laboratory is open to the public.
(See "Museums")

MOLINARD
60, boulevard Victor Hugo,
06130 Grasse. Tel: (16) 93 36 03 91
The real Habanita enthusiasts go to Grasse to buy this perfume, because that is where it was created. Because of its size, the Molinard perfume house is more like an exhibition hall than a boutique, but its ochre-colored walls and the Provençal furniture used for displaying the perfumes lend it warmth. Here one can purchase scented furniture polish, delightful concretes presented in small, black, hand-painted cases and of course the original toilet waters so highly prized by Queen Victoria.
(See "Museums")

AUX PARFUMS DE GRASSE
10, rue Saint Gaëtan,
06000 Nice. Tel: (16) 93 85 60 77
This minute boutique nestles in one of the narrow, picturesque streets in the old part of Nice. This is the domain of jasmine, violet and lavender essences, of rose-water and perfumed soaps smelling sweetly of Provence. All the products come from Grasse and the surrounding countryside.

England

THE BODY SHOP
Head Office: Watersmead, Littlehampton,
West Sussex BN17 6LS. Tel: (1903) 731500
Since it was founded by Anita Roddick in 1976, The Body Shop has expanded steadily and, as of February 1995, has a total of 1,120 retail outlets worldwide. The Body Shop supplies a comprehensive range of thirty-one fragrances, from the best-selling White Musk and Dewberry, to the more novel but extremely popular Vanilla. There is also a full range of scented soaps, perfume oils, bath and shower gels and a line of unfragranced toiletries which can be perfumed to customer specification.

CRABTREE & EVELYN
6, Kensington Church Street,
London W8. Tel: (171) 937 9335
This perfume house, founded in the 1970s, has developed with exceptional rapidity, and currently boasts around 250 boutiques throughout the world. Their fragrances are regularly updated, the latest ones including lavender, lilac, carnation and violet.
(See "Perfume Stores, Paris")

CZECH AND SPEAKE
39c, Jermyn Street,
London SW1Y 6DN. Tel: (171) 439 0216
Initially founded in 1979 as a purveyor of bathroom fittings and accessories, Czech and Speake has diversified and now specializes in perfumes, bath oils, colognes and other luxury fragrance products.

FLORIS PERFUMERS
89, Jermyn Street,
London SW1Y 6JH. Tel: (171) 930 2885
This boutique has been in the same premises since it was founded by Juan Floris in 1730. The building was severely damaged during the Second World War, but was restored to its original splendor with magnificent wood paneling and mahogany showcases displaying a collection of antique perfume bottles and presentation cases. The perfume range includes eleven fragrances for women, three men's fragrances and three traditional lavender, moss rose and hyacinth toilet waters. Bouvardia, a recent creation with oriental notes, and Zinnia, a rose, violet and iris accord with a woody base note, are popular with the ladies, while gentlemen favor JF (the founder's initials) with its fresh mandarin and cypress notes.

GEO F. TRUMPER
9, Curzon Street,
London WIY 7FL. Tel: (171) 499 1850
In 1875, Geo F. Trumper opened one of the most elegant barber shops in Curzon Street and rapidly set about creating a range of colognes. There are now two establishments, each with an old-fashioned barber shop interior. A wide choice of colognes is available, including Eau de Cologne, Eau de Portugal and Eau de Quinine, which can be worn by both men and women.

MARY CHESS PERFUMES
Manufactured by Fine Fragrances
&, Cosmestics Ltd.
6, Kingsway Business Park, Oldfield Road,
Hampton, Middlesex. Tel: (181) 979 8156
Mary Chess fragrances are available by mail order. They were created in London at the beginning of the 1930s by the American Grace Mary Chess Robinson, and given the royal warrant by Queen Elizabeth, the Queen Mother, in 1977. Two new complementary lines, Austère and Tapestry, have recently been added to the exist-

ing range. The former, a floral fragrance with rose, tuberose and gardenia notes, is available in toilet water, soap and lotion form, while Tapestry, an opulent floral fragrance with an amber and moss theme, comes not only as a toilet water, but also in the form of perfumed moss essence for the bath and as a home fragrance.

NEAL'S YARD REMEDIES
5, Golden Cross, Cornmarket Street,
Oxford OX1 3EU. Tel: (1865) 245436
Although more famous for its exclusive range of aromatic and aromatherapy oils, the company also sells a wide selection of essential oils and its own aftershave and cologne. The latter is a blend of selected oils from the range, among others: lemon, petulia, coriander and cinnamon. Since its foundation in 1981, the company has expanded rapidly, and currently has ten shops and franchises, 250 stockists in the UK and a network of distributors throughout North America, Europe, Australia and Japan.

NORFOLK LAVENDER
Caley Mill,
Heacham. Tel: (148) 557 0384
Since the time when Queen Victoria used to visit the lavender fields in Surrey, accompanied by the official Royal Purveyor of Lavender Essence, English lavender, of which the queen was an unconditional devotee, has been considered by the English as the best in the world. It is available at the Queen's Gallery, the Buckingham Palace gift shop. Here they sell lavender grown on land belonging to the royal family in every conceivable form: eau de Cologne, essential oil, concretes, soap, bath products, fragrant sachets, room fragrances, potpourris and candles, to name just a few.

PENHALIGON'S PERFUMERS LTD
41, Wellington Street,
London WC2E 7BN Tel: (171) 836 2150
This famous perfume house was founded in 1870 and for the last twenty years has been based in a former florist's shop in Covent Garden. Hammam Bouquet, which is still Penhaligon's best-selling men's fragrance, was created in 1870 along with the establishment itself. Female clients favor Cornubia, a bouquet of exotic flowers and woods. All the fragrances are presented in Penhaligon's original perfume bottle with its spherical stopper. The toll-free telephone numbers for obtaining the perfume catalogue and for placing orders are: 0800 716 108 (inside the UK); 44 181 880 2050 (outside the UK).
(See under "Perfume Stores, Paris")

ALSO:
CULPEPPER THE HERBALISTS
21, Bruton Street, Berkeley Square,
London W1X 7DA. Tel: (171) 629 4559
LIBERTY
210–220, Regent Street,
London W1R 6AH. Tel: (171) 734 1234

DEPARTMENT STORES:
THE CONRAN SHOP
81, Fulham Road, London SW3 6RD.
Tel: (171) 589 7401
HEALS
196, Tottenham Court Road, London W1A 1BJ.
Tel: (171) 636 1666

HARRODS
87–135, Brompton Road, Knightsbridge,
London SW1X 7XL. Tel: (171) 730 1234
SELFRIDGES
400, Oxford Street, London W1A 1AB.
Tel: (171) 629 1234

Italy

OFFICINA PROFUMO-FARMACEUTICA DI SANTA MARIA NOVELLA
Via della Scala, 16,
50123 Florence. Tel: (55) 216276
This is an exclusive address hidden away in an unassuming street near the railroad station. Behind an unmarked door is the breathtaking magnificence of the Renaissance, with bronze candelabras in the form of vestal virgins casting their soft light over the polychrome marble floor, Gothic-style vaulting and sixteenth-century frescoes by Paolino Sarti. Nothing has changed since the establishment was founded. Today perfumed soaps still emerge from machines which were developed in the seventeenth century and they are still stocked for two months in airing cupboards before being wrapped by hand. The toilet waters and handkerchief extracts, presented in delightful Art Nouveau bottles, are composed entirely of natural products, hence their incomparable subtlety. In order to maintain their traditions, this perfume house organizes introductory courses in Medicean cosmetology.

LORENZO VILLORESI
Via de' Bardi, 14,
50125 Florence. Tel: (55) 234 11 87

SIGNATURE FRAGRANCES
Perfumers who are willing to devote their precious time to a fragrance which will only be worn by a single person are few and far between. In France, special mention should be made of Annick Goutal (see p. 202), Patricia de Nicolaï (see p. 204), Monique Schlienger (see "Perfume Schools") and Nicolas Mamounas (see address below). These perfumers consider custom-made fragrances (known as "signature fragrances") as an extension of their own research. Prospective clients should arm themselves with patience and an ample wallet, as an exclusive fragrance often requires several weeks waiting, and several thousand dollars.

NICOLAS MAMOUNAS
Chemin de Châteauneuf,
06620 Bar-sur-Loup. Tel: (16) 93 42 57 76
This perfumer of Greek origin left his job as perfumer for the Rochas perfume house in Paris and settled in Provence, not far from Grasse. Working in an independent capacity, he creates exclusive perfumes for those in whom he recognizes a kindred spirit. The first step, therefore, is to meet him . . . which is also a good opportunity to admire the wonderful collection of old roses in his garden.

To reach this talented perfumer's studio, one only has to cross the Ponte Vecchio curving over the Arno, walk for a few minutes along the Via de' Bardi and then climb to the top floor of a handsome building. Lorenzo Villoresi creates men's and women's fragrances, often with the spicy trails typical of the Medici tradition, and a range of home fragrances. His perfumes are presented in cut crystal perfume bottles and leather cases made by Florentine craftsmen. People come from all over the world to place orders for his exclusive perfumes. All you need to do is to make an appointment—what better reason for a trip to Florence.

The United States

Variety is the name of the game here. Not only do New York and Beverly Hills have outlets for the prestigious European designer names (Chanel, Yves Saint Laurent, etc.) and the traditional English fragrances, but there is also the high glamour of the department stores on Fifth Avenue and Rodeo Drive, with their ground floors transformed into veritable olfactory temples, where demonstrations are never-ending and lavish . . . and headaches frequent. Most of the classic European fragrances are available here, but the majority of products are American—a treat for European visitors who can discover fragrances which are not available in Europe. Then there are the smaller boutiques in New York's downtown SoHo, which offer alternative products which emphasize natural, environmentally friendly materials.

SPECIALTY STORES IN NEW YORK:
AVEDA LIFESTYLE STORE
509, Madison Avenue,
New York, NY 10022. Tel: (212) 832 2416
Aveda indigenous plant "Pure-fumes" are an exploration of the beauty of pure, natural essences. "Pure-fumes" are available in sixteen different aromas derived exclusively from flowers and plants. Also available are Single Notes, individual flower extracts used for fragrance and aromatherapy, and Purifying Mists, used for environmental scent. Products can be bought at the fifty Aveda Lifestyle stores in the U.S. and worldwide.

AVON PRODUCTS
9 West Fifty-seventh Street,
New York, NY 10019. Tel: 1-800-FOR-AVON
Direct sales by representatives both within the U.S. and internationally. Avon offers an array of floral and exotic fragrances, and an Ultra line, as well as a selection of men's colognes. Customers can call the 800 number given above to locate their nearest representative.

AYURVEDA
129 First Avenue,
New York, NY 10003. Tel: (212) 260 1218
This store sells body care products, books and vitamins—all animal and cruelty free. It carries an array of oriental perfume essences, such as Santal Blanc, Reve D'Orient and Khadija, aromatherapy oils including jasmine, rose and neroli, as well as essential oils including lavender, tea tree and coriander.

L'ARTISAN PERFUMEUR
870 Madison Avenue.
New York, NY 10021. Tel: (212) 517 8665
In a setting reminiscent of a nineteenth-century French perfumer's cabinet, one can admire the impressive selection of original eaux de toilette offering both men and women an opportunity to discover their own signature scent. Additional home fragrances are also available, including amber balls, room sprays and drawer sachets, characterized by the natural aromas of flowers, fruits, spices and woods.

ORIGINS
402 West Broadway
New York, NY 10012. Tel: (212) 219 9764
A division of Estée Lauder International, Origins Natural Resources, Inc. carries over one hundred therapy oils and gels, such as Energy Boost and Sleep Time, as well as its own fragrance. Spring Fever. Their products can be found in over two hundred department and specialty stores, as well as in eighteen of their own retail shops across the country.

DEPARTMENT STORES:
Fine fragrances by top designers are best found at a number of department stores in New York and across the country.
New York:
BARNEY'S NEW YORK
106, Seventh Avenue,
New York, NY 10011. Tel: (212) 826 8900
BERGDORF-GOODMAN
1, West Fifty-seventh Street
New York, NY 10019. Tel: (212) 753 7300
BLOOMINGDALE'S
Fifty-ninth Street & Lexington Avenue
New York, NY 10022. Tel: (212) 705 2000
HENRY BENDEL
712, Fifth Avenue,
New York, NY 10019. Tel: (212) 247 1100
LORD & TAYLOR
424, Fifth Avenue,
New York, NY 10018. Tel: (212) 391 3344
MACY'S
Herald Square,
New York, NY 10001. Tel: (212) 695 4400
SAKS FIFTH AVENUE
611, Fifth Avenue,
New York, NY 10022. Tel: (212) 753 4000

SPECIALTY STORES IN BEVERLY HILLS:
BIJAN
421, North Rodeo Drive Penthouse
Beverly Hills, CA, 90210. Tel: (310) 371 1122
A menswear couturier for 25 years, Bijan now produces perfumes and body care products for both men and women under the name Bijan—a "Floriental composition" for women—and in the DNA range which features triple helix shaped bottles. Working with designers such as Baccarat for his flacons, Bijan has accumulated numerous awards for both the perfumes themselves and their packaging and advertising. Bijan's showrooms can be visited by appointment only, and are also at: 699 Fifth Avenue, New York, NY 10022. Tel: (212) 758 7500.

The following stores are also outside New York: Neiman Marcus; Nordstrom's; Dayton-Hudson; Dillard's; Filene's; and Jordan Marsh.

FASHION DESIGNER
PERFUMERS

It would be an impossible task to list all the names and addresses of the fashion designers who have created a perfume, as it gets longer every day. We have therefore only included the addresses (where possible in Paris, London and New York) of those designers mentioned in the text who have boutiques where the reader can find their range of fragrances, as well as certain exclusive creations which are not available either in department stores or in perfume stores.

GIORGIO ARMANI
6, place Vendôme, 75001 Paris.
Tel: (1) 42 61 55 09
178, Sloane Street, London SW1X 9QL.
Tel: (171) 235 6232
110, Fifth Avenue, New York, NY 10011.
Tel: (212) 727 3240
LORIS AZZARO
65, rue du Faubourg-St-Honoré, 75008 Paris.
Tel: (1) 42 66 92 06
PIERRE BALMAIN
237, rue St-Honoré, 75001 Paris.
Tel: (1) 42 60 68 38
99, Baker Street, London W1M 1FB.
Tel: (171) 486 7833
CACHAREL
5, place des Victoires, 75001 Paris.
Tel: (1) 42 33 29 88
CHANEL
(see "Perfume Salons, Paris")
19, Old Bond Street, London W1X 3DA.
Tel: (171) 493 3836
5, East Fifty-seventh Street, New York, NY 10022. Tel: (212) 355 5050
CHRISTIAN DIOR
(See "Perfume Salons, Paris")
13, Grosvenor Crescent, London SW1X 7EE.
Tel: (171) 235 9411
703, Fifth Avenue, New York, NY 10022.
Tel: (212) 223 4646
JEAN-PAUL GAULTIER
30, rue du Faubourg-Saint-Antoine,
75012 Paris. Tel: (1) 42 86 05 05
171, Draycott Avenue, London SW3 3AJ.
Tel: (171) 584 4648
GIVENCHY
3, avenue George V, 75008 Paris.
Tel: (1) 44 31 50 06
11, Old Esher Road, Hersham KR12 4RL.
Tel: (1932) 245111
KENZO
3, place des Victoires, 75001 Paris.
Tel: (1) 40 39 72 03
15, Sloane Street, London SW1 9NB.
Tel: (171) 235 4021
KARL LAGERFELD
17, rue du Faubourg-Saint-Honoré,
75008 Paris. Tel: (1) 42 66 64 64
173, New Bond Street, London W1Y 9PB.
Tel: (171) 493 6277
LANVIN
5, rue du Faubourg-Saint-Honoré, 75008 Paris.
Tel: (1) 42 68 05 21
88, Brompton Road, London SW3 1ER.
Tel: (171) 581 4401

GUY LAROCHE
29, avenue Montaigne, 75008 Paris.
Tel: (1) 40 69 69 50
65, New Bond Street, London W1Y 9DF.
Tel: (171) 493 1362
36, East Fifty-seventh Street, New York, NY 10022.. Tel: (212) 759 2301
RALPH LAUREN
2, place de la Madeleine, 75008 Paris.
Tel: (1) 44 77 53 50
143, New Bond Street, London W1Y 9FD.
Tel: (212) 581 3760
867, Madison Avenue, New York, NY 10021.
Tel: (212) 606 2100
ISSEY MIYAKE
3, place des Vosges, 75004 Paris.
Tel: (1) 48 87 01 86
270, Brompton Road, London SW3 2AW.
Tel: (171) 581 3760
992, Madison Avenue, New York, NY 10021.
Tel: (212) 439 7822
CLAUDE MONTANA
313, rue de Grenelle, 75007 Paris.
Tel: (1) 45 49 13 02
THIERRY MUGLER
49, avenue Montaigne, 75008 Paris.
Tel: (1) 47 23 37 62
PACO RABANNE
23, rue du Cherche-Midi, 75008 Paris.
Tel: (1) 42 22 87 80
NINA RICCI
17-19, rue François 1er, 75008 Paris.
Tel: (1) 49 52 56 00
6, Brook Street, Hanover Square, London W1Y 9FA. Tel: (171) 493 8232
MARCEL ROCHAS
33, rue François 1er, 75008 Paris.
Tel: 47 23 54 56
YVES SAINT LAURENT
(See "Perfume Salons, Paris")
137, New Bond Street, London W1Y 9FA.
Tel: (171) 493 1800
855, Madison Avenue, New York, NY 10021.
Tel: (212) 472 5299
JIL SANDER
52, avenue Montaigne, 75008 Paris.
Tel: 44 95 06 70
EMANUEL UNGARO
2, avenue Montaigne, 75008 Paris.
Tel: (1) 47 23 61 94
36, Sloane Street, London SW1 XLP.
Tel: (171) 259 6111
782, Madison Avenue, New York, NY 10021.
Tel: (212) 249 4090
YVES SAINT LAURENT
(See "Perfume Salons, Paris")
857, Madison Avenue, New York, NY 10021.
Tel: (212) 472 5299

HOME FRAGRANCES

Fragrances designed for the home can help to create a harmonious environment which will be appreciated by family and friends alike. These fragrances should not be used in every room of the house, as it is important to preserve areas of "olfactory silence." The kitchen and dining room have their own odors, so home fragrances should be avoided here (a strong fragrance can spoil the taste of food), but they are well suited to the hall, the living room, or the study.

Real fragrance-lovers do not privilege just one method of perfuming rooms, but on the contrary use a whole variety of techniques: perfumed candles and oils, potpourris, and atomizers, which diffuse differently and have varying lengths of life.

POTPOURRIS
Decorative and fragrant objects, potpourris should on no account be placed in the corner of a room and then forgotten. They should be regularly revived with the appropriate perfumed oils. Making them yourself can be great fun. Jean-François Laporte, the first perfumer to introduce English potpourris and home perfumes in France, proposes the following fresh potpourri recipe, inspired by those concocted in the eighteenth century. Clean a receptacle with alcohol and line the base with six ounces of sea salt to act as a disinfectant and preserver. Add about a quarter of an ounce of odorous seeds, fresh pepper, vanilla pods, laurel leaves, thyme, myrtle, mint and nutmeg. Add petals of wild, fragrant roses and jasmine, clove flowers and elderberry blossom, avoiding bulbs such as narcissus. Cover the recipient and leave the mixture to rest for a while. Mix gently every day with a disinfected wooden spoon. Add fresh flowers. It takes about five or six weeks for the potpourri to reach maturity.

CANDLES
Perfumed candles diffuse a pleasant fragrance, immediately creating an inviting atmosphere which lasts several hours. The candles created by Dyptique are marvelous, while those made by Rigaud never go out of fashion. The perfumed candles created by Jean-François Laporte, Maître Parfumeur et Gantier, plunge us into idyllic atmospheres, such as that of geranium mixed with amber, Atlas cedar and peony.

PEBBLES, STONES AND RINGS
Any object can be impregnated with fragrance which will in turn perfume the atmosphere. There are hundreds of perfumed articles waiting to be discovered, such as sachets containing delicate little perfumed pebbles, which, when placed near a source of heat, gently diffuse fragrances; or perfumed rings which fit round light bulbs, an efficient, even if not particularly attractive, way of perfuming the air, as the heat ensures the fragrance is rapidly diffused.

SPRAY PERFUMES
Spray perfumes immediately create an atmosphere and are easy to use. You can spray carpets, wall coverings and any materials which are not too fragile.

PERFUMED LINEN
Nothing is more refined than perfumed linen. Natural perfumes are the most appropriate ones for linen. Sachets filled with lavender or other dried flowers are ideal for linen cupboards. Alternatively there are little muslin sachets of iris, or cornflower, which are particularly suited to small items of linen; charming coat-hangers covered in floral-patterned material impregnated with lavender, rose, cinnamon, lily of the valley and orchid; perfumed shelf liners for closets, cupboards and drawers; and sachets filled with fragrant powders to slip between articles of clothing. Catherine Memmi of Maison Douce in

Paris, has filled large sachets and immaculately white percale pouches with armfuls of lavender. Grain de Beauté stocks a whole range of perfumed accessories intended for linen: ravishing belts covered with floral material impregnated with lavender, rose and cinnamon-orange, lily of the valley or orchid. Guerlain, for its part, has created pretty blue perfumed flannels, either in the classic form of a square or cut in the shape of the famous Guerlain perfume bottles, such as Shalimar, L'Heure Bleue and Jardins de Bagatelle.

PARIS:
ANNICK GOUTAL (See above)
L'ARTISAN PARFUMEUR (See above)
CATHERINE MEMMI, LA MAISON DOUCE
34, rue Saint-Sulpice, 75006 Paris.
Tel: 44 07 22 26
CIR
22, rue Saint-Sulpice, 75006 Paris.
Tel: 43 26 46 50
This boutique offers, in addition to the famous classic candles by Rigaud, a beautiful choice of incenses, one of the most delightful of which is Pontifical.
CONRAN SHOP
117, rue du Bac, 75006 Paris. Tel: 42 84 10 01
CRABTREE & EVELYN (See above)
DYPTIQUE (See above)
GUERLAIN (See above)
LE SAPONIFERE
59, rue Bonaparte, 75006 Paris.
Tel: 46 33 98 43
This pretty store with its white façade, its pine interior and its angled corners is the first shop in Paris to stock products and accessories for the bath. Here you can find Rigaud candles, concentrated potpourris which perfume a room for two or three months (and which can be renewed), silk sachets for linen perfumed with cedar, vanilla or gardenia, sprays, such as the beautiful Original, and decorative bunches of dried flowers which are specially treated so that they perfume your living room over a long period.

LONDON:
THE CONRAN SHOP (See above)
CULPEPER HERBALISTS
8, The Market, Covent Garden Piazza, London WC2. Tel: 171 379 6698
PENHALIGON'S (See above)

BOTTLES

Auctions and experts — antiques and boutiques

When buying old perfume bottles, it is advisable to proceed with caution. Interest in the field is such, that in some non-specialized secondhand stores it is not uncommon to find perfume bottles of brands which are under one year old. In order to start a real collection, it is best to turn to the specialists. If you already own rare or old perfume bottles and wish to find out more about them, the simplest solution is to consult an expert who will be able to give you an idea of their quality and value. Below is a list of the best auction houses and experts:

AUCTION HOUSES:
HOTEL DROUOT
9, rue Drouot, 75009 Paris. Tel: (1) 48 00 20 20
GALERIE DE CHARTRES
1 bis, place du Général de Gaulle, 28000 Chartres. Tel: 37 36 04 33
HOTEL DES VENTES DE CORBEIL-ESSONNES
10, quai de l'Essonne, 91000 Corbeil-Essonnes.
In Paris most international transactions are concluded at six-monthly auctions, organized by Maître Couteau-Bégarie at the Hôtel Drouot in Paris and Maîtres Lelièvre, Maiche and Paris at the Galerie de Chartres. The objects sold at auction in these sales rooms are always of the highest quality.

BONHAM'S
Montpelier Street, Knightsbridge, London.
Tel: (171) 393 3930
Many fine perfume bottles can be found across the Channel in the prestigious English auction houses. Bonham's in London is located a mere stone's throw from Harrods. It does not hold auctions exclusively for perfume bottles, but every October they organize a special sale of objects by Lalique, the creator of some of the most beautiful perfume bottles, notably those he designed for Houbigant, Coty, Worth, Molinard, Lubin, Volnay, Roger & Gallet, Rochas, D'Orsay and Guerlain. Perfume bottles also appear in the decorative arts sales. The catalogues of these auctions are of great interest for collectors.

CHRISTIE'S
85, Old Brompton Road, London.
Tel: (171) 839 9060
Christie's Decorative Arts Department is located in the South Kensington branch of this prestigious auction house. It organizes six sales a year where you can find glassware, ceramics and, among other things, perfume bottles, potpourris, perfume censers, etc. For the most part, the bottles on offer are by Lalique. For those interested, Christie's publishes a brochure indicating the year's sales calendar, together with detailed and richly illustrated catalogues for individual sales. For information, contact Jane Haye, an expert who, if you send her a photograph, is also happy to give you information about your perfume bottles and an evaluation.

SOTHEBY'S
34–35, New Bond Street, London W1A 1AA.
Tel: (171) 493 8080
Perfume bottles dating from the eighteenth century to the present day, variously made from precious metals and hard stone and often embellished with jewels and enamel, are sold in Objects of Vertu sales in London, while the coveted scent bottles of Fabergé are included in the twice yearly sales of Russian works of art in Geneva. For further information, contact Julia Clarke on (171) 408 5324.

EXPERTS:
JEAN-MARIE MARTIN-HATTEMBERG
28, rue Mansart, 78160 Marly-le-Roi.
Tel: 39 58 86 57
Jean-Marie Martin-Hattemberg is an expert at the Court of Appeal in Versailles specializing in twentieth-century decorative art. Besides his expertise in the field of antique toilet articles, he is also an expert on exceptional contemporary perfume bot-

tles. He has a passion for one-off bottles or limited series, which are beginning to interest private collectors, museums and foundations.

CLARENCE DUCHESNE
35, rue Marbeuf, 75008 Paris. Tel: (1) 45 62 93 33
For several years now, Clarence Duchesne has been helping prestigious perfume houses reconstitute and evaluate their heritage. Perfume bottles, posters, glass artists, illustrators and designers hold no secrets for this enthusiastic expert. She is also a specialist on glasswork and is familiar with all the creations by crystal and glass craftsmen who were working at the turn of the century. A mine of information.

RÉGINE DE ROBIEN (see "Boutiques")
BOUTIQUES:
BEAUTÉ DIVINE
Régine de Robien
40, rue Saint-Sulpice, 75006 Paris.
Tel: (1) 43 26 25 31
This romantic boudoir-style boutique, a temple of antique perfume bottles, situated near the Saint-Sulpice church, is a must for any collectors visiting Paris. The most beautiful and rare perfume bottles in the world find their way into this store, such as unique pieces by René Lalique and bottles by Paul Poiret or Lanvin, and stocks are regularly renewed as collectors quickly snap them up. Régine de Robien knows collectors of perfume bottles from many countries and has in fact been the instigator of many a vocation in this domain. She officiates at the major perfume bottle auctions in France and has a long-standing reputation. Her expert eye detects the slightest flaw and she is able to appraise any perfume bottle with accuracy. Well-edited catalogues are available and allow one to follow the fluctuations of market prices.

BELLE DE JOUR
7, rue Tardieu, 75008 Paris.
Tel: (1) 46 06 15 28
At this little boutique, situated at the foot of the funicular railway in Montmartre, you can consult one of the finest specialists in the restoration of perfume bottles, Yann Schalburg. He has the gift of transforming a defective flacon into one that looks brand new and he is the only person who repairs antique perfume sprays. One can also purchase good-quality perfume bottles which he makes in his boutique.

VIA ANTICA
11, rue Jacob, 75006 Paris. Tel: (1) 40 51 77 79
Soraya Feder left the Saint-Ouen flea market and now displays the Baccarat and Lalique perfume bottles dating from the 1920s, limited editions, and similar objects which fascinate her, in a boutique located in the heart of Paris. An interesting place to go and browse!

Further addresses for perfume bottles in Paris:
CIRCÉ AEA
1, rue Saint-Philippe-du-Roule, 75008 Paris.
Tel: (1) 42 89 39 13
LALIQUE
11, rue Royale, 75008 Paris.
Tel: (1) 42 66 52 40
LES CRISTALLERIES DE SAINT-LOUIS
13, rue Royale, 75008 Paris.
Tel: (1) 40 17 01 74

BACCARAT
30 bis, rue de Paradis, 75010 Paris.
Tel: (1) 47 70 64 30

DANENBERG
Le Louvre des Antiquaires
2, place du Palais Royal, 75001 Paris.
Tel: (1) 42 61 57 19

GLASSWORKS
The valley of the river Bresle in Normandy, northwest France, has been famous for its glassworks since the Gallo-Roman period. For bottle collectors traveling in France, a visit to these wonderful factories is a must.
LE VIEUX-ROUEN, Tel: 35 92 45 06. The factory which produced the bottle for L'Air du Temps by Nina Ricci.
COURVAL, in Hodeng-au-Bosc. Tel: 35 93 50 68
NESLE-NORMANDIE. For guided tours and reservations contact the tourist office in Eu.
Tel: 35 86 04 68
WALTERSPERGER, in Blangny. Tel: 35 93 52 48. Houses one of the last workshops where glass is still blown in the traditional way. Visits by appointment. Closed in August.

FRAGRANCE GAMES

When the French perfumer Véronique Debroise created a series of fragrance games, produced by the Sentosphère company, her aim was to teach both children and adults to recognize everyday odors and to test and develop the most neglected of the human senses, the sense of smell. The games are available in France in the chain of stores called Nature et Découverte, the Chantelivre bookstore at 3, rue de Sèvres in Paris, and at all major department stores and toy stores. In the United States, the games are

---

ATOMIZERS AND BOTTLES

Antique or contemporary perfume atomizers, with their pear-shaped bulb attachments, can be found in secondhand or gift stores. They are charming but unreliable. Not being airtight, there is more danger of oxidation and it is therefore best to leave them empty, or only fill them with sufficient perfume for one week's use. On the other hand, the atomizers manufacturers use for eau de parfum and toilet water are perfectly airtight. The fragrance is ejected by means of a propulsive gas which is added in equal proportions to the perfumed solution. Atomizers are considered to be the most reliable container available on the market, although aesthetically they cannot rival with the beauty and diversity of the extract bottles. After use, the stoppers of the latter should be replaced with care to avoid damaging the neck, and the bottle returned to its presentation case. Extract bottles are sedentary creatures and when traveling it is preferable to use an eau de parfum atomizer. If, however, you cannot bear to be separated from your bottle, it should travel in its original presentation box in your hand luggage.

---

sold and represented by Scenterprises, a division of Susan Phillips Enterprises Ltd, an innovative company that specializes in and markets a variety of intriguing products from the world of scents. For information, please contact Scenterprises, tel: (212) 580 5309, or fax (212) 721 3954.

FOLLOW YOUR NOSE
Children are fascinated by odors and love this game, which can be played by alert children from the age of six up. It illustrates thirty different foods, edibles, flowers and everyday smells, such as chocolate, milk, biscuits, grass and the sea, on easy-to-handle boards, and contains matching aromas.

THE PERFUMEMAKER
This game is designed for children from the age of six up. It comprises eight natural, single floral essences, including sandalwood, bergamot and lavender, three compound bases to be dissolved in water, blotter strips and a set of instructions. Children can create their own perfumes in total safety. This fascinating game brings them into contact with a whole new world of creativity and also gives them the chance them to offer special, personalized gifts to those they love.

MUSEUMS

Museums devoted exclusively to perfumery are few and far between, but those that do exist house such exceptional objects that, when in Paris or Grasse, a visit is essential for all perfume aficionados.

MUSÉE BACCARAT
30 bis, rue de Paradis,
75010 Paris. Tel: 47 70 64 30
The Baccarat Museum is enchantingly decorated in Napoleon III style, with wood paneling and a glazed roof. The museum, entered through a vast boutique full of wonderful crystal objects, has recently been renovated and houses a large collection of perfume bottles which testify to the refined talent and creativity of one of the greatest crystal manufacturers of our time. Since 1898, the Compagnie des Cristalleries de Baccarat has manufactured perfume bottles for Guerlain, François Coty, Houbigant, Jean Patou, Elsa Schiaparelli, Elizabeth Arden and many others. Here you can admire Elsa Schiaparelli's Le Roy Soleil designed by Salvador Dali, It's You by Elizabeth Arden, in the form of a white, opaline glass hand holding a gold flacon topped by a rose, the diamond-shaped perfume bottle for Molinard, and Guerlain's turtle-shaped bottle for Champs Elysées. The objects are skillfully displayed to enable the visitor to appreciate the technique, skill and talent involved in this craft. (See "Perfume Bottles")

MUSÉE FRAGONARD
20, boulevard Fragonard, 06130 Grasse.
Tel: 93 36 44 65
9, rue Scribe, 75009 Paris. Tel: 47 42 04 56
39, boulevard des Capucines, 75002 Paris.
Tel: 42 60 37 14
In 1975, Jean-François Costa, the owner of the

Fragonard perfume house (named after the painter Jean-Honoré Fragonard, who lived for a time Grasse and whose father was a perfumer), started to collect a few objects connected with perfumery. They now form part of the largest private collection in France comprising more than three thousand objects. More than five thousand years of perfume history and extremely rare objects, dating from antiquity to modern times, take visitors on a journey across the centuries and around the world. All the most remarkable aspects of perfume art are exhibited here, such as ointment pots, fragrance lamps and perfume vessels in terra cotta, glass, crystal and precious metals. The collection is divided between three museums, one in Grasse and two in Paris: the Grasse museum evokes the pleasant atmosphere of a typical Provençal property which imparts a particular intensity to each of the objects; the museum in the rue Scribe in Paris owes its distinctive style to the romantic paintings from the Napoleon III era which grace the walls; finally, the museum in the rue des Capucines, opened two years ago, is located in a former theater which dates from the end of the last century and provides a rich setting for a remarkable collection, which includes several very beautiful pomanders.

MUSÉE MOLINARD
60, boulevard Victor Hugo,
06130 Grasse. Tel: 93 36 01 62
Molinard, the famous Grasse perfumer, started creating fragrances as early as 1849. Jean-Pierre Lerouge-Benard, the founder's great-grandson and president of Molinard, decided to relate the history of perfumery in a Provençal setting—decorated with superb sixteenth-, seventeenth- and eighteenth-century Provençal furniture, tapestries and paintings—where one can admire the most beautiful Molinard perfume bottles created by Lalique, such as the famous Baiser du Faune, Iles d'Or, Calendal and Madrigal. There is also a wonderful collection of labels and perfume cards testifying to a charming and exceptionally inventive art. One can follow the various stages in the creation of a fragrance, from the perfume organ to distillation and maceration. Introductory courses in the art of perfume for groups of not more than five people can be arranged by appointment with Madame Chanson-Lebel. Participants have the opportunity of creating their own perfume.

MUSÉE INTERNATIONAL DE LA PARFUMERIE
8, place du Cours,
06130 Grasse. Tel: 93 36 80 20
The idea of creating an international perfume museum dates from the 1900 World Fair, but it was not until 1989 that this museum finally opened. It is located in a magnificent town house in the heart of Grasse. The museum owes its existence to the determination of Georges Vindry, a historian fascinated by perfume, and curator of the museum for several years. A series of magnificent objects trace the various stages in the preparation of a fragrance and every aspect of perfumery is represented: perfume bottles, posters, labels and promotional objects. Mademoiselle Grasse, the present curator, pays particular attention to the variety of the objects on show and to the acquisition of new exhibits. Visitors can study, for example, the material for koh-do, the traditional Japanese art of identifying incense, or admire Marie-Antoinette's toiletries trunk which she took with her when traveling.

In addition to the exhibits, there are screenings of perfume commercials and, on the top floor, many of the magnificent plants and flowers used in perfumery, such as lavender, roses, jasmine, vanilla, vetiver and ylang-ylang, are cultivated under glass. The museum also runs an introductory course in the creation of a toilet water. Visitors should not miss "La Visite de Grenouille," which takes them around Grasse on the trail of the hero of Süskind's novel, *Perfume.*

CHÂTEAU-PROMENADE
DES PARFUMS DE CHAMEROLLES
45170 Chilleurs-aux-Bois. Tel: 38 39 84 66
The Château de Chamerolles, near Orléans, with its drawbridge and exquisitely proportioned main courtyard, offers visitors what is charmingly called a "perfume walk." After five years of restoration, this superb Renaissance château opened its doors to the public in 1992, revealing a delightful museum incorporating a series of small, beautifully decorated salons, each of which sets the scene for one use of the various ways perfume was used from the sixteenth to the eighteenth centuries. Visitors can admire an extremely interesting collection of perfume bottles displayed using skillful lighting, which sets off the glass, crystal and magic of the perfume bottles to their best advantage. There is a store where you can purchase traditional posters and perfumed objects, fragrance sachets for perfuming wardrobes and pretty soaps. This idyllic walk continues in the grounds, where one can visit the gardens and the herb gardens, and admire the fine collection of old roses.

L'OSMOTHÈQUE DE VERSAILLES
36, rue du Parc de Clagny,
78000 Versailles. Tel: 39 55 46 99
Visits by appointment only.
The Osmothèque in Versailles is a veritable fragrance library, a sort of olfactory conservatory which is absolutely unique. It was created in 1990 by Jean Kerléo, the perfumer for Jean Patou, and its vocation is to preserve and perpetuate the perfume heritage. There are six hundred contemporary perfumes assembled here, their ranks constantly swelled by new acquisitions. In addition, Osmothèque perfumers have been able to gain access to certain secret formulas, enabling them to reconstitute one hundred long-forgotten perfumes for presentation to the public. A perfumer is in charge of each session, which is attended by about thirty participants. He presents the perfumes in their minute phials and, using blotter strips, the participants can smell perfumes such as Eau de la Reine de Hongrie, Le Trèfle Incarnat created by L.T. Piver in 1896, Le Fruit Défendu by Les Parfums de Rosine (created by Paul Poiret in 1918), Sous le Vent de Guerlain created in 1933, A Suma by Coty dating from 1936, Jacques Fath's Iris Gris created in 1947 and the eau de Cologne which Napoleon used in Saint Helena.

ODORAMA
Presented in conjunction with the series of exhibitions, "Expressions et Comportements," Musée Explora, Niveau 1, La Villette, Cité des Sciences et de l'Industrie, 30, avenue Corentin Cariou, 75019 Paris. Tel: 40 05 70 00
Open daily except Mondays.
The powerful fragrance of the orchid which slipped down into Odette's cleavage and which Swann passionately sought with his lips is quite irresistible! In Odorama's small projection room, the scent of the orchid contributes to the emotion of the audience watching this scene in Schlöndorff's movie, Swann's Way. When the images and sounds of scenes on the screen are accompanied by odors, they seem far more real. In another scene, a delicious aroma heralds the appearance of a bowl of hot chocolate. The Cinéma Odorant game, in which the spectator chooses the movie sequence he wants to see and smell, is the only one so far open to the public, but Odorama, which was opened in 1986 and is the highlight of the Explora Museum, will be opening two more in 1996.

LE MUSÉE DES ARÔMES ET DU PARFUM
La Chavêche, petite route du Grès,
13690 Graveson-en-Provence. Tel: 90 95 81 55
For fifteen years now, Nelly Grosjean, who is descended from a long line of traditional aromatherapists, has chosen to share her love of plants and her passion for essential oils with the public. Today, her creations are enjoyed in France and abroad. Aromatherapy opens up an enchanting aromatic world centered around nature and contributes to personal well-being and an improved lifestyle. In addition to the museum, there is a store where one can purchase essential oils, perfumes, and antique perfume bottles, etc.

PERFUME SCHOOLS

Whether you are looking for an introduction to the world of perfumery or wanting to improve existing skills, the best schools and the most prestigious training centres in the world are to be found in France. Details of these are given below, along with addresses of institutions in the United States offering courses on various aspects of perfumery.

France

ÉCOLE GIVAUDAN-ROURE
57, avenue Pierre Semard,
06332 Grasse Cedex. Tel: (16) 93 40 10 60
This school was founded by the perfumer Jean Carles in 1947. It is known throughout the world and has trained most of the greatest perfumers of our age. According to the perfumer Françoise Marin, who took over the management of the school in 1990, the principal qualities required in this profession are patience, enthusiasm and perseverance. The entire course lasts six years and comprises eighteen months of theory in Grasse, eighteen months training abroad and, finally, three years of apprenticeship. This school provides the best chances for

those aspiring to the highest posts in the perfume industry.

ISIPCA
Institut Supérieur International du Parfum, de la Cosmétique et de l'Aromatique Alimentaire,
36, rue du parc de Clagny,
78000 Versailles. Tel: 39 54 85 82
This school, known throughout the world for the quality of its training, is unique. The curriculum for the three-year training period is drawn up in conjunction with the management of the industries concerned, and students are in direct contact with established members of the profession.

CINQUIEME SENS
18, rue de Montessuy,
75007 Paris. Tel: 47 53 79 16
Monique Schlienger, a talented perfumer, has decided to share her passion with all those, amateur or professional, who wish to learn about perfume, or to broaden their existing knowledge. Neophytes can become initiated in the rudiments of perfume, learn to decode fragrances and recognize the main olfactory families. People with more experience are given the opportunity to review their existing knowledge, explore new trends and analyze the most recent creations. This institution offers a flexible, personalized training course attended by groups of no more than ten people in a professional and welcoming atmosphere. Courses in English can be arranged on request.

EMANESCENCE
18, rue de Montessuy, 75007 Paris.
Tel: 47 53 00 86
The aim of this association, presided over by Monique Schlienger, is to permit amateurs to discover the art of perfumery. The training course, which is both fun and educational, enables participants to explore the world of perfume, to develop their olfactory perception and to become acquainted with the raw materials used by perfumers. Courses are organized all year round. English-language courses for groups can be arranged on demand.

USA

Ms. Peg Smith
FASHION INSTITUTE OF TECHNOLOGY
227, West Twenty-seventh Street, New York,
NY 10001.
Tel: (212) 760 7850
Ms. Bonnie M. Scheid
TOBE COBURN SCHOOL FOR FASHION CAREERS
686, Broadway, New York, NY 10021.
Tel: (212) 460 9600

Ms. Terry Reynolds
COSMETIC & FRAGRANCE MKTG. & MERCHANDISING DIV.
Parsons Midtown Campus,
560, Seventh Avenue, New York, NY 10018.

FAIRLEIGH DICKINSON UNIVERSITY
College of Science and Engineering,

PERFUMED FABRICS
Who will be able to resist the materials of the future which combine the pleasures of sight, touch and smell, such as a silk scarf perfumed with one's favorite Guerlain or Patou fragrance?
It is thanks to the dynamic and talented young chemist Sandra Vogt that Jean-François Perrin, an industrialist from the Dauphiné region in France, was able to produce the first perfumed fabric. In order to create this revolutionary object, Sandra Vogt had to accomplish the technical feat of introducing minute particles saturated with essential oils into the molecules of the material. The success of the operation has paved the way for materials perfumed with all kinds of fragrances. Sandra Vogt, who loves Samsara and Shalimar, already dreams of new ways of dressing, "A garment enclosing a fragrance could be an original way of wearing a perfume." What could be simpler? The natural movements of the body magnify the aromas and fragrances of the material. "Furthermore," explains the inventor of the process, "after several weeks the perfumed material will continue to perfume the wardrobe."
Although in its early stages, we are sure this is not the last we shall hear of this invention.
For more information, contact: Groupe Perrin, 202, Chemin du Violet, 38690 Le Grand-Lemp. Tel: (16) 76 55 59 20.

Department of Chemistry, Hackensack Campus,
Teaneck, NJ 07666. Tel: (201) 692 2330

FAIRLEIGH DICKINSON UNIVERSITY
The Continuing Education Center,
P.O. Box 1605, South Hackensack, NJ 07606.
Tel: (201) 836 4652

Ms. Jeanne O. Leonard
FASHION INSTITUTE OF DESIGN & MERCHANDISING
818, West-Seventh Street, Los Angeles, CA 90017–3407.
Tel: (213) 624 1200

Dean Stack
INTERNATIONAL FINE ARTS COLLEGE
1737, N. Bayshore Drive, Miami, FL 33132.
Tel: (305) 373 4684

FOOD AND FRAGRANCE

Some of the great French chefs like Michel Bras have revived the French gastronomic tradition of using herbs and creating daring accords. However, to our knowledge, Maurice Maurin is the only chef to have gone as far as incorporating essences used by perfumers into his dishes. This perfumer and gourmet decided to give the public the opportunity of trying the various dishes he had concocted for his friends. After a series of dinners on the theme of fragrance, organized in conjunction with Gaston Lenôtre, he decided to open his own restaurant. This unique establishment offers exquisite dishes seasoned with essential oils, such as the consommé of velvet swimming crab and langoustine with lemon leaves and neroli essence, which has to be tasted to be believed. A must for perfume-lovers visiting Paris!

MACIS ET MUSCADE
110, rue Legendre, 75017 Paris.
Tel: (1) 42 26 62 26

WEARING PERFUME

The art of perfuming oneself is a pleasure accessible to all. There are, however, a few rules and secrets which one should be aware of in order to fully appreciate fragrances and their powers of attraction.

SKIN TYPES

Everyone has had occasion to notice that perfumes vary depending on the wearer's skin, to such an extent that it is sometimes impossible to recognize your favorite fragrance when it is worn by someone else. Four factors determine the way in which perfume changes once it is applied:
– perspiration favors perfume evaporation, in other words the more a person perspires the less lasting the perfume;
– skin acidity, known as the pH, affects the quality of the odorous molecules, thus altering the harmony of the accords;
– the skin's profile, i.e. its smoothness or roughness, which is visible under the microscope, influences the persistence of perfume; rough skin retains fragrances, whereas smooth skin allows them to escape more rapidly;
– the skin's fat content also affects duration: those with greasy skins are in luck because they retain perfume the longest!

IN THE SUN

It is not advisable to wear perfume on the beach or when exposed to the sun for long periods because of the numerous cutaneous reactions which ultraviolet rays can provoke when in contact with the carbon content of the alcohol which is used in perfume. In the heat of the summer it is therefore advisable to use nonalcoholic perfumes, such as lotions, creams and perfumed talcs.

HOW TO APPLY PERFUME

Coco Chanel used to say that one could perfume oneself where one would like to be kissed. This idea is appealing, but needs to be adapted to suit the range of perfume products now available. How and where a perfume is applied depends on whether one uses an extract, eau de parfum, or toilet water.

The extract, which is lasting and heady, but can also be intrusive, requires precision and discretion. It should be dabbed on the pulse points (where the pulse of the heartbeat is closest to the skin), i.e. the base of the throat, behind the ear lobes, between the breasts, the underside of the wrists and behind the knees. Hair is a wonderful captor of odors and one drop applied to the roots is sufficient to create a trail. The extract is effective for six hours.

Eau de parfum, generally sold in atomizers, can be applied more generously, for example to the shoulders, the nape of the neck and the bust, and can be renewed during the day. It is a product which is well adapted to professional life, for the fragrance it diffuses is noticeable but discreet. Its fragrance lasts for four hours.

The lightness and transience of toilet water enable it to be used in the morning, or after sport or physical exertion. It is not very concentrated and leaves a subtle, fragrant veil on the skin which lasts for two hours. It is particularly favored by men, who appreciate its invigorating effect. It is true that toilet water is ideally suited

---

SOLID PERFUMES

Nothing is more pleasant and convenient, when traveling or working at the office, than colognes and fragrances in solid form, like the charming concretes now coming back into fashion. Perfume in this minimal form has great diffusive power. A concrete obtained from flower waxes produces a single floral fragrance of, for example, rose, jasmine, lavender, vetiver, sandalwood, vanilla or patchouli. When derived from perfume essences, it assumes the identity of the perfume used. Ever since Molinard produced the first concretes in the 1920s, numerous perfumers have followed in his footsteps, including Fragonard and Norfolk Lavender (see "Perfume Stores, England").

---

to the somewhat haphazard way men have of perfuming themselves and has an immediate revivifying effect.

Lotions, creams and perfumed talc, the body collections, offer a more sensual and lasting way of perfuming oneself. Whereas perfume is applied to strategic points, these products envelop the skin, clothing the body. The association of cream and talc is just as effective as the extract, as the talc acts as a fixative. The average perfume concentration is 9% for talcs, 8% for creams and 3–5% for lotions.

PERFUMING CLOTHES

In Japan, clothes were always the principal medium for perfume. The refined Japanese woman never perfumed her skin directly, for fear of compromising her purity, or of being taken for a woman of easy morals, but instead stitched odorous wood shavings into the hem of her kimono. This sophisticated use of perfume might appeal to western women, but they should be extremely

---

HOW TO KEEP YOUR PERFUME

Fragrances deteriorate if kept more than three years. This especially applies to the extract, which, even if it is closed and sealed by the baudruchage process, is more sensitive to light than other perfumed products. The first piece of advice, which applies to all perfumed products irrespective of their concentration, is to keep them in a cool place away from direct light. Light, along with heat, damp and variations in temperature, is damaging to all perfumes. As soon as they are opened, they start to suffer the effects of the environment. If badly stored, fragrances become unusable after only a few months. It is therefore preferable to buy them in minimal quantities, that is to say 15 ml. of extract, 25 ml. of eau de parfum and 50 ml. of toilet water, which significantly reduces the risk of deterioration.

---

wary of it. "Perfuming one's clothes can lead to disaster," explains Madame Lesêche, who runs a dry cleaner's in Paris. It is to her that the leading fashion designers bring their valuable creations. "When I started this trade in 1936, the stains caused by perfumes were not as damaging as they are today, which is due to the artificial coloring now used. The marks cannot be removed from certain materials; the most vulnerable materials are silk, satin, synthetic fibers, all white and pastel-colored materials and white fur; the stain turns yellow and then brown if the garment is left hanging in the wardrobe for several days under a dust cover. I advise all my clients to perfume themselves before dressing. In the event of an accident, the sooner I receive the garment, the better my chances of saving it." On the other hand, there is no risk with dark-colored wool, cashmere and soft materials such as tweed, whose heavy fibers capture the perfume without sustaining any damage. The "fur" perfumes are heady fragrances with balsam and animal notes, but you should avoid saturating astrakhans, minks and fox furs with them, especially if they are white. Fur, like silk or crepe, is fragile, so only the lining should be perfumed. Prudence is also recommended with leather and suede garments which can also be stained by perfume. Finally, if you wear pearls they should be removed when applying perfume, as they too can stain.

PERFUME CONCENTRATES

Perfumes are available in more or less concentrated forms and their designations are governed by two criteria: the degree of concentration of the perfume base and the strength of the alcohol added to it. These two quantities vary considerably depending on the make and the raw materials employed. The proportions of raw materials used in the formula also vary, depending on whether it is for the extract or its derivatives.

The **extract** (sometimes improperly termed "perfume"), the ultimate in perfumery, contains the highest percentage, i.e. 20–30% of perfumed concentrate diluted in very pure, 96% proof alcohol. This is the most lasting and intense means of perfuming oneself.

Eau de parfum (sometimes called coeur de parfum, fleur de parfum, etc., by certain manufacturers—the terms are as varied as they are poetic), is generally sold in atomizers and is the most popular product on the market today. Its concentration is lower than that of the extract, i.e. 10–20% concentrate, diluted in 90% proof alcohol.

Toilet water suits those who are looking for something light and discreet. It contains less than 10% of perfumed concentrate diluted in 90% proof alcohol. In order to provide maximum freshness, the top notes are accentuated.

Eau de Cologne is derived from a specific formula based on the cologne first introduced by Giovanni Paolo Feminis. It is dominated by fresh, citrus notes, which are blended with floral or spicy notes, depending on the formula. Its concentration never exceeds 8%, diluted in 85% proof alcohol.

CLASSIFYING PERFUMES

Prompted by the fact that perfumes are becoming more numerous every day and their olfactory characteristics are constantly evolving, in 1990 a group of perfumers from the Société Française des Parfumeurs, led by Jean Kerléo, Jean Patou's perfumer, decided to draw up a classification of perfume types. Seven large olfactory families were defined. These seven families have been subdivided into smaller families, allowing a more precise identification of the personality of each fragrance. The classification includes all the men's and women's fragrances on the market, the oldest being Eau de Cologne 4711 by Mülhens. Some perfumes which are no longer available, such as Chypre by Coty, are also included because they are key olfactory reference points. This classification is very useful, of course, to the profession, in that it provides a panorama of contemporary and past creations, but it also provides the consumer with a guide when choosing a new fragrance among the myriad creations—a notoriously difficult task! The classification by family makes your choice less complicated: if you have a perfume you like, but want a change, you can find ideas for new fragrances in the same family. In this way you can be sure of finding the same basic notes which you like so much in your usual perfume, but with a subtle difference, that key touch which makes each fragrance so individual.

The classification is updated once a year, which explains why some of the very latest creations have not yet been included. Moreover, perfumers do not consider the classification as definitive: frequent changes are made to ensure that it evolves with the times and fits consumers' tastes. The American Fragrance Foundation follows a slightly different method of classification, including not seven but nine fragrance families: single floral, floral bouquet, spicy, oriental blend, green, fruity, citrus, aldehyde and woody-mossy. For a full description of fragrances available on the American market, consult *The Fragrance Foundation Reference Guide* (see Bibliography). Here, the French classification system has been used.

CITRUS
This category covers the original eaux de Cologne, which are citrus waters made from the essential oils of bergamot, lemon and mandarin, combined with bitter orange blossom. It also includes all the contemporary colognes used by both men and women.

FLORAL
This is the largest of the seven fragrance families. It comprises the fragrances centered around one flower, known as single florals, the floral bouquets and all perfumes with predominantly floral notes. A few men's fragrances, such as Grey Flannel by Geoffrey Beene and Christian Dior's Fahrenheit, figure in this category.

FOUGERE
Although the French word fougère means fern, these fragrances do not evoke a fern odor, but an accord of lavender, woody, oakmoss, coumarin and bergamot notes. The best-known woman's fragrance in this category is Jicky by Guerlain. The most popular men's fragrances fall into this category, such as Azzaro pour Homme, Paco Rabanne pour Homme and Drakkar Noir by Guy Laroche.

CHYPRE
The perfume called Chypre created by François Coty in 1917, an accord of oakmoss, labdanum, patchouli and bergamot, was the source of this family, which mainly contains women's fragrances, such as the prestigious Mitsouko by Guerlain, Femme by Rochas and Christian Dior's Miss Dior.

WOODY
This group is dominated by men's fragrances. The woody notes are generally provided by sandalwood and cedar essences, as well as patchouli and vetiver with their fresh and invigorating top notes. All the vetiver fragrances created by Guerlain, Carven, Lanvin and Givenchy belong to this family.

AMBER
This family is generally known as "the orientals." These fragrances have a soft, powdery personality with vanilla accents. This group is dominated by women's fragrances, including some superb creations like Opium by Yves Saint Laurent, Estée Lauder's Cinnabar, Samsara by Guerlain, Coco by Chanel, but it also contains a few men's fragrances, such as Guerlain's sensual Habit Rouge.

LEATHER
This family stands somewhat apart from the others and is the smallest of the seven, comprising only about ten perfumes. Their unique, extremely dry notes are obtained from tobacco and from birch essences, which have a smoky fragrance. Tabac Blond by Caron, Cuir de Russie by Chanel and Bel Ami by Hermès all figure in this category.

THE SEVEN FRAGRANCE FAMILIES

The first column gives the name of the perfume, the second, in capitals, the name of its creator and the year of creation.
M: men's fragrance W: women's fragrance

CITRUS

CITRUS

W
Eau Folle	GUY LAROCHE (1970)
Eau de Patou	JEAN PATOU (1976)
Bulgari	BULGARI (1992)

M
Kölnisch Wasser	FARINA GEGENUBER (1714)
Kölnisch Wasser 4711	MÜLHENS (1792)
Eau de Lubin	LUBIN (1798)
Gold Medal Cologne	ATKINSONS (1799)
Jean-Marie Farina	ROGER & GALLET (1806)
Eau de Cologne Impériale	GUERLAIN (1853)
Eau Fraîche	CHRISTIAN DIOR (1953)
Monsieur de Givenchy	GIVENCHY (1959)
Messire	JEAN D'ALBRET (1961)
Monsieur Balmain	PIERRE BALMAIN (1964)
Signoricci	NINA RICCI (1965)
Eau de Guerlain	GUERLAIN (1974)
Eau d'Hadrien	ANNICK GOUTAL (1980)
Ungaro II	UNGARO (1992)

M
Eau Fraîche	LEONARD (1974)
Monsieur Lanvin	LANVIN (1964)
Eau Sauvage	CHRISTIAN DIOR (1966)
Eau Neuve	LUBIN (1968)
Bravas	SHISEIDO (1969)
Eroika	KANEBO (1970)
Eau de Cologne d'Hermès	HERMES (1979)
Trophée Lancôme	LANCOME (1982)
Eau Sauvage Extrême	CHRISTIAN DIOR (1984)
Eau du Caporal	L'ARTISAN PARFUMEUR (1985)
Boucheron	BOUCHERON (1991)

CITRUS FLORAL CHYPRE

W
Ô de Lancôme	LANCOME (1968)
Eau de Rochas	ROCHAS (1970)

CITRUS SPICY

M
Eau de Lanvin	LANVIN (1933)
Eau d'Hermès	HERMES (1951)
Lime Old Spice	SHULTON (1965)
Royal Regiment	MAX FACTOR (1969)
Cacharel pour Homme	CACHAREL (1981)

CITRUS WOODY

M
Eau de Sport Lacoste	JEAN PATOU (1968)
Drakkar	GUY LAROCHE (1972)

Halston D 12	HALSTON (1972)
Masculin 2	BOURJOIS (1975)
Signoricci 2	NINA RICCI (1975)
Armani	ARMANI (1984)
Eau de Sport Santos	CARTIER (1989)
1881	NINO CERRUTI (1990)
Eau de Rochas	ROCHAS (1993)

CITRUS AROMATIC

W	Eau de Courrèges	COURREGES (1974)
M	Dunhill for Men	DUNHILL (1936)
	Green Water	JACQUES FATH (1947)
	Eau Cendrée	JACOMO (1971)
	Lanvin for Men	LANVIN (1979)
	Ebène	PIERRE BALMAIN (1983)
	Byblos Uomo	BYBLOS (1992)

FLORAL

SINGLE FLORAL
ROSE

W	Rose	MOLINARD (1860)
	Rose Jacqueminot	COTY (1904)
	La Rose d'Orsay	D'ORSAY (1908)
	Tea Rose	THE PERFUMER'S WORKSHOP (1976)
	A Rose is a Rose	HOUBIGANT (1976)

JASMINE

W	Jasmin	MOLINARD (1860)
	Jasmin de Corse	COTY (1906)
	Jasmin	LE GALION (1940)

LILY OF THE VALLEY

W	Le Muguet des Bois	COTY (1942)
	Lily of the Valley	LE GALION (1950)
	Le Muguet du Bonheur	CARON (1952)
	Premier Muguet	BOURJOIS (1955)
	Diorissimo	CHRISTIAN DIOR (1956)

CARNATION

| W | Bellodgia | CARON (1927) |

NARCISSUS

| W | Narcisse Noir | CARON (1912) |

LILAC

| W | Apple Blossom | HELENA RUBINSTEIN (1948) |

GARDENIA

| W | Gardénia | CHANEL (1925) |
| | Gardénia | LE GALION (1937) |

TUBEROSE

W	Tubéreuse	LE GALION (1939)
	Fracas	PIGUET (1948)
	Crescendo	LANVIN (1965)
	Chloé	KARL LAGERFELD (1975)
	Jontue	REVLON (1976)
	Pavlova	PAYOT (1976)
	Spectacular	JOAN COLLINS (1989)

VIOLET

W	Vera Violetta	ROGER & GALLET (1892)
	Violette Pourpre	HOUBIGANT (1907)
	Violette de Toulouse	BERDOUES (1937)
	Violette	LE GALION (1950)

SINGLE FLORAL LAVENDER

M	English Lavender	ATKINSONS (1910)
	Old English Lavender	YARDLEY (1913)
	Pour un Homme	CARON (1934)
	Agua Lavanda	PUIG (1940)

FLORAL BOUQUET

W	L'Idéal	HOUBIGANT (1900)
	Floramye	L.T. PIVER (1903)
	Pompéia	L.T. PIVER (1907)
	Quelques Fleurs	HOUBIGANT (1912)
	Narcisse Bleu	MURY (1920)
	My Sin	LANVIN (1925)
	Rêve d'Or	L.T. PIVER (1926)
	Amour Amour	JEAN PATOU (1928)
	Moment Suprême	JEAN PATOU (1931)
	Je Reviens	WORTH (1932)
	Fleurs et Rocaille	CARON (1933)
	Blue Grass	ELIZABETH ARDEN (1935)
	Joy	JEAN PATOU (1935)
	Fame	CORDAY (1937)
	Brumes	LE GALION (1939)
	L'Air du Temps	NINA RICCI (1947)
	Le Dix	BALENCIAGA (1947)
	Snob	LE GALION (1952)
	Le Dé	GIVENCHY (1956)

Capricci	NINA RICCI (1960)
Princesse d'Albret	JEAN D'ALBRET (1964)
Super Estée	ESTEE LAUDER (1969)
Super Moondrops	REVLON (1970)
1000	JEAN PATOU (1972)
Charlie	REVLON (1973)
Yendi	CAPUCCI (1975)
Unspoken	AVON (1975)
Cardin	PIERRE CARDIN (1976)
Flamme	BOURJOIS (1976)
Blasé	MAX FACTOR (1977)
Valentino	VALENTINO (1978)
White Linen	ESTEE LAUDER (1978)
Anaïs Anaïs	CACHAREL (1979)
Métal	PACO RABANNE (1979)
Madame de Carven	CARVEN (1979)
Symbiose	STEBDHAL (1980)
Giorgio	GIORGIO BEVERLY HILLS (1981)
Or Noir	PASCAL MORABITO (1981)
Guirlandes	CARVEN (1982)
Clair de Jour	LANVIN (1983)
Fleurs d'Orlane	ORLANE (1983)
Les Jardins de Bagatelle	GUERLAIN (1983)
Paris YSL	YVES SAINT LAURENT (1983)
Azzaro 9	LORIS AZZARO (1984)
Lumière	ROCHAS (1984)
Création	TED LAPIDUS (1984)
Barynia	HELENA RUBINSTEIN (1985)
Gian Franco Ferre	GIAN FRANCO FERRE (1985)
Maxim's	MAXIM'S (1985)
Intrigue	CARVEN (1986)
Insolent	CHARLES JOURDAN (1986)
Rose de Rouge	GEMEY (1986)
Mon Classique	MORABITO (1987)
Trouble	REVLON (1988)
Eternity	CALVIN KLEIN (1988)
Vie Privée	YVES ROCHER (1989)
Parfum d'Elle	MONTANA (1990)
Trésor	LANCOME (1990)
Fantasme	TED LAPIDUS (1992)
Très Jourdan	JOURDAN (1992)
Volupté	OSCAR DE LA RENTA (1992)
Wines	GIORGIO BEVERLY HILLS (1992)
Zoa	REGINE (1992)
360°	PERRY ELLIS (1993)

GREEN FLORAL

W	Vent Vert	PIERRE BALMAIN (1945)
	Grafitti	CAPUCCI (1963)
	Câline	JEAN PATOU (1964)
	Belle de Rauch	MADELEINE DE RAUCH (1966)
	Fidji	GUY LAROCHE (1966)
	Masumi	COTY (1967)
	Chanel N° 19	CHANEL (1970)
	Norell	NORELL (1970)
	Geoffrey Beene	GEOFFREY BEENE (1971)
	Alliage	ESTEE LAUDER (1972)
	Cialenga	BALENCIAGA (1973)
	Inouï	SHISEIDO (1976)
	Shocking You	SCHIAPARELLI (1976)
	Silence	JACOMO (1978)
	Vôtre	CHARLES JOURDAN (1978)
	Murasaki	SHISEIDO (1980)
	Eau de Givenchy	GIVENCHY (1980)
	Must du Jour	CARTIER (1981)
	Alix	GRES (1982)

	Fleur de Fleurs	NINA RICCI (1982)
	Le Jardin	MAX FACTOR (1983)
	Sung	A. SUNG (1989)
	Safari	RALPH LAUREN (1989)
	Cabotine	GRES (1990)
	Private Number	AIGNER (1991)
	Parfum d'Eté	KENZO (1992)
	DNA for Women	BIJAN (1993)
	Must II	CARTIER (1993)
	Nature	YVES ROCHER (1993)
	Pour la Femme	ROGER & GALLET (1993)

FLORAL ALDEHYDE

W	Chanel N° 5	CHANEL (1921)
	Le Dandy	D'ORSAY (1923)
	L'Aimant	COTY (1927)
	Arpège	LANVIN (1927)
	Liu	GUERLAIN (1929)
	Sortilège	LE GALION (1937)
	Cœur de Joie	NINA RICCI (1947)
	Robe d'un Soir	CARVEN (1947)
	Magie	LANCOME (1949)
	Detchema	REVILLON (1953)
	Fath de Fath	JACQUES FATH (1953)
	Casaque	JEAN D'ALBRET (1956)
	L'Interdit	GIVENCHY (1957)
	Topaze	AVON (1959)
	Madame Rochas	ROCHAS (1960)
	Parce Que	CAPUCCI (1963)
	Dédicace	CHERAMY (1966)
	Climat	LANCOME (1967)
	Calandre	PACO RABANNE (1969)
	Kiku	FABERGE (1969)
	Evasion	BOURJOIS (1970)
	Infini	CARON (1970)
	Chicane	JACOMO (1971)
	Rive Gauche	YVES SAINT LAURENT (1971)
	Farouche	NINA RICCI (1974)
	Gucci I	GUCCI (1974)
	Aviance	MATCHABELLI (1975)
	First	VAN CLEEF & ARPELS (1976)
	Tamango	LEINARD (1977)
	Cléa	YVES ROCHER (1981)
	Gauloise	MOLYNEUX (1981)
	Ombre Rose	JEAN-CHARLES BROSSEAU (1981)
	Un Jour	CHARLES JOURDAN (1982)
	Saso	SHISEIDO (1987)
	Nina	NINA RICCI (1987)
	Loulou	CACHAREL (1987)
	Unhibited	CHER (1988)
	Joop! le Bain	JOOP! (1989)
	Ferré de Ferré	FERRE (1991)
M	Tabac Original	MAURER & WIRTZ (1955)
	Jovan Musk for Men	JOVAN (1974)

WOODY FLORAL

M	Grey Flannel	GEOFFREY BEENE (1976)
	Lauder for Men	ESTEE LAUDER (1985)

	Fahrenheit	CHRISTIAN DIOR (1988)
	Insensé	GIVENCHY (1993)
W	Amarige	GIVENCHY (1991)
	Laguna	DALI (1991)
	Lalique	LALIQUE (1992)
	Magnetic	GABRIELA SABATINI (1992)
	Charlie Red	REVLON (1993)
	Touch	FRED HAYMAN (1993)
	Vendetta	VALENTINO (1993)
	Fashion	LEONARD (1993)

WOODY FRUITY FLORAL

W	Iris Gris	JACQUES FATH (1947)
	Amazone	HERMES (1974)
	Quartz	MOLYNEUX (1977)
	Lauren	RALPH LAUREN (1978)
	Nahéma	GUERLAIN (1979)
	Molinard	MOLINARD (1979)
	Eau de Fleurs	NINA RICCI (1980)
	Envol	TED LAPIDUS (1980)
	Ivoire	PIERRE BALMAIN (1980)
	Turbulences	REVILLON (1981)
	Armani	GIORGIO ARMANI (1982)
	K	KRIZIA (1982)
	Nombre Noir	SHISEIDO (1982)
	Courrèges in Blue	COURREGES (1983)
	Filly	CAPUCCI (1983)
	Bambou	WEIL (1984)
	Niki de St-Phalle	NIKI DE SAINT-PHALLE (1984)
	Clandestine	GUY LAROCHE (1986)
	Jardin d'Amour	MAX FACTOR (1986)
	Tiffany	TIFFANY (1987)
	Calyx	ESTEE LAUDER (1987)
	Kenzo	KENZO (1988)
	273	FRED HAYMAN (1989)
	Red	GIORGIO BEVERLY HILLS (1989)
	Rose Cardin	PIERRE CARDIN (1990)
	Realities	LIZ CLAIBORNE (1990)
	Anthracite	JACOMO (1991)
	Giò	GIORGIO ARMANI (1992)
	Narcisse	CHLOE (1992)
	Senso (2)	UNGARO (1992)
	Catalyst	HALSTON/BORGHESE (1993)
	Il Bacio	PRINCESSE MARCELLA BORGHESE (1993)
	Sweet Courrèges	COURREGES (1993)
	Tribu	BENETTON (1993)
M	Ténéré	PACO RABANNE (1988)
	Cool Water	DAVIDOFF (1988)
	Eternity	CALVIN KLEIN (1989)
	Photo	KARL LAGERFELD (1990)
	Night Flight	JOOP!/LANCASTER (1992)

OCEANIC FLORAL

W	New West for Her	ARAMIS (1990)
	Wrappings	CLINIQUE (1990)
	Escape	CALVIN KLEIN (1991)
	L'Eau d'Issey	ISSEY MIYAKE (1992)
	Sunflowers	ELIZABETH ARDEN (1992)

FOUGERE

FOUGERE

W	Jicky	GUERLAIN (1889)
	Le Trêfle Incarnat	L.T. PIVER (1896)
	Maia	MYRURGIA (1925)
	Flor de Blason	MYRURGIA (1927)
	20 Carats	DANA (1933)
	Canoé	DANA (1935)
M	Fougère Royale	HOUBIGANT (1882)
	Moustache	ROCHAS (1949)
	Heno de Pravia	GAL (1955)
	That Man	REVLON (1961)
	YSL	YVES SAINT LAUREN (1975)
	Il pour Homme	DIPARCO (L'OREAL) (1977)
	AZTEC	YVES ROCHER (1993)

SWEET AMBER FOUGERE

M	Skin Bracer	MENNEN (1941)
	Equateur	BOURJOIS (1993)

FLORAL AMBER FOUGERE

M	Varon Dandy	PARERA (1924)
	Jade East	SWANK (1964)
	Brut for Men	FABERGE (1964)
	Arden for Men (Sandalwood)	ELIZABETH ARDEN (1965)
	Hai Karate	LEEMING PACQUIN (1967)
	Blue Stratos	SHULTON (1975)
	Para Hombre	LOEWE (1978)

SPICY FOUGERE

M	Ice Blue Aqua Velva	WILLIAMS (1935)
	Old Spice	SHULTON (1935)

Monsieur Rochas	ROCHAS	(1969)
Equipage	HERMES	(1970)
Ho Hang	BALENCIAGA	(1971)
Anthracite	JACOMO	(1991)
Enigme	PIERRE CARDIN	(1992)

AROMATIC FOUGERE

M	Men's Club	HELENA RUBINSTEIN	(1966)
	Balafre	LANCOME	(1967)
	Rabanne pour Homme	PACO RABANNE	(1973)
	Juvena Men	JUVENA	(1974)
	Captain	MOLYNEUX	(1975)
	Bogart	BOGART	(1976)
	Marbert Man	MARBERT	(1977)
	Azzaro pour Homme	LORIS AZZARO	(1978)
	Chaps	WARNER COSMETICS	(1979)
	L'Homme	ROGER & GALLET	(1980)
	Calvin	CALVIN KLEIN	(1981)
	Stetson	STETSON COTY	(1981)
	Drakkar Noir	GUY LAROCHE	(1982)

Lacoste	LACOSTE	(1984)
Tuscany	ARAMIS LAUDER	(1984)
Bleu Marine	PIERRE CARDIN	(1986)
Boss	BOSS H. BETRIX	(1986)
Smalto	FRANCESCO SMALTO	(1987)
Jazz	YVES SAINT LAURENT	(1988)
Gucci Nobile	GUCCI	(1988)
Tsar	VAN CLEEF & ARPELS	(1989)
Red	GIORGIO BEVERLY HILLS	(1991)
Versus	VERSACE	(1991)
Elements	HUGO BOSS	(1993)
Egoïste Platinum	CHANEL	(1993)
Horizon	GUY LAROCHE	(1993)
Molto Smalto	FRANCESCO SMALTO	(1993)
Ungaro III	UNGARO	(1993)
Eau Fresh	JACQUES BOGART	(1993)

FRUITY FOUGERE

M	Escape for Men	CALVIN KLEIN	(1993)

CHYPRE

CHYPRE

M	Pour Monsieur	CHANEL	(1955)
	Sagamore	LANCOME	(1985)
W	Chypre	COTY	(1917)

FLORAL CHYPRE

M	Chromatics	ESTEE LAUDER	(1973)
	Giorgio for Men	GIORGIO BEVERLY HILLS	(1984)
	Davidoff	DAVIDOFF	(1984)
	Zino Davidoff	DAVIDOFF	(1986)
	Dali pour Homme	SALVADOR DALI	(1987)
	Furyo	JACQUES BOGART	(1988)
	Ungaro pour Homme	UNGARO	(1991)
	Héritage	GUERLAIN	(1992)
	Escada for Men	ESCADA	(1993)
W	Donna Trussardi	TRUSSARDI	(1993)

FLORAL ALDEHYDIC CHYPRE

W	Crêpe de Chine	MILLOT	(1925)
	Zibeline	WEIL	(1928)
	Fruit Vert	FLOREL	(1930)
	Nuit de Longchamp	LUBIN	(1937)
	Carnet de Bal	REVILLON	(1937)
	Aphrodisia	FABERGE	(1938)
	Antilope	WEIL	(1945)
	Ma Griffe	CARVEN	(1946)
	Réplique	RAPHAEL	(1947)
	Glamour	BOURJOIS	(1953)
	Mémoire Chérie	ELIZABETH ARDEN	(1957)
	Calèche	HERMES	(1961)
	Chant d'Arômes	GUERLAIN	(1962)
	Fashion	LEONARD	(1970)
	Vivre	MOLYNEUX	(1971)
	Coriande	JEAN COUTURIER	(1973)
	Complice	COTY	(1976)
	Halston	HALSTON	(1974)
	Mystère de Rochas	ROCHAS	(1978)
	Versace	GIANNI VERSACE	(1982)
	Diva	UNGARO	(1983)
	Schéhérazade	JEAN DESPREZ	(1983)
	Diamella	YVES ROCHER	(1984)
	Trussardi	TRUSSARDI	(1984)
	Paloma Picasso	PALOMA PICASSO	(1985)
	Catherine Deneuve	CATHERINE DENEUVE	(1986)
	Fendi	FENDI	(1987)
	JCC2	JEAN-CHARLES CASTELBAJAC	(1988)
	Knowing	ESTEE LAUDER	(1988)

FRUITY CHYPRE

W	Mitsouko	GUERLAIN	(1919)
	Cinq de Molyneux	MOLYNEUX	(1925)
	Rumeur	LANVIN	(1932)
	Femme	ROCHAS	(1944)
	Diorama	CHRISTIAN DIOR	(1949)

Canasta	JACQUES FATH	(1950)
Quadrille	BALENCIAGA	(1955)
Fête	MOLYNEUX	(1962)
Y	YVES SAINT LAURENT	(1964)
Diorella	CHRISTIAN DIOR	(1972)
Cristalle	CHANEL	(1974)
Azzaro	LORIS AZZARO	(1975)
Choc	PIERRE CARDIN	(1981)
Cerruti	NINO CERRUTI	(1987)
Bleu de Chine	MARC DE LA MORANDIERE	(1987)
V.E.	GIANNI VERSACE	(1990)
Yves Saint Laurent	YVES SAINT LAURENT	(1993)

	(Champagne) Le Parfum	SONIA RYKIEL	(1993)
M	Sables	ANNICK GOUTAL	(1982)
	Halston Limited	HALSTON	(1987)

GREEN CHYPRE

W	Miss Dior	CHRISTIAN DIOR	(1947)
	Intimate	REVLON	(1955)
	Vert et Blanc	CARVEN	(1958)
	Vivara	PUCCI	(1956)
	Givenchy III	GIVENCHY	(1970)
	Timeless	AVON	(1974)
	Sophia	COTY	(1980)
	Senchal	CHARLES OF THE RITZ	(1981)
	Halston Couture	HALSTON	(1988)
M	Grès pour Homme	GRES	(1965)
	Polo	RALPH LAUREN	(1978)
	Polo Crest	RALPH LAUREN	(1978)
	Chevignon	CHEVIGNON	(1992)

AROMATIC CHYPRE

M	Snuff	SCHIAPARELLI	(1938)
	Sir Irish Moos	MÜLHENS 4711	(1969)
	Yaragan	CARON	(1976)
	Halston 714	HALSTON	(1976)
	Révillon pour Homme	REVILLON	(1977)
	Jules	CHRISTIAN DIOR	(1980)
	Léonard pour Homme	LEONARD	(1980)
	Oscar pour Lui	OSCAR DE LA RENTA	(1980)
	Kouros	YVES SAINT LAURENT	(1981)
	Sander for Men	SANDER	(1981)
	Quorum	PUIG	(1982)
	Trussardi Uomo	TRUSSARDI MONTEIL	(1984)
	Borsalino	DIS PRA SPA	(1984)
	Philéas	NINA RICCI	(1984)
	Lapidus pour Homme	TED LAPIDUS	(1987)
	Lord	MOLYNEUX	(1988)
	New West for Him	ARAMIS	(1988)
	Street Life	HELENE BETRIX	(1990)
	White Water	REVLON	(1993)

LEATHER CHYPRE

W	Sous le Vent	GUERLAIN	(1993)

Emir	DANA	(1935)
Bandit	PIGUET	(1944)
Ramage	BOURJOIS	(1951)
Jolie Madame	PIERRE BALMAIN	(1953)
Cabochard	GRES	(1959)
Celui	DESSES	(1959)
Diorling	CHRISTIAN DIOR	(1963)
Zen	SHISEIDO	(1964)
Unforgettable	AVON	(1965)
Imprévu	COTY	(1966)
Miss Balmain	PIERRE BALMAIN	(1967)
Cachet	MATCHABELLI	(1970)
Empreinte	COURREGES	(1971)
Sikkim	LANCOME	(1971)
Red	GEOFFREY BEENE	(1976)
Ungaro	UNGARO	(1977)
J-L Scherrer	JEAN-LOUIS SCHERRER	(1980)
Norell 2	NORELL	(1980)
Missoni	MISSONI	(1982)

	Paradoxe	PIERRE CARDIN	(1983)
	La Nuit	PACO RABANNE	(1985)
	Parfum Rare	JACOMO	(1985)
	Montana	MONTANA	(1986)
	With Love	GALE HAYMAN	(1991)
	L'Arte di Guicci	GUICCI	(1991)
	Donna Karan	KARAN	(1992)
M	Aramis	ARAMIS/LAUDER	(1966)
	Kanon	SCANNON	(1966)
	Braggi	REVLON	(1966)
	Aigner Numéro 1	AIGNER	(1975)
	Van Cleef & Arpels Homme	VAN CLEEF & ARPELS	(1978)
	Party	HELENE BETRIX	(1980)
	Antaeus	CHANEL	(1981)
	Or Black	MORABITO	(1982)
	French Line	REVILLON	(1984)
	Iquitos	ALAIN DELON	(1987)
	Vendetta	VALENTINO	(1993)
	Zegna	A. PUIG	(1993)

WOODY

WOODY

M	Vetiver	CARVEN	(1957)
	Vetiver	GIVENCHY	(1959)
	Vetiver	LANVIN	(1964)
	Vetiver	LE GALION	(1969)
	Monsieur Venet	PHILIPPE VENET	(1969)
	Teck	MOLINARD	(1990)

CONIFER CITRUS WOODY

M	Aqua di Selva	VICTOR	(1949)
	Pino Sylvestre	VIDAL	(1955)
	Agua Brava	PUIG	(1968)
	Halston 101	HALSTON	(1984)
	Essencia Loewe	LOEWE	(1988)

AROMATIC WOODY

M	Executive	ATKINSONS	(1972)
	Gucci pour Homme	GUCCI	(1976)
	Devin	ARAMIS	(1978)
	Cerruti pour Homme	NINO CERRUTI	(1979)
	Tactics	SHISEIDO	(1979)
	Delon	ALAIN DELON	(1980)
	Macassar	ROCHAS	(1980)
	One Man Show	JACQUES BOGART	(1980)
	Versace l'Homme	VERSACE	(1984)
	Xeryus	GIVENCHY	(1986)
	Sport	PACO RABANNE	(1986)
	Métropolis	ESTEE LAUDER	(1987)
	Samarkande	YVES ROCHER	(1988)
	Vetiver Dry	CARVEN	(1988)
	Globe	ROCHAS	(1990)
	Ocean Rain	VALENTINO	(1990)
	Biagiotti Uomo	BIAGIOTTI	(1990)
	Ice Water	PINO SYLVESTRE	(1992)
	Minotaure	PALOMA PICASSO	(1992)
	Monsieur Léonard	LEONARD	(1992)
	Pasha	CARTIER	(1992)
	Safari for Men	RALPH LAUREN	(1992)
	Basala	SHISEIDO	(1993)

SPICY WOODY

M	Vetiver	GUERLAIN	(1959)
	Jacomo de Jacomo	JACOMO	(1980)
	Open	ROGER & GALLET	(1985)
	Kipling	WEIL	(1986)
	Bois Noir	CHANEL	(1987)
	Colors	BENETTON	(1988)
	Montana Homme	MONTANA	(1989)
	Ricci Club	NINA RICCI	(1989)
	Egoïste	CHANEL	(1990)
	Balenciaga pour Homme	BALENCIAGA	(1990)
	Pancaldi Uomo	PANCALDI	(1990)
	Gengis Khan	MORANDIERE	(1991)
	Herrera for Men	HERRERA	(1991)
	Land	LACOSTE	(1991)
	Salvador	SALVADOR DALI	(1992)
	Witness	JACQUES BOGART	(1992)

SPICY LEATHER WOODY

M	Acteur	LORIS AZZARO	(1989)

AMBER WOODY

M	Bill Blass for Men	BLASS	(1970)
	Gentleman	GIVENCHY	(1974)
	Patou pour Homme	PATOU	(1980)
	Santos	CARTIER	(1981)
	Le Troisième Homme	CARON	(1985)
	Ferré Uomo	GIAN FRANCO FERRE	(1986)
	Maxim's pour Homme	MAXIM'S	(1988)
	Sybaris	PUIG	(1988)
	Caractère	DANIEL HECHTER	(1989)
	Moods	KRIZIA	(1989)
	Background	JIL SANDER	(1993)

OCEANIC WOODY

M	Kenzo pour Homme	KENZO	(1991)
	Nautica	REVLON	(1992)

FRUITY WOODY

W	Féminité du Bois	SHISEIDO	(1992)

AMBER

FLORAL WOODY AMBER

W	Un Air Embaumé	RIGAUD	(1912)
	Nuit de Noël	CARON	(1922)
	Habanita	MOLINARD	(1924)
	Toujours Moi	CORDAY	(1924)
	Bois des Iles	CHANEL	(1926)
	Prétexte	LANVIN	(1937)
	Shocking	SCHIAPARELLI	(1937)
	Chamade	GUERLAIN	(1969)

Vu	TED LAPIDUS	(1975)
Expression	JACQUES FATH	(1977)
Magie Noire	LANCOME	(1978)
Must du Soir	CARTIER	(1981)
Nocturnes	CARON	(1981)
Parfum Hermès	HERMES	(1984)
Salvador Dali	SALVADOR DALI	(1984)
Ysatis	GIVENCHY	(1984)
Dans la Nuit	WORTH	(1985)

	Obsession	CALVIN KLEIN (1985)
	Venise	YVES ROCHER (1986)
	Colors	BENETTON (1987)
	Bijan	BIJAN (1987)
	Passion	ELIZABETH TAYLOR (1987)
	Roma	LAURA BIAGIOTTI (1988)
	Ambré	TAN GIUDICELLI (1988)
	Joop!	JOOP! (1989)
	Samsara	GUERLAIN (1989)
	Régine's	REGINE (1989)
	Only	JULIO IGLESIAS (1989)
	Stéphanie	BOURJOIS (1989)
	Ungaro	UNGARO (1990)
	Casmir	CHOPARD (1991)
	Dune	CHRISTIAN DIOR (1991)
	Krazy	KRIZIA (1991)
	White Diamonds	ELIZABETH TAYLOR (1991)
	Angel	THIERRY MUGLER (1992)
	Guess	REVLON (1992)
	Maroussia	ZAITSEV (1992)
	Tuscany para Donna	TUSCANY (1992)
	Venezia	LAURA BIAGIOTTI (1992)
	Jean-Paul Gaultier	JEAN-PAUL GAULTIER (1993)
M	Lagerfeld	KARL LAGERFELD (1978)
	Obsession for Men	CALVIN KLEIN (1978)
	Passion for Men	ELIZABETH TAYLOR (1989)
	Homme	JOOP! (1989)

FLORAL SPICY AMBER

W	L'Origan	COTY (1905)
	Après L'Ondée	GUERLAIN (1906)
	Cœur de Jeannette	HOUBIGANT (1912)
	L'Heure Bleue	GUERLAIN (1912)
	Maderas de Oriente	MYRURGIA (1924)
	Soir de Paris	BOURJOIS (1928)
	Vol de Nuit	GUERLAIN (1933)
	Chasse Gardée	CARVEN (1950)
	Bal à Versailles	JEAN DESPREZ (1962)
	Oscar de la Renta	OSCAR DE LA RENTA (1977)
	Raffinée	HOUBIGANT (1982)
	Balahé	LEONARD (1983)
	Poison	CHRISTIAN DIOR (1985)
	Panthère	CARTIER (1987)
	Senso	UNGARO (1987)
	Byzance	ROCHAS (1987)
	Red Door	ELIZABETH ARDEN (1989)
	C'est la Vie	CHRISTIAN LACROIX (1990)

	Initiation	MOLYNEUX (1990)
	Parfum Sacré	CARON (1990)
	Escada	MARGARETA LEY (1990)
	Spellbound	ESTEE LAUDER (1991)

SWEET AMBER

W	Ambre Antique	COTY (1905)
	Emeraude	COTY (1921)
	Shalimar	GUERLAIN (1925)
	Tabu	DANA (1931)
	Chantilly	HOUBIGANT (1941)
	Royal Secret	MONTEIL (1960)
	Anna Klein II	ANNA KLEIN (1986)
	Lyra	ALAIN DELON (1993)

CITRUS AMBER

M	Mouchoir de Monsieur	GUERLAIN (1904)
	Habit Rouge	GUERLAIN (1965)
	Cardin pour Monsieur	PIERRE CARDIN (1972)
	KL Homme	KARL LAGERFELD (1986)
W	Courant d'Air	AGNES B (1992)

FLORAL SEMI-AMBER

W	Youth Dew	ESTEE LAUDER (1952)
	Bird of Paradise	AVON (1969)
	Private Collection	ESTEE LAUDER (1973)
	J'ai Osé	GUY LAROCHE (1977)
	Opium	YVES SAINT LAURENT (1977)
	Cinnabar	ESTEE LAUDER (1978)
	Dioressence	CHRISTIAN DIOR (1979)
	KL	KARL LAGERFELD (1982)
	Prélude	BALENCIAGA (1982)
	Kéora	JEAN COUTURIER (1983)
	Coco	CHANEL (1984)
	Fétiche	L.T. PIVER (1986)
	Gem	VAN CLEEF & ARPELS (1987)
	Ma Liberté	JEAN PATOU (1987)
	Capucci	CAPUCCI (1987)
	Boucheron	BOUCHERON (1988)
	Sublime	JEAN PATOU (1992)
	Oh Là Là	AZZARO (1993)
	Van Cleef	VAN CLEEF & ARPELS (1993)
M	JHL	ARAMIS/LAUDER (1982)
	M	MORABITO (1989)

WOODY AMBER

M	Relax	DAVIDOFF (1990)

LEATHER

LEATHER

W	Tabac Blond	CARON (1919)
	Cuir de Russie	CHANEL (1924)
	Scandal	LANVIN (1932)
	Karako	BOURJOIS (1936)
M	Derby	GUERLAIN (1985)
	Bel Ami	HERMES (1986)

FLORAL LEATHER

M	Knize Ten	KNIZE (1924)
	Cuir de Russie	LE JARDIN RETROUVE (1987)
W	Delicious	GALE HAYMAN (1993)
	Ombre de la Nuit	UNGARO (1993)

TOBACCO LEATHER

M	English Leather	MEM COMPANY (1949)
	Royal Copenhagen	SWANK (1970)

GLOSSARY

Although it is difficult to describe odors with words, perfumery nevertheless has its own specific language to designate its raw materials, along with technical terms and expressions deriving from the history of perfumery. The most important terms are listed below.

ABSOLUTE (OR ABSOLUTE OIL): Strongly odorous raw material, very pure and viscous, which is obtained after the elimination of the waxy part of the concrete by purification in alcohol. It imparts a richness and an inimitable texture. In the case of jasmine, it takes twelve thousand pounds of flowers to produce two pounds of oil . . . which accounts for the very high prices.

ACCORD: The harmonious association of several raw materials, and the resulting olfactory effect.

ALCOHOL: Denatured ethyl alcohol, generally 96% proof, is used as a neutral solvent in the preparation of a fragrance. It is added to the concentrate as a vehicle for the fragrance oil, modifying its intensity and making it more easily applicable to the skin.

ALDEHYDE: An organic chemical containing the group carbon, hydrogen and an oxygen atom that can be derived from natural or synthetic materials. Aldehydes have a powerful diffusive effect. Ernest Beaux used them profusely in Chanel N° 5, which gave birth to the so-called aldehydic-type fragrances, also known as modern blends, which are characterized by a rich opulent top note.

AMBER: Perfume family. See under ORIENTAL BLEND.

AMBERGRIS: Very odorous substance expelled by the sperm whale and which can weigh tens of pounds. Because of its rarity and consequently its price, in modern perfumery it is usually replaced by synthetic products.

ANOSMIA: The inability to detect odor. One can suffer from temporary anosmia as a result of a nose infection, selective anosmia, which only concerns a certain type of odors, and total anosmia, which deprives individuals of all olfactory pleasure.

AQUA MIRABILIS (MIRACLE WATER): The ancestor of eau de Cologne. A type of light fragrance with an alcohol base, which appeared after the Renaissance. Renowned for their therapeutic properties, they were the subject of lively competition on the part of perfumers. Their popularity was such that Napoleon issued a decree in 1810 obliging perfumers to divulge their formulas, but they managed to circumvent it by renaming them "fragrance waters."

BASE: Elementary olfactory structure composed of a limited number of raw materials and which forms the matrix of the perfume.

BASE NOTE: Base notes are responsible for the underlying tones of the fragrance and its lasting quality, and can be heavy, persistent animal notes from civet, for example, or enveloping notes from patchouli or vanilla.

BAUDRUCHAGE: Manual operation which consists of covering the perfume bottle neck with a fine natural membrane (usually pig's intestine) tied with a cotton thread and knotted four times in order to ensure that the flacon is perfectly airtight. A few rare perfume houses still employ this method for their extract bottles.

BIOTECHNOLOGY: The use of micro-organisms to create synthetic odorous molecules. Progress is now also being made in genetics: plant cells producing essential oils have been successfully cultivated in vitro.

BLIND-TEST: Method of evaluating a new perfume's potential popularity in relation to its competitors. The operation consists of having a group of volunteers smell a series of fragrances, including the new creation, which are presented in identical unlabeled bottles, so as to guarantee impartial judgment.

BLOTTER STRIP: Narrow strips of special absorbent, glue-free paper, used by perfumers and professionals to test blends, follow their evolution and assess their quality. Scent strips are also used in perfume stores to enable clients to sample fragrances.

BOUQUET: Dominant theme that expresses well-known flowers. As a description, bouquet denotes a subtle, well-rounded blend of two or more fragrance complexes. In France in the nineteenth century, the term designated "fine and sweet" floral compositions, which were in line with the moral precept of the period forbidding honest women to wear heady perfumes.

CASTOREUM: Substance secreted by the glands of the Canadian and Russian beaver, recognizable by its inky or tar-like odor, and which is used to create chypre and leather notes.

CHARACTER: Trait which distinguishes and personalizes a note, an accord or a perfume; e.g. the white flowers accord has a suave character.

CHROMATOGRAPHY: Method of scientific analysis enabling one to identify and calculate the extent of a molecule's presence in essential oils and finished products. Chromatography enables researchers to discover new odorous molecules, but is sometimes used fraudulently to produce counterfeit copies of popular fragrances.

CHYPRE: Perfume family. (See p. 212).

CIVET: Yellowish-brown substance secreted by the anal scent glands of the Ethiopian civet cat and stored in a sac near the genital region. In its natural state the odor is nauseous and only when diluted does it acquire its sensual aroma.

CONCENTRATE: All the odorous components of a fragrance whose proportions are defined in the perfumer's formula and which are subsequently mixed with alcohol to produce the fragrance.

CONCRETE: Solid substance made up of wax and essential oil representing the closest odor duplication of the raw materials (flower, bark, leaves, etc.) from which it has been extracted by volatile solvents. Concretes can be further concentrated to produce absolutes.

CYPRESS: An essential oil traditionally distilled in Provence and which liberates the amber and balsam widely used in oriental, chypre and woody accords.

DIFFUSION: The ability of a fragrance to develop its notes harmoniously around the wearer, leaving an impression of unity and volume in the air.

DIGESTION: Ancient extraction method consisting of immersing natural odorous raw materials in hot or cold oil or fats. Used since antiquity in Mediterranean countries and in India, and used in the west until the nineteenth century.

DISSONANCE: A rupture in the harmony between the notes. When skillfully handled, it can impart a certain liveliness to the fragrance.

DISTILLATION: Ancient method of extraction based on the principle of using a steam. It was used in Mesopotamia as early as 5000 BC It was rediscovered by Avicenne in the year AD 1000 and has undergone constant improvements.

DOMINANT (NOTE OR ACCORD): Olfactory effect of a perfume which is present throughout its diffusion, e.g. floral accord with a dominant jasmine note.

EAU DE COLOGNE: fresh, invigorating formula composed of lemon, bergamot, rosemary and neroli, created in Italy in the seventeenth century and which owes its name to the German town of Cologne where the product first became commercially successful at the end of the eighteenth century.

EAU DE PARFUM: Perfumed product whose concentration varies from 10 to 20% depending on the brand and the quality of the raw materials. It is diluted in 90% proof alcohol. Many manufacturers choose to use more fanciful designations such as cœur de parfum, fleur de parfum, etc., in order to distinguish themselves from other brands.

ENFLEURAGE: Ancient method for processing natural raw materials which exploits the properties of certain unheated purified fats to absorb and retain fragrances. A pomade is obtained which yields the essential oil after washing in alcohol. This particular method was developed in the town of Grasse in the eighteenth century, but for many years previously the inhabitants had used similar processes involving vegetable or mineral powders, sesame seeds and oleaginous kernels such as almonds or hazelnuts.

ESSENTIAL OIL (OR ESSENCE): Fragrant volatile extracts obtained from aromatic plant elements by various methods, i.e. distillation, expression, extraction, enfleurage, maceration or headspace technology. Essential oils are the basic ingredients employed by the perfumer in the preparation of a fragrance and are mixed with 96% proof alcohol in strictly prescribed proportions.

EXPRESSION: Extraction of essential oils from citrus fruits obtained by rupturing the small cells containing these oils, which are situated in the peel. Until the Second World War leather gloves with inlaid pumice stone chips were employed, whereas nowadays machines have replaced this traditional method resulting increased output.

EXTRACT: Commonly called perfume, this is the most concentrated and consequently noblest perfumed product, with a 20 to 30% odorous concentration, depending on the make and the quality of the raw material; it is diluted in very pure 96% proof alcohol. The persistence and diffusion of the extract are far superior to those of other perfumed products.

EXTRACTION: A very effective process developed in the nineteenth century for extracting the odorous principles of raw materials, such as rose, jasmine and orange blossom. Flower petals, leaves and/or roots are placed on perforated trays in vast sealed containers and a volatile solvent is run through them at a low temperature, causing the oils to be released without the use of harmful heat. The solvent is then evaporated to obtain the concrete, a waxy odorous paste, which, after purification by alcohol, yields the absolute.

FAMILIES: Fragrances are divided into seven families according to the raw materials used to make them (see p. 212).

FLORAL: Perfume family. (See p. 212).

FLORAL (NOTE): All perfumes, even those for men, contain flowers. The rose-jasmine-lily of the valley accord in Lanvin's Arpège is one of the great classics, like the rose-jasmine-narcissus accord in Amazone created by Hermès. The floral notes in masculine perfumes are more discreet but sometimes identifiable, as in the case of the violet note which can be detected in Christian Dior's Fahrenheit, or the rose note in Acteur by Azzaro.

FORMULA: Very precise list of raw materials and quantities, to the nearest milligram, which compose a fragrance, and known only to the perfumer himself. The formula, like a musical score, is the result of the creator's sensibility and experience and is the key to the preparation of the fragrance. However it is not protected by any patent and is sometimes the object of poor counterfeit copies which are immediately recognizable to professions.

FOUGERE: Perfume family. (See p. 212).

FRAGRANCE: Derived from the Latin fragrare (to smell), it denotes a pleasant odor or skillful association of harmonious odors. In perfumery terminology, it denotes the various concentrations such as extract, eau de parfum, toilet water or cologne.

FRUITY (NOTE): The first was the peach note, a synthetic evoking the odor of this fruit, produced at the beginning of the century and used in Mitsouko by Guerlain and Femme by Rochas. Today there are a considerable number of fruity notes reminiscent of red fruit, exotic fruit and berries. The attractive odor of these new molecules gave new impetus to contemporary creativity by introducing the so-called gourmand perfumes.

FUMIGATION: Action of producing aromatic smoke and vapors by burning odorous woods, resins, powders or fragrance waters. Originally fumigations were used for ritual and sacred purposes. From antiquity to the seventeenth century, they were used to mask bad odors and to combat epidemics since certain ingredients were considered to have purifying properties.

GLOVER–PERFUMER: The symbolic power of the glove gracing the hand of the mighty inspired the name of corporation of master glover–perfumers, which was an integral part of the tanning trade. In those days heady perfumes served to mask the unpleasant odors which persisted on tanned leather. In 1614 the master glovers became separate from the tanners and received a patent letter from Louis XIII authorizing them to "se nommer et qualifier tant maistres gantiers que parfumeurs" (be called and qualify as master glovers and perfumers). The newly independent corporation found itself in a monopoly position in the perfume trade and supplanted the existing apothecaries, distillers and alchemists.

GOURMAND (NOTE): Note evoking ripe fruit or honey and even the tempting smell of chocolate, vanilla and cinnamon, transforming fragrances into an olfactory extension of the pleasures of taste.

GREEN (NOTE): A fresh invigorating note evoking freshly cut grass, leaves or branches. Fragrances in this category generally contain a large proportion of violet leaf essences, Pistacia lentiscus, commonly known as the mastic tree, or galbanum, an extract from the root of a large wild carrot. Vent Vert by Balmain is considered by perfumers as the archetype of green perfumes.

HEADSPACE (TECHNOLOGY): A method for analyzing odors present in the air, involving chromatography, which was developed about twenty years ago. The process consists of capturing the perfumed aura of a flower, or any other odorous substance, by means of an apparatus resembling a bell-jar. After analysis by a chromatograph, an identity card, or fingerprint, corresponding to this odor is drawn up, which after interpretation by the perfumer enables him to reconstitute the odor. Headspace enlarged the perfumer's palette by providing fresher raw materials, very close to nature, and more openings for his creativity, since it enabled him to capture not only the odor of coffee, leather, or a garden in autumn, but also that of flowers, like lily of the valley, from which it is impossible to extract essential oil by any other method.

HEADY: An odor or fragrance with a powerful, intoxicating appeal.

INCENSE: Resinoid obtained from the natural sap of a shrub growing wild in the Arabian desert and in the high plains of Somalia. In hot temperatures the bark bursts allowing the sap to escape. The sap then hardens in the atmosphere to form small pebbles, which when distilled in steam produce an essential oil sometimes used in oriental notes.

INCENSE: Various combinations of resins, odorous woods and dried plants, combined with gum or honey, and used for sacred fumigations. The image of the "heavenly staircase" associated with incense is common to the Catholic, Orthodox, Taoist and Buddhist religions.

INFUSION: A process of dissolving the solid, odorous parts of certain products in pure unheated alcohol for several months. These products can be derived from animals such as musk or amber, or from plants such as tonka beans, iris rhizomes or mosses. Very refined products are obtained by this technique.

KOH-DO: a Japanese ceremony (meaning "the way of incense"), which is as complex and refined as the traditional bouquet or tea rituals. This ancient art, whose rules were laid down in the sixteenth century, consists of creating links between poetry and fragrances. The master of ceremonies associates each sequence of a poem with a specific mixture of odorous woods, which he proffers to the participants. They are subsequently presented a second time in a different order and the participants have to identify them and classify them in the original order.

LEATHER: Perfume family. (See p. 212).

LINE: Range of perfumed products deriving from a fragrance and which denotes the various concentrations in which it is available, e.g. the extract, eau de parfum, toilet water and nonalcoholic fragrance waters which are recommended for use in the summer. The term is also used to designate various perfumed products for the body, such as creams, milks, soaps, bubble baths and deodorants.

LINEAR: Term used to describe a perfume whose top, middle or base notes present the same olfactory characteristics throughout its evaporation.

MACERATION: One of the last stages in the preparation of a perfume which consists of leaving the concentrate to rest in 96% proof alcohol for several weeks or even months in order to optimize its olfactory qualities, as in the case of wine. It is only after having been subjected to a temperature of between 0 and −10° Celsius and then filtered to eliminate the insoluble residues that the perfume can finally be bottled.

MATURITY: The stage when the various perfume components have reached their equilibrium at the end of the maceration period.

MIDDLE NOTES: A harmonious blend of the fragrance ingredients, also considered as the heart notes. They are slower and more voluptuous than the top note. The dominant notes designate the fragrance family, e.g. floral (rose, jasmine, tuberose, etc.) chypre, green, spicy, oriental, etc. It usually takes about ten minutes for the middle or heart notes to develop fully on the skin.

NOSE: Colloquial term for a perfumer. Although his nose is indeed his principal tool, the art of the perfumer is by no means limited solely to smelling. It is above all with his judgment, refined taste and memory that he creates a perfume.

NOTE: Term borrowed from music designating an olfactory impression of a single smell in a raw material or a composition, or to indicate the three parts of a fragrance, the top, middle and base notes. The plural form, e.g. musk notes, designates all the odorous products which are more or less closely associated with musk.

OCEANIC: A synthetically produced fragrance evoking ocean-like qualities, such as kelp and briny sea air. This olfactory family became popular at the end of the eighties with the widespread enthusiasm for escape and wide open spaces. New West for Her by Aramis, which conjures up a sun-drenched beach on the west coast of the United States, and Kenzo pour Homme, evoking the invigorating Atlantic coast, are eloquent examples.

ODOR: Volatile chemicals emanating from various elements which stimulate the olfactory system. Odor is an objective and quantitative description, unlike perfume, which is the fruit of reflection and subjective intention.

OLFACTORY MEMORY: A particularly highly developed faculty in the case of an experienced perfumer, who is capable of memorizing several hundred, or even several thousand, odors. This is due to the fact that he is constantly exercising this faculty and also to his irrepressible curiosity, for in addition to the odorous raw materials he uses in his compositions, a perfumer uses complex fragrances he has come across during walks, encounters and journeys and which enrich his personal palette.

ORIENTAL BLEND, ALSO KNOWN AS AMBER: A perfume family (see p. 212) dominated by soft, powdery, vanilla notes over discreet animal base notes. Shalimar by Guerlain (1925) is regarded by perfumers as the archetypal oriental perfume.

OXIDATION: The chemical change or deterioration of the fragrance and/or its color when exposed to air, light or heat. Perfumers stock the most fragile odorous raw materials away from direct light at a constant temperature of about 15° Celsius.

PACKAGING: The presentation case or box protecting the perfume bottle, and also the art of designing them. Packaging plays an essential marketing role, as it conveys the personality and style of the brand and the spirit of the fragrance.

PALETTE: The complete range of raw materials used by a perfumer. These are his favorite materials and notes, which, like a painter's palette, reflect his personality and particular characteristics.

PERFUME: Commonly used to designate the extract, the most concentrated form of fragrance. Perfume is a work of art in that it is the result of a creative gesture and an aesthetic intention, the harmonious combination of many components. The word is derived from the Latin *per fumum* (through smoke).

PERFUME ORGAN: Traditional term for a fan-shaped wooden unit reminiscent of the musical instrument, and which formerly contained, and afforded easy access to, all the essential raw materials used by the perfumer.

POMADE: Combination of perfumed, purified fats and oils resulting from enfleurage. Formerly when the women from Grasse were on their way to work at the enfleurage of jasmine or tuberose in the summer, they were said to be going to *faire pommade* (literally, "make pomade").

POWDERY: Characteristic trait of fragrances with a very tangible, velvety softness, evoking voluptuous materials like mohair. Iris and tonka bean, and also synthetics such as vanillin, heliotropin and coumarin, which evokes the odor of hay, provide this powdery element which can be found in Chanel N° 22 and Jean-Charles Brosseau's Ombre Rose.

PRESERVATIVE: Chemical agent sometimes added to perfume to delay the effects of oxidation and which is indispensable in nonalcoholic fragrances used notably used for children.

RAW MATERIALS: The odorous products which compose the perfumer's palette. About one hundred natural raw materials exist in plants and animals, in the form of essential oils, absolutes, resinoids, etc. and several thousand raw materials are derived from synthesis.

RESINOID: Resinous product obtained after extraction by volatile solvents, from gums, balsams, resins or roots and which, like the concrete obtained by the same process, can be further concentrated to yield the absolute after purification by alcohol and freezing between 0 and –10° Celsius. Resinoids generally serve as fixatives in perfume compositions.

SCENT STRIPS: Bands of paper sprinkled with microscopic perfumed capsules, which liberate the fragrance immediately the protective membrane is removed. This technique is frequently used in magazine advertisements.

SINGLE FLORAL: These fragrances have the recognizable scent of a single flower, such as rose, violet, lily of the valley or lilac, although this impression may be created by numerous ingredients. This type of perfume was very popular at the end of the last century, but is not so common nowadays, except in England, where simple, refined fragrances evoking gardens are very popular.

SPICY (NOTE): An olfactory effect reminiscent of the smell of cinnamon, cloves, nutmeg and pepper, and which gives depth to certain floral, amber or woody compositions, such as Coco by Chanel.

STILL: Distillation apparatus, composed of a still surmounted by a sealed head or neck linking it to a double tube condenser which cools and condenses the odorous vapours by means of running water. The most ancient stills which were made of earthenware and date from 5000 BC. After being perfected by the Arabs in the tenth century, stills were introduced in Europe at the time of the Crusades.

SYNTHESIS: Chemical process by which new raw materials are obtained. As Edmond Roudnitska explains, "These are elements which already existed in nature and that man has reconstituted for his own purposes". Nowadays there are thousands of synthetic products which have contributed to a new style of perfumery.

THEME: The basic idea which inspired a perfume and forms the dominant accord developed by the perfumer during the various stages of the composition. Fragrances are described as having a floral, violet, underwood or white garden theme, to name just a few, for they are as unlimited as the perfumer's inspiration.

TOILET WATER: Perfumed product whose odorous concentration is inferior to 10%. It is diluted in 8% or 9% proof alcohol depending on the brand.

TOP NOTE: The first scent impression immediately after the bottle has been opened or after the fragrance has been applied to the skin. Top notes are designed to be light and volatile, such as the essences of lemon, bergamot or orange, and set the sensory stage for the development of middle and base notes.

TRAIL: A fragrant aura persisting in the air after somebody wearing a perfume has gone by and which is the characteristic of perfumes rich in balsams, odorous woods and animal notes.

UNGUENT OR OINTMENT: Oily or fatty substance saturated with odors or fragrances and used in bygone days for perfuming oneself. From the Middle Ages they were used exclusively in therapeutic preparations.

VOLATILE: The property of an odor or a perfume possessing little persistence and which evaporates rapidly. The most volatile notes in a perfume are the citrus top notes whose fragrance diminishes in the space of a few minutes.

WARM: Ample olfactory effect generating emotional warmth and conveying a sensation of intimacy and well-being, which is obtained with labdanum, patchouli, and by animal notes such as musk and spicy notes.

WOODY: Perfume family (see p. 212).

B I B L I O G R A P H Y

This bibliography is not exhaustive. We have selected the best works on perfume, which are listed under various categories. Readers can choose the aspect of perfume which interests them the most: the history of perfume, perfumes described by great writers, the fascinating world of perfume bottles, and many more. Works in French have been included when they are of particular historical interest, unique in their field, or cited by the authors and have not, to our knowledge, been published in English.

SPECIALIST LIBRARIES

The Fragrance Foundation
145, East Thirty-second Street,
New York, NY 10016
Tel: (212) 725 2755
The Fragrance Foundation has a Research Information Center which holds a collection of current books and articles on fragrance, along with prints and videos relating to the perfume industry.

Bibliothèque des parfums
(at the Société Française des Parfumeurs)
36, rue du Parc de Clagny,
78000 Versailles
Tel: (1) 39 55 46 99 (by appointment)
The largest library of its kind in France, with a collection of over 800 books on all areas of the perfume industry (history, techniques, economy, style, etc.).

REFERENCE

Dictionnaire des Parfums. Paris: Editions Patrick Sermadiras, 1981–1991.
The Fragrance and Olfactory Dictionary. New York: The Fragrance Foundation, 1994.
The Fragrance Foundation Reference Guide. New York: The Fragrance Foundation, 1995.

THE HISTORY OF PERFUME

BARBE, Simon. *Le Parfumeur royal* [1699]. Paris: Klincksieck, 1992.
DELBOURG-DELPHIS, Marylène. *Le Sillage des élégantes*. Paris: Jean-Claude Lattès, 1983.
FICIN, Marcile. *Antidotes des maladies pestilentes*. Cahors, 1595.
FREEMAN, John F. and Roger L. WILLIAMS. *Citizens and Clergy of Grasse. How Modernity came to a Provençal Town*. E. Mellen (USA), 1989.
HAARMAN & REIMER. *The Book of Perfume*. 5 vols. R. Gloss & Co. (Germany), 1989.
LYNNE, Mary. *Galaxy of Scents: The Ancient Art of Perfume Making*. Kila, USA: Kessinger Publishing Company, 1994.
MORRIS, Edwin T. *Fragrance, The Story of Perfume from Cleopatra to Chanel*. New York: Macmillan, 1984.
PIESSE, Septimus. *Histoire des parfums*. Paris: J.B. Baillière et fils, 1890.

RIMMEL, Eugène. *Le Livre des parfums*. Le Lavandou: Editions du Layet. Copy of 1870 edition by C. Muquardt.
VINDRY, Georges. *Aimer Grasse et le parfum*. Editions Ouest France, 1992.

TREATISES AND TECHNIQUES

BAILES, Edith G. *An Album of Fragrance*. Richmond, USA: Cardomom Press, 1993.
CALKIN, Robert R. and J. Stephen JELLINEK. *Perfumes: Techniques and Technology*. New York: John Wiley & Sons, 1994.
CURTIS, Tony and David WILLIAMS. *Introduction to Perfumery: Technology and Marketing*. Hemel Hempstead, UK: Horwood (Ellis) Ltd, 1994.
HASLEWOOD, Louis, ed. *Perfume Manufacture. A Bibliography*. London: Clarke, 1990.
HOWARD, George and W.E. ARNOLD-TAYLOR. *Principles and Practice of Perfumery and Cosmetics*. Philadelphia: Trans-Atlantic Publications, 1987.
JOUHAR, A.J. *The Raw Materials of Perfumery*. New York: Chapman & Hall, 1989.
LAMPARSKY, D., ed. *Perfumes: Art, Science and Technology*. New York: Elsevier Science, 1991.
LE FLORENTIN, René. *Les Parfums* Desforges, Girardot et Cie, 1927.
PARRY, E.J. *Encyclopedia of Perfumery*. 2 vols. New York: Gordon Press, 1992.
POUCHER, W.A. *The Production, Manufacture and Application of Perfumes*. New York: Chapman & Hall, 1994.
THOMPSON, C.J. *The Mystery and Lure of Perfume*. New York: Gordon Press Publishers, 1981.
Traité des parfums. Le parfumeur royal, 1761.
WELLS, F.V. and Marcel BILLOT. *Perfumery Technology: Art, Science, Industry*. Hemel Hempstead: E. Horwood, 1981.

MONOGRAPHS

BARILLE, Elisabeth. *Coty*. Editions Assouline, 1995.
CHARLES-ROUX, Edmonde. *Chanel*. Translated by Nancy Amphoux. London: Collins, 1989.
COLARD, Grégoire. *Le Charme secret d'une maison parfumée*. Caron. Paris: Editions Jean-Claude Lattès, 1984.
DEMORNEX, Jacqueline. *Lancôme*. Paris: Editions du Regard, 1985.
DESLANDRES, Yvonne. *Paul Poiret*. Paris: Editions du Regard, 1986.
ETHERINGTON-SMITH, Meredith. *Patou*. New York: St. Martin's/Marek, 1983.
FELLOUS, Colette. *Guerlain*. Paris: Denoël, 1987.
GALANTE, Pierre. *Mademoiselle Chanel*. Translated by Eileen Geist and Jessie Wood. Chicago: H. Regenery Co., 1973.
GUILLAUME, Valérie. *Jacques Fath*. Paris: Editions Paris-Musées, Adam Biro, 1993.
HAEDRICH, Marcel. *Coco Chanel; her life, her secrets*. Translated by Charles L. Markmann. Boston: Little, Brown, 1972.

LE MAGUET, Jocelyne and Jean-Paul. *Sous le signe du parfum: Edmond Roudnitska, Compositeur de Parfum*. L'Albaron, 1992.
LEYMARIE, Jean. *Chanel*. Geneva: Skira, 1987.
POCHNA, Marie-France. *Nina Ricci*. Paris: Editions du Regard, 1992.
———. *Christian Dior*. Paris: Flammarion, 1994.

THE PERFUMER'S PALETTE, PLANTS AND AROMATHERAPY

ACKERMAN, Diane. *Natural History of the Senses*. London: Chapmans Publishers, 1991.
BOSSCHERE, Jean de. *La Fleur et son parfum*. Paris: Stock, 1942.
CHARABOT, Eugène. *Les Parfums artificiels*. Paris: J.B. Baillière et fils, 1900.
CHARABOT, Eugène and C.L. GATIN. *Le Parfum chez la plante*. Paris: O. Doin, 1908.
CUNNINGHAM, Scott. *Encyclopaedia of Magical Herbs*. St Paul, Minn.: Llewellyn Publications, 1985.
———. *Magical Aromatherapy. The Power of Scent*. St Paul, Minn.: Llewellyn Publications, 1985.
DEBAY, A. *Les Parfums et les fleurs*. Paris: E. Dentu, 1882.
DUFF, Gail. *Outdoor Scents for Indoor Uses*. London: Sidgwick & Jackson, 1989.
———. *The Book of Pot Pourri*. London: Merehurst, 1987.
FETTNER, Ann Tucker. *Potpourri, Incense and Other Fragrant Concoctions*. London: Hutchinson, 1983.
FRICHET, Henri. *Plantes et parfums magiques*. 1937.
GENDERS, Roy. *Scented Flora of the World*. London: Robert Hale Limited, 1977.
KAISER, Roman. *The Scent of Orchids*. Givaudan-Roure, Editions Roche, 1993.
KING, Janine. *Scents*. Chic Simple Components. London: Thames & Hudson, 1993.
LAKE, Max. *Scents and Sensuality: The Essence of Excitement*. London: Futura Publications, 1991.
MACKENZIE, Dan. *Aromatics and the Soul*. London: William Heinemann, 1923.
MAETERLINCK, Maurice. *L'Intelligence des fleurs*. Editions d'Aujourd'hui, 1977.
MILLER, Richard A. and Iona MILLER. *Magical and Ritual Use of Perfumes*. Rochester, USA: Inner Traditions International, 1990.
MONTESQUIOU, Robert de. *Pays des aromates*. Report on the Universal Exhibition, Paris 1900.
MORGAN, Jan. *Fabulous Fragrances: How To Select Your Fragrance Wardrobe*. Beverly Hills: Crescent House Publishing, 1994.
MORITA, Kiyoko. *The Book of Incense*. Tokyo: Kodansha International Ltd., 1984.
SECONDI, Olindo. *Handbook of Perfumes and Flavors*. New York: Chemical Publishing Company, 1990.
WEBB, David A. *Easy Potpourri*. Blue Ridge Summit: TAB Books, 1991.
WILDWOOD, Christine. *Creative Aromatherapy*. London: Thorsons, 1993.

THE SENSE OF SMELL

ARISTOTLE. *On the Soul*. Translated by H.L. Tancred. Harmondsworth: Penguin, 1987.
DEJEAN, Antoine. *Traité des odeurs*. Paris, 1788.
DUMENIL, H. Auguste. *Des odeurs, de leur nature et de leur action physiologique*. Paris, 1843.
ENGEN, Trygg. *The Perception of Odours*. London: Academic Press, 1982.
KITTREDGE, Mary. *The Senses*. Chelsea House Publishers, 1990.
OHLOFF, Gunther. *Scent and Fragrances: The Fascination of Odors and their Chemical Perspectives*. Translated by W. Pickenhagen. New York: Springer-Verlag, 1994.
POLYCARPE PONCELET. *La Chimie du goût et de l'odorat*. Paris, 1776.
SULLY, Nina. *Looking at the Senses*. London: Batsford, 1982.
THEIMER, Ernst T., ed. *Fragrance Chemistry. The Science of the Sense of Smell*. San Diego: Academic Press, 1982.
TOLLER, S. VAN and George H. DODD. *Perfumery. The Psychology and Biology of Fragrance*. London: Chapman & Hall, 1987.

GLASSMAKING AND THE ART OF PERFUME BOTTLES

Baccarat Perfume Bottles. Editions Baccarat. H. Addor, 1988.
BAYER, Patricia and Mark WALLER. *The Art of René Lalique*. London: Bloomsbury Publishing Ltd., 1988.
CURTIS, Jean-Loup. *Baccarat*. Editions du Regard, 1991.
DUBBS BALL, Joanne and Dorothy HEHL. *Commercial Fragrance Bottles*. Pennsylvania: Schiffer Publishing, 1993.
DINAND, Pierre. *Les formes du parfum. 30 ans de design*. Paris: Editions Belfond, 1990.
FONTAN, Geneviève and Nathalie BARNOUIN. *Parfums d'exception*. Paris: Editions Milan, 1993.
MAYER LEFKOWITH, Christie. *The Art of Perfume*. New York: Thames & Hudson, 1994.
NORTH, J. Jones. *Perfume, Cologne and Scent Bottles*. Pennsylvania: Schiffer Publishing Ltd., 1987.
———. *Commercial Perfume Bottles*. Pennsylvania: Schiffer Publishing Ltd.,1988.
SLOAN, Jean. *Perfume and Scent Bottle Collecting*. Wallace-Hamstead Book Company (USA), 1990.
UTT, Mary Lou, et al. *Lalique Perfume Bottles*. London: Thames & Hudson, 1991.

PERFUMES AND LITERATURE

BALZAC, Honoré de. *César Birotteau*. Translated by Robin Buss. Harmondsworth: Penguin, 1994.
BAUDELAIRE, Charles. *Les Fleurs du Mal*. Translated by Richard Howard. London: Pan Books, 1987.
COLETTE. *Break of Day, a Novel*. Translated by Enid McLeod. New York: Farrar, Strauss and Cudahy, 1961.

ESTEVE, Louis. *Les parfums dans la littérature moderne.* Poésie, 1905.

FLAUBERT, Gustave. *Madame Bovary.* Translated by Francis Steegmuller. New York, 1992.

———. *Sentimental Education.* Translated by G.Hopkin. Oxford University Press, 1981.

———. *Salammbô.* Translated by A.J. Karilsheimer. Harmondsworth: Penguin, 1977.

HUYSMANS, Joris Karl. *Against Nature.* Translated by Robert Baldick. Harmondsworth: Penguin, 1959. New ed. 1974.

———. *The Cathedral.* Translated by Clara Bell. London: K. Paul, Trench, Trübner & co., ltd. New York: E.P. Dutton, 1925.

LORRIS, Guillaume de, and Jean de MEUN. *The Romance of the Rose.* Translated by Charles Dahlberg. Princeton, New Jersey: Princeton University Press, 1971.

MONTAIGNE, Michel de. *Essays and Selected Writings.* Bilingual edition. Translated by Donald M. Frame. New York: St. Martin's Press, 1963.

PROUST, Marcel. *Remembrance of Things Past.* 3 vols. Translated by C.K. Scott Moncrieff and Terence Kilmartin. New York: Random House, 1981.

ROUSSEAU, Jean-Jacques. *Emile.* London: J.M. Dent & Sons, ltd. New York: E.P. Dutton & co., 1933.

Sillages. Texts and poems on perfume, chosen by Guy Laroche. Paris: Editions Saint-Germain des Près, 1983.

SÜSKIND, Patrick. *Perfume, the Story of a Murderer.* Translated by John E. Woods. Harmondsworth: Penguin, 1987.

TENNYSON, Alfred. *Poems and Plays.* Oxford University Press, 1975.

WILDE, Oscar. *The Picture of Dorian Gray.* From *The Complete Works of Oscar Wilde.* London and Glasgow: Collins, 1989.

EXHIBITIONS

3000 ans de Parfumerie à Grasse. Musée d'Art et d'Histoire. Grasse, July 22–October 22, 1980.

Autour du parfum du XVIᵉ au XIXᵉ siècle. Le Louvre des Antiquaires. Paris, May 31–September 15, 1985.

Heavenly Scent. Exhibition organized by the Comité Français du Parfum. Paris. Royal College of Art. London, March 24–April 17, 1995.

Hymne au parfum, deux siècles d'histoire dans les arts décoratifs et la mode. Musée des Arts de la Mode. Paris, October 16–February 3, 1991.

La Parfumerie française et l'Art de la Présentation. Paris, 1925.

Parfums de plantes. Musée d'Histoire Naturelle. Paris, December 1987–June 1988.

Rose, Rosa, Rosae. Musée International de la Parfumerie. Grasse, May 18–September 15, 1991.

Plantes et Parfums. Société Nationale d'Horticulture de France. Paris, November 19–27, 1994.

Scents of Smell. Museum of the City of New York. New York, 1988.

Seeing Scents. Fashion Institute of Technology. New York, 1989.

PICTURE CREDITS

Front jacket: © Emilio F. Simion, Milan/Luisa Ricciarini, Milan; Cover (vignette): Photo Flammarion; Page 1: © Photo RMN; Pages 2–3: Stedelijk Museum, Amsterdam; Page 4: © Wendi Schneider; Page 6: Photo Flammarion; Page 9: By kind permission of Quest; Page 10: © Wendi Schneider; Page 11: Bibliothèque Nationale de France; Page 12: © Cyril Le Tourneur d'Ison/CHANEL; Page 13: © Cyril Le Tourneur d'Ison/CHANEL; Page 14: © Cyril Le Tourneur d'Ison/CHANEL; Page 15: © Gérard Sioen/VISA; Pages 16–17: © Cyril Le Tourneur d'Ison/CHANEL; Page 18: © Cyril Le Tourneur d'Ison/CHANEL Page 19: © Cyril Le Tourneur d'Ison/CHANEL; Page 20: SIP/Côté Sud/H. del Olmo; Page 21: Hoaqui/E. Valentin; Page 22: © Cyril Le Tourneur d'Ison/CHANEL; Page 23: © Cyril Le Tourneur d'Ison/CHANEL; Page 24 (top left): © Cyril Le Tourneur d'Ison/CHANEL; Page 24 (top right): © Cyril Le Tourneur d'Ison/CHANEL; Page 24 (middle left): © Cyril Le Tourneur d'Ison/CHANEL; Page 24 (middle right): © Cyril Le Tourneur d'Ison/CHANEL; Page 24 (bottom left): © Cyril Le Tourneur d'Ison/CHANEL; Page 24 (bottom right): © Cyril Le Tourneur d'Ison/CHANEL; Page 25: SIP/Côté Sud/N. Mackenzie; Page 26: © Cyril Le Tourneur d'Ison/CHANEL; Page 27 (top): © Cyril Le Tourneur d'Ison/CHANEL; Page 27 (bottom): © Cyril Le Tourneur d'Ison/CHANEL; Page 28: (top): G. Véron and M. Skinner; Page 28 (bottom): Peter Eaton (Booksellers) Ltd, London; Page 29: © Elkouby/VISA; Page 30: Givaudan-Roure; Page 31: Weiss/Rapho; Page 32: Corporate Image/Jack Burlot; Page 33: Gérard Sioen/Rapho; Page 34: SIP/Côté Sud/Bernard Touillon; Page 36: Robertet; Page 37: The Bettmann Archive; Pages 38–9; © Guy Bouchet; Page 40: © Perri/Cosmos; Page 41: G. Véron & M. Skinner; Page 42: Hulton Deutsch Collection Limited; Page 43: Marie-Claire Beauté/Gilles de Chabaneix; Page 44: UPI/Bettmann; Page 45: Collection Molinard/Photo Michel Cresp; Page 46: Lipnitzki-Viollet; Page 47: Edouard Boubat for Hermès; Page 48: Annick Goutal; Page 49: B. Pellerin/Imapress; Page 50: Collection Molinard; Page 51: Musée d'Art et d'Histoire, Grasse; Page 52: Nicolas Bruant/Caroline Lebeau/Vogue Decoration; Page 53: Nicolas Bruant; Page 54: Collection Musée International de la Parfumerie, Grasse, France; Page 55 (top): © Collection Viollet; Page 55 (bottom): Collection Molinard; Page 56 (top left): Muelhens GmbH & Co., Cologne; Page 56 (top right): Photo Flammarion; Page 56 (bottom): Muelhens GmbH & Co., Cologne; Page 57 (top) : Muelhens GmbH & Co., Cologne; Page 57 (middle): Muelhens GmbH & Co., Cologne; Page 57 (bottom): Muelhens GmbH & Co., Cologne; Page 58 (top): Photo Flammarion; Page 58 (bottom): Roger et Gallet; Page 59 (top): Muelhens GmbH & Co., Cologne; Page 59 (middle): Muelhens GmbH & Co., Cologne; Page 59 (bottom): Photo Flammarion; Page 60 (top): Anthony Blake Photo Library; Page 60 (bottom): Santa Maria Novella; Page 61: Anthony Blake Photo Library; Page 62 (top): J. Floris Ltd.; Page 62 (bottom): Peter Aprahamian; Page 63: Ghislaine Bavoillot; Pages 64–5: Harrods Ltd.; Page 66 (top left): Penhaligon's; Page 66 (top middle): Penhaligon's; Page 66 (top right): Penhaligon's; Page 66 (bottom): Penhaligon's; Page 67: E. T. Archive; Page 68 (top): © Martin Breese/Retrograph Archive 1995; Page 68 (bottom): © Martin Breese/Retrograph Archive 1995; Page 69: Photo Flammarion/Collection L. T. Piver; Page 70 (top): Photo Flammarion; Page 70 (bottom): Collection Fragonard; Page 71 (top): Photo Flammarion/Collection L. T. Piver; Page 71 (bottom): Photo Flammarion/Collection L. T. Piver; Page 72: Parfums Guerlain; Page 73: Photo Flammarion; Page 74 (top): Photo Ali von Bothner; Page 74 (bottom): Document Parfums Guerlain; Page 75 (top): Document Parfums Guerlain; Page 75 (bottom): Document Parfums Guerlain; Page 76 (top): Collection Molinard/ Photo Michel Appollot; Page 76 (bottom): Lauros-Giraudon; Page 77 (top): Collection Molinard; Page 77 (middle): Collection Molinard; Page 77 (bottom, left): Collection Molinard; Page 77 (bottom middle): Photo Flammarion; Page 77 (bottom right): Collection Molinard/Photo Michel Appollot; Page 78 (top): Archives Parfums Caron; Page 78 (bottom): Photo Flammarion/Archives Parfums Caron; Page 79: Photo Ali von Bothner; Page 80 (top): © Harlingue-Viollet; Page 80 (bottom): © Martin Breese/Retrograph Archive, 1995; Page 81: Photo Flammarion/Collection Musée de Suresnes; Page 82 (top left): © Jacques Boulay/Editions du Regard; Page 82 (top, right): © Jacques Boulay/Editions du Regard; Page 82 (middle right): Jacques Boulay/Editions du Regard; Page 82 (bottom): Musée International de la Parfumerie, Grasse, France; Page 83 (top): © Lipnitzki-Viollet; Page 83 (bottom left): Photo Flammarion; Page 83 (bottom right): Photo Flammarion; Page 84: Archive Photos; Page 85: Ali von Bothner; Page 87: Ali von Bothner; Page 88: Jacques Boulay; Page 90: Ali Von Bothner; Page 91: Photo Christian Moser for Kenzo; Page 92: Ali Von Bothner; Page 93: Ali Von Bothner; Page 94: Ali Von Bothner; Page 96: Marc Arbeit; Page 97: Giraudon; Page 98: Sotheby's London; Page 99: Christopher Wood Gallery, London; Bridgeman/Giraudon; Page 100: Musée Carnavalet/Photothèque des Musées de la Ville de Paris; Page 101: Collection Famille Masana; Page 102: Collection Molinard/Photo Cédric Lerouge-Bénard; Page 103: © Wendi Schneider; Page 104: EDIMEDIA; Page 105: The Metropolitan Museum of Art, The Alfred Stieglitz Collection, 1933 (33 43 141); Page 106: Masan Family Collection; Page 107: Photo de Sheila Metzner/Fendi; Page 108 (top): © Martin Breese/Retrograph Archive, 1995; Page 108 (bottom): Roger & Gallet; Page 109: Léonard de Selva-Tapabor; Page 110: Giraudon; Page 111: Photo: Nimatallah/Luisa Ricciarini, Milan; Page 112: ©

Leslie Ellison/Barnaby's Picture Library; Page 113: Collection Fragonard; Page 114: © Martin Breese/Retrograph Archive, 1995; Page 115: Sterling & Francine Clark Art Institute, Williamstown, USA; Page 116: © Martin Breese/Retrograph Archive, 1995; Page 117: Sotheby's, London; Page 118: © Martin Breese/Retrograph Archive, 1995; Page 121 (top): The Kobal Collection; Page 121 (bottom): © Martin Breese/Retrograph Archive, 1995; Page 122: George Holz © 1984 Courtesy Harper's Bazaar; Page 123: J-P Dieterlin; Page 124: Photo by Robert Rubic/Science & Technology Research Center; Science, Industry & Business Library; The New York Public Library; Astor, Lenox & Tilden Foundation; Page 125: Photo F. Kollar, Ministry of Culture, France; Page 126: 100 Idées/B. Jarret/Lajouanie. Cop. Bibliothèque Centrale/M.N.H.N. Paris; Page 127: Collection Musée International de la Parfumerie, Grasse, France; Page 128: Parfums Christian Dior; Page 129: Photo Flammarion; Page 130: Bibliothèque Forney; Page 131: Photo Flammarion/Archives Parfums Caron; Page 132: Collection Molinard; Page 133: Document Parfums Guerlain/ Aquarelle de Thierry Marchal; Page 134: Parfums Christian Dior; Page 135: Photo Paolo Roversi/Courtesy French Vogue; Page 136: © Martin Breese Retrograph Archive, 1995; Page 137: Photo by Robert Rubic/Science & Technology Research Center; Science, Industry & Business Library; The New York Public Library; Astor, Lenox & Tilden Foundations; Page 137 (bottom): Photo Flammarion; Page 138: Photo F. Kollar, Ministry of Culture, France; Page 139: Bibliothèque Forney; Page 140: Photo Flammarion; Page 141: UPI/Bettmann; Page 142 (top): The Kobal Collection; Page 142 (bottom): Archives Lancôme; Page 143: B.F.I., STILLS, POSTERS & DESIGNS; Page 144: The Kobal Collection; Page 145: UPI/Bettmann; Page 146 (top): B.F.I., STILLS, POSTERS & DESIGNS; Page 146 (bottom): Photo Flammarion; Page 148: Ali von Bothner; Page 149: Galerie Vallois, Paris; Page 151: Ali von Bothner; Page 152: Ali von Bothner; Page 153: Ali von Bothner; Page 154: Photo Jacques Dirand; Page 155: Jacques Boulay; Page 156: Jacques Boulay; Page 157: Chris-

tie's, London/Bridgeman-Giraudon; Page 158 (top): Cristalleries Saint Louis; Page 158 (bottom, left): Cristalleries Saint Louis; Page 158 (bottom, right): Cristalleries Saint Louis; Page 159: Roger et Gallet; Page 160 (top): Bonham's, London; Page 160 (bottom): Bonham's, London; Page 161 (top): Collection Lalique; Page 161 (bottom): Bonham's, London; Page 162: Photo Flammarion; Page 163 (top): Archives Parfums Caron; Page 163 (bottom): Archives Parfums Caron; Page 163: Archives Parfums Caron; Page 164: CHANEL; Page 164: © J.M. Charles/Rapho; Page 165: Ali von Bothner; Page 167: Ali von Bothner; Page 168: Photo Flammarion; Page 169: Jacques Boulay; Page 170: Ali von Bothner; Page 172: Magnum/Salgado; Page 174: Jacques Dirand; Page 175: Jacques Dirand; Page 176: J.-P. Dieterlin; Page 177: Ali von Bothner; Page 178: Collection Nina Ricci; Page 179: Ali von Bothner; Page 179: © COSM'ART/Photo Fabrice Nageotte; Page 180: Photo Steve Hiett/Parfums Jean-Louis Scherrer; Page 181: Rochelle Redfield photographed by Lothar Schmid for Yves Saint Laurent; Page 182: © Martin Breese/Retrograph Archive, 1995; Page 183: Lanvin Page 184 (top): Photo Flammarion; Page 184 (bottom): © Léonard de Selva-Tapabor; Page 185: Ali von Bothner; Page 186: Document Parfums Guerlain; Page 187 (top left): Archives Parfums Caron; Page 187 (top right): Archives Parfums Caron; Page 187 (bottom): Photo Flammarion; Page 188 (top): Parfums Nina Ricci; Page 188 (bottom): Archives Parfums Caron; Page 189: Lanvin; Page 190 (left): Léonard de Selva/ Tapabor; Page 190 (top right): Collection Musée de la Publicité, Paris; Page 190 (bottom right): © Martin Breese/Retrograph Archive, 1995; Page 191: Photo Flammarion; Page 192 © Martin Breese/Retrograph Archive, 1995; Page 192 (bottom): Photo Flammarion; Page 193: Parfums Christian Dior; Page 195: Photo by Sarah Moon for Cacharel; Page 197: Photo by Patrick Demarchelier for Armani Perfumes; Page 198: Yves Saint Laurent; Page 199: Parfums Guy Laroche; Page 200: © Wendi Schneider; Page 201: © Martin Breese/Retrograph Archive, 1995; back jacket: Jacques Boulay.

ACKNOWLEDGMENTS

We wish to express our warmest thanks to the team at Flammarion for enabling us to produce this work, and in particular to Nathalie Bailleux for her patient help and invaluable advice during the writing of the book. We would also like to thank Claire Both for her kind collaboration on the picture research.

We also wish to thank our perfumer friends: Maurice Maurin, the late and sadly missed Jean-François Blayn, Françoise Caron (Quest), Jacques Cavallier (Firmenich), Jean Garnero, Max Gavary (IFF), Olivia Giacobetti (Iskia), Annick Goutal, Jean-Paul Guerlain, Sophia Grosjman (IFF), Jean Guichard (Givaudan-Roure), Jean Kerléo (Jean Patou), Jean-François Laporte (Maître Parfumeur et Gantier), Monsieur Lepage (ISIPCA Library), Nicolas Mamounas, Jeannine Mongin, Patricia de Nicolaï (Parfums Nicolaï), Louis Peyron, Jacques Polge (Chanel), Maurice Roucel (Quest), Edmond Roudnitska, Monique Schlienger (Cinquième Sens), Lorenzo Villoresi, Jean-Louis Sieuzac and Dominique Ropion (Florasynth).

Not forgetting all those who shared their professional knowledge and memories with us, and kindly put their archives at our disposal. This book owes them a great deal: Mr Al Fayed (Chairman of Harrods), Eric Amouyal (L.T. Piver), Jérome Bartau (Parfums et Beauté / Prestige et Collections), Eliane de la Béraudière and Nathalie Huet (Christian Dior), Alain and Michelle Blondel (Galerie Blondel, Paris), Yves Broché and Chantal Evrard (Caron-Revillon), Catherine Calevras (Estée Lauder), Messrs. Colonna and Varlet (Pochet et du Courval), Agnès Costa (Fragonard), Olivier Creed (Creed), Jessie Daniel (IFF), Jacqueline Demornex and Monique Sarras (Lancôme), Joël Desgrippes (Desgrippes-Gobé and Associates), Pierre Dinand (designer), Clarence Duchesne (Cosm'Art), Valérie Dufournier (Jean Patou), Philippe Dupin de Lacoste and Elisabeth Sirot (Guerlain), Danièle Escher (Lalique), Didier Fourmy and Odile Fraigneau (Musée Lanvin), Jolanda Gallarotti, Marie-Hélène Gourmelon and Mme Guespin (Comité Français du Parfum), Robert Granai (designer), Cliff Harris (Floris, London),

Marianne Honvault (Yves Saint Laurent), François Huygues-Despointes (Givaudan-Roure), Bridget Kinally (B.F.I., Stills, Posters and Design), Marie-Claude Lalique (Lalique), Ariane Lasson (Musée International de la Parfumerie, Grasse), Serge Lutens (Shiseido), Jean-Pierre Lerouge-Benard (Molinard), Patrick MacLeod and Macha Magaloff (Nina Ricci), Serge Mansau (designer), Christopher March (Floris, London), Jean-Marie Martin-Hattemberg (expert), Rosandra Masana and Christophe Maubert (Robertet), Marie-Claude Mayer (Publicis), Lyliane Menard (Shiseido), Michèle Meyer (Quest), Danièle Michelet and Laurence Balland (Fédération Française de la Parfumerie), Lauren Munton (Penhaligon's, London), Carole Nairne and Jean-Pierre Petitdidier (Hasslauer), Ioana Ratiu (Groupe Payot–4711), Caroline Regin (Roger & Gallet), Ariel Ricaud-Barsi and Tessa Guilloux (ARB), Bérengère Ridoux (Chanel), Régine de Robien (Beauté Divine), Daphné de Saint-Marceaux (Montana), Marie-Hélène Rogeon (Les Parfums de Rosine), Michèle Samuel (Club des Créateurs), Dany Sautot (Baccarat), Alexandra Schamis (Caron), Alexander Von Solodkoff (Hermitage Gallery, London), Laura Straus (Abbeville Press, New York), Marie-Laure Tiné (Givaudan-Roure), Martine Thorel (Bourjois), Yves Tillon (Roger & Gallet), Alain Trophardy (Saint Gobain Desjonquères), Francis Touyarou-Grabe and Anne Van Latum (Centre du Verre).

The editor would like to thank in particular: Marianne Honvault (Yves Saint Laurent), Patricia Dupond and Karen Bonneau (Guerlain) and Liliane Wickersheim (Comité Français du Parfum), for their vital help during the presentation of this publication to the French and American markets; Hannah Goring (Bonham's, London), and Tessa Trethowan and Jane Hay (Christie's) for the numerous documents they sent us to complement our research; Marie-Hélène Gourmelon (Comité Français du Parfum) for her invaluable information and advice.

We would also like to thank the team who helped to create this book: Marc Walter, Olivier Canaveso, Barbara Kekus, Margerita Mariano, Murielle Vaux, Safia Bendali, and Topaz le Tourneau; also Veronique Manssy, Vincent Guillemard, Elsa Tardif and Sophie Alibert.

INDEX